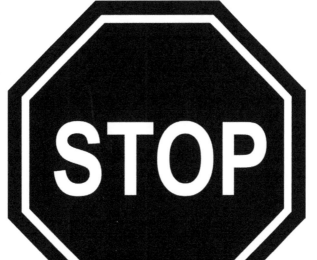

FREE Test Taking Tips Video/DVD Offer

To better serve you, we created videos covering test taking tips that we want to give you for FREE. **These videos cover world-class tips that will help you succeed on your test.**

We just ask that you send us feedback about this product. Please let us know what you thought about it—whether good, bad, or indifferent.

To get your **FREE videos**, you can use the QR code below or email freevideos@studyguideteam.com with "Free Videos" in the subject line and the following information in the body of the email:

    a. The title of your product

    b. Your product rating on a scale of 1-5, with 5 being the highest

    c. Your feedback about the product

If you have any questions or concerns, please don't hesitate to contact us at info@studyguideteam.com.

Thank you!

NAPLEX 2023 and 2024 Review Prep

NAPLEX Study Guide Book with Practice Test Questions
[Includes Detailed Answer Explanations]

Joshua Rueda

Interested in buying more than 10 copies of our product? Contact us about bulk discounts: bulkorders@studyguideteam.com

ISBN 13: 9781637750452
ISBN 10: 1637750455

Table of Contents

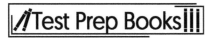

Area 5 – Compounding, Dispensing, or Administering Drugs, or Managing Delivery Systems....................................61

Area 6 – Developing or Managing Practice or Medication-Use Systems to Ensure Safety and Quality....................................71

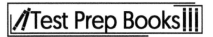

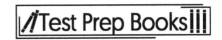

Quick Overview

As you draw closer to taking your exam, effective preparation becomes more and more important. Thankfully, you have this study guide to help you get ready. Use this guide to help keep your studying on track and refer to it often.

This study guide contains several key sections that will help you be successful on your exam. The guide contains tips for what you should do the night before and the day of the test. Also included are test-taking tips. Knowing the right information is not always enough. Many well-prepared test takers struggle with exams. These tips will help equip you to accurately read, assess, and answer test questions.

A large part of the guide is devoted to showing you what content to expect on the exam and to helping you better understand that content. In this guide are practice test questions so that you can see how well you have grasped the content. Then, answer explanations are provided so that you can understand why you missed certain questions.

Don't try to cram the night before you take your exam. This is not a wise strategy for a few reasons. First, your retention of the information will be low. Your time would be better used by reviewing information you already know rather than trying to learn a lot of new information. Second, you will likely become stressed as you try to gain a large amount of knowledge in a short amount of time. Third, you will be depriving yourself of sleep. So be sure to go to bed at a reasonable time the night before. Being well-rested helps you focus and remain calm.

Be sure to eat a substantial breakfast the morning of the exam. If you are taking the exam in the afternoon, be sure to have a good lunch as well. Being hungry is distracting and can make it difficult to focus. You have hopefully spent lots of time preparing for the exam. Don't let an empty stomach get in the way of success!

When travelling to the testing center, leave earlier than needed. That way, you have a buffer in case you experience any delays. This will help you remain calm and will keep you from missing your appointment time at the testing center.

Be sure to pace yourself during the exam. Don't try to rush through the exam. There is no need to risk performing poorly on the exam just so you can leave the testing center early. Allow yourself to use all of the allotted time if needed.

Remain positive while taking the exam even if you feel like you are performing poorly. Thinking about the content you should have mastered will not help you perform better on the exam.

Once the exam is complete, take some time to relax. Even if you feel that you need to take the exam again, you will be well served by some down time before you begin studying again. It's often easier to convince yourself to study if you know that it will come with a reward!

Test-Taking Strategies

1. Predicting the Answer

When you feel confident in your preparation for a multiple-choice test, try predicting the answer before reading the answer choices. This is especially useful on questions that test objective factual knowledge. By predicting the answer before reading the available choices, you eliminate the possibility that you will be distracted or led astray by an incorrect answer choice. You will feel more confident in your selection if you read the question, predict the answer, and then find your prediction among the answer choices. After using this strategy, be sure to still read all of the answer choices carefully and completely. If you feel unprepared, you should not attempt to predict the answers. This would be a waste of time and an opportunity for your mind to wander in the wrong direction.

2. Reading the Whole Question

Too often, test takers scan a multiple-choice question, recognize a few familiar words, and immediately jump to the answer choices. Test authors are aware of this common impatience, and they will sometimes prey upon it. For instance, a test author might subtly turn the question into a negative, or he or she might redirect the focus of the question right at the end. The only way to avoid falling into these traps is to read the entirety of the question carefully before reading the answer choices.

3. Looking for Wrong Answers

Long and complicated multiple-choice questions can be intimidating. One way to simplify a difficult multiple-choice question is to eliminate all of the answer choices that are clearly wrong. In most sets of answers, there will be at least one selection that can be dismissed right away. If the test is administered on paper, the test taker could draw a line through it to indicate that it may be ignored; otherwise, the test taker will have to perform this operation mentally or on scratch paper. In either case, once the obviously incorrect answers have been eliminated, the remaining choices may be considered. Sometimes identifying the clearly wrong answers will give the test taker some information about the correct answer. For instance, if one of the remaining answer choices is a direct opposite of one of the eliminated answer choices, it may well be the correct answer. The opposite of obviously wrong is obviously right! Of course, this is not always the case. Some answers are obviously incorrect simply because they are irrelevant to the question being asked. Still, identifying and eliminating some incorrect answer choices is a good way to simplify a multiple-choice question.

4. Don't Overanalyze

Anxious test takers often overanalyze questions. When you are nervous, your brain will often run wild, causing you to make associations and discover clues that don't actually exist. If you feel that this may be a problem for you, do whatever you can to slow down during the test. Try taking a deep breath or counting to ten. As you read and consider the question, restrict yourself to the particular words used by the author. Avoid thought tangents about what the author *really* meant, or what he or she was *trying* to say. The only things that matter on a multiple-choice test are the words that are actually in the question. You must avoid reading too much into a multiple-choice question, or supposing that the writer meant something other than what he or she wrote.

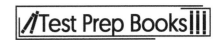

5. No Need for Panic

It is wise to learn as many strategies as possible before taking a multiple-choice test, but it is likely that you will come across a few questions for which you simply don't know the answer. In this situation, avoid panicking. Because most multiple-choice tests include dozens of questions, the relative value of a single wrong answer is small. As much as possible, you should compartmentalize each question on a multiple-choice test. In other words, you should not allow your feelings about one question to affect your success on the others. When you find a question that you either don't understand or don't know how to answer, just take a deep breath and do your best. Read the entire question slowly and carefully. Try rephrasing the question a couple of different ways. Then, read all of the answer choices carefully. After eliminating obviously wrong answers, make a selection and move on to the next question.

6. Confusing Answer Choices

When working on a difficult multiple-choice question, there may be a tendency to focus on the answer choices that are the easiest to understand. Many people, whether consciously or not, gravitate to the answer choices that require the least concentration, knowledge, and memory. This is a mistake. When you come across an answer choice that is confusing, you should give it extra attention. A question might be confusing because you do not know the subject matter to which it refers. If this is the case, don't eliminate the answer before you have affirmatively settled on another. When you come across an answer choice of this type, set it aside as you look at the remaining choices. If you can confidently assert that one of the other choices is correct, you can leave the confusing answer aside. Otherwise, you will need to take a moment to try to better understand the confusing answer choice. Rephrasing is one way to tease out the sense of a confusing answer choice.

7. Your First Instinct

Many people struggle with multiple-choice tests because they overthink the questions. If you have studied sufficiently for the test, you should be prepared to trust your first instinct once you have carefully and completely read the question and all of the answer choices. There is a great deal of research suggesting that the mind can come to the correct conclusion very quickly once it has obtained all of the relevant information. At times, it may seem to you as if your intuition is working faster even than your reasoning mind. This may in fact be true. The knowledge you obtain while studying may be retrieved from your subconscious before you have a chance to work out the associations that support it. Verify your instinct by working out the reasons that it should be trusted.

8. Key Words

Many test takers struggle with multiple-choice questions because they have poor reading comprehension skills. Quickly reading and understanding a multiple-choice question requires a mixture of skill and experience. To help with this, try jotting down a few key words and phrases on a piece of scrap paper. Doing this concentrates the process of reading and forces the mind to weigh the relative importance of the question's parts. In selecting words and phrases to write down, the test taker thinks about the question more deeply and carefully. This is especially true for multiple-choice questions that are preceded by a long prompt.

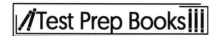

9. Subtle Negatives

One of the oldest tricks in the multiple-choice test writer's book is to subtly reverse the meaning of a question with a word like *not* or *except*. If you are not paying attention to each word in the question, you can easily be led astray by this trick. For instance, a common question format is, "Which of the following is…?" Obviously, if the question instead is, "Which of the following is not…?," then the answer will be quite different. Even worse, the test makers are aware of the potential for this mistake and will include one answer choice that would be correct if the question were not negated or reversed. A test taker who misses the reversal will find what he or she believes to be a correct answer and will be so confident that he or she will fail to reread the question and discover the original error. The only way to avoid this is to practice a wide variety of multiple-choice questions and to pay close attention to each and every word.

10. Reading Every Answer Choice

It may seem obvious, but you should always read every one of the answer choices! Too many test takers fall into the habit of scanning the question and assuming that they understand the question because they recognize a few key words. From there, they pick the first answer choice that answers the question they believe they have read. Test takers who read all of the answer choices might discover that one of the latter answer choices is actually *more* correct. Moreover, reading all of the answer choices can remind you of facts related to the question that can help you arrive at the correct answer. Sometimes, a misstatement or incorrect detail in one of the latter answer choices will trigger your memory of the subject and will enable you to find the right answer. Failing to read all of the answer choices is like not reading all of the items on a restaurant menu: you might miss out on the perfect choice.

11. Spot the Hedges

One of the keys to success on multiple-choice tests is paying close attention to every word. This is never truer than with words like *almost*, *most*, *some*, and *sometimes*. These words are called "hedges" because they indicate that a statement is not totally true or not true in every place and time. An absolute statement will contain no hedges, but in many subjects, the answers are not always straightforward or absolute. There are always exceptions to the rules in these subjects. For this reason, you should favor those multiple-choice questions that contain hedging language. The presence of qualifying words indicates that the author is taking special care with his or her words, which is certainly important when composing the right answer. After all, there are many ways to be wrong, but there is only one way to be right! For this reason, it is wise to avoid answers that are absolute when taking a multiple-choice test. An absolute answer is one that says things are either all one way or all another. They often include words like *every*, *always*, *best*, and *never*. If you are taking a multiple-choice test in a subject that doesn't lend itself to absolute answers, be on your guard if you see any of these words.

12. Long Answers

In many subject areas, the answers are not simple. As already mentioned, the right answer often requires hedges. Another common feature of the answers to a complex or subjective question are qualifying clauses, which are groups of words that subtly modify the meaning of the sentence. If the question or answer choice describes a rule to which there are exceptions or the subject matter is complicated, ambiguous, or confusing, the correct answer will require many words in order to be expressed clearly and accurately. In essence, you should not be deterred by answer choices that seem

4

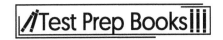

excessively long. Oftentimes, the author of the text will not be able to write the correct answer without offering some qualifications and modifications. Your job is to read the answer choices thoroughly and completely and to select the one that most accurately and precisely answers the question.

13. Restating to Understand

Sometimes, a question on a multiple-choice test is difficult not because of what it asks but because of how it is written. If this is the case, restate the question or answer choice in different words. This process serves a couple of important purposes. First, it forces you to concentrate on the core of the question. In order to rephrase the question accurately, you have to understand it well. Rephrasing the question will concentrate your mind on the key words and ideas. Second, it will present the information to your mind in a fresh way. This process may trigger your memory and render some useful scrap of information picked up while studying.

14. True Statements

Sometimes an answer choice will be true in itself, but it does not answer the question. This is one of the main reasons why it is essential to read the question carefully and completely before proceeding to the answer choices. Too often, test takers skip ahead to the answer choices and look for true statements. Having found one of these, they are content to select it without reference to the question above. Obviously, this provides an easy way for test makers to play tricks. The savvy test taker will always read the entire question before turning to the answer choices. Then, having settled on a correct answer choice, he or she will refer to the original question and ensure that the selected answer is relevant. The mistake of choosing a correct-but-irrelevant answer choice is especially common on questions related to specific pieces of objective knowledge. A prepared test taker will have a wealth of factual knowledge at his or her disposal, and should not be careless in its application.

15. No Patterns

One of the more dangerous ideas that circulates about multiple-choice tests is that the correct answers tend to fall into patterns. These erroneous ideas range from a belief that B and C are the most common right answers, to the idea that an unprepared test-taker should answer "A-B-A-C-A-D-A-B-A." It cannot be emphasized enough that pattern-seeking of this type is exactly the WRONG way to approach a multiple-choice test. To begin with, it is highly unlikely that the test maker will plot the correct answers according to some predetermined pattern. The questions are scrambled and delivered in a random order. Furthermore, even if the test maker was following a pattern in the assignation of correct answers, there is no reason why the test taker would know which pattern he or she was using. Any attempt to discern a pattern in the answer choices is a waste of time and a distraction from the real work of taking the test. A test taker would be much better served by extra preparation before the test than by reliance on a pattern in the answers.

FREE Videos/DVD OFFER

Doing well on your exam requires both knowing the test content and understanding how to use that knowledge to do well on the test. We offer completely FREE test taking tip videos. **These videos cover world-class tips that you can use to succeed on your test.**

To get your **FREE videos**, you can use the QR code below or email freevideos@studyguideteam.com with "Free Videos" in the subject line and the following information in the body of the email:

   a. The title of your product

   b. Your product rating on a scale of 1-5, with 5 being the highest

   c. Your feedback about the product

If you have any questions or concerns, please don't hesitate to contact us at info@studyguideteam.com.

Thanks again!

Introduction to the NAPLEX

Background of the NAPLEX

The North American Pharmacist Licensure Examination (NAPLEX) is an examination created to assess the knowledge and competence of recent college of pharmacy graduates. The National Association of Boards of Pharmacy (NABP) was established to help develop uniform education and licensure standards for potential pharmacists. The NAPLEX exam is one part of the licensure process that helps determine whether candidates are qualified to practice as pharmacists.

The NAPLEX is offered to graduates of the Accreditation Council for Pharmacy Education (ACPE)-accredited entry level pharmacy schools soon after they complete their degree and to foreign-educated pharmacists who have recently completed their Foreign Pharmacy Graduate Examination Committee (FPGEC) Certification. Each individual state board of pharmacy may have unique requirements for the licensure process.

Test Administration

Candidates must apply for exam eligibility and pay an application fee. Application fees and processing timelines vary by state. Candidates must have their transcripts submitted by their college of pharmacy before they are eligible to purchase the exam and receive an Authorization to Test (ATT). Testing appointments are able to be scheduled through Pearson VUE once eligibility requirements have been met.

During the application process, an armed forces discount can be requested if applicable. Candidates with disabilities may submit a Request for Testing accommodations form with their online application.

Candidates may retake the NAPLEX exam if they do not pass, but they must complete the eligibility process each time they choose to retake it. Candidates must also wait 45 days after failing the exam to retake it. Candidates are limited to three attempts in a period of twelve months. Also, there is a maximum of five attempts allowed to pass the NAPLEX unless approval is received from the board of pharmacy for further attempts.

Test Format

The NAPLEX exam consists of 225 questions presented in a computerized, fixed format and lasts 6 hours. 200 of the questions from the exam are used to calculate results, and the other 25 are pretest items. These questions are spaced throughout the exam and do not affect exam results because they are being evaluated for use on future exams.

Most questions are based on scenarios that should be read first. Additional information such as sample patient profiles or medical records may be included as well. Test takers will need to scroll through all such information provided before being allowed to answer. The exam also includes stand-alone questions that are not connected to the information in the scenarios. All questions must be answered, and test takers will be unable to return to previous questions to change any answers. Question types on the exam include multiple-choice, multiple-response, and constructed-response.

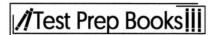

The questions on the exam relate to the following competency statements:

Area	Competency Statement	Percentage of Exam
Area 1	Obtain, Interpret, or Assess Data, Medical, or Patient Information	18%
Area 2	Identify Drug Characteristics	14%
Area 3	Develop or Manage Treatment Plans	35%
Area 4	Perform Calculations	14%
Area 5	Compound, Dispense, or Administer Drugs, or Manage Delivery Systems	11%
Area 6	Develop or Manage Practice or Medication-Use Systems to Ensure Safety and Quality	7%

Two 10-minute breaks are available during the examination, but they are optional. At timed intervals, the computer will alert the test taker when breaks are allowed. Other unscheduled breaks will use part of the test taker's allotted time for taking the exam.

Scoring

Candidates will receive pass or fail results within approximately seven business days if the primary jurisdiction where they tested participates in the NABP's online exam result interface. Candidates who fail the exam will receive a performance report with additional information related to performance in each of the competency areas of the exam. Exam results will also be sent to the board of pharmacy indicated by a candidate on their NAPLEX application. The passing standard for the NAPLEX exam is set by a panel of pharmacy experts, and the standard is consistent for all NAPLEX administrations. According to the NABP, the all time pass rate (which includes first and subsequent attempts) for graduates from the various schools of pharmacy ranged from 53% to 100% for 2021 graduates.

Candidates may also use the score transfer program to submit their scores to multiple states in addition to their primary state to accelerate the licensure process in these states. The cost for a score transfer is $75 per state. Requests can be submitted up to 89 days after taking the NAPLEX.

Study Prep Plan for the NAPLEX

1   **Schedule** - Use one of our study schedules below or come up with one of your own.

2   **Relax** - Test anxiety can hurt even the best students. There are many ways to reduce stress. Find the one that works best for you.

3   **Execute** - Once you have a good plan in place, be sure to stick to it.

One Week Study Schedule		
Day 1	Area 1 – Obtaining, Interpreting, or...	
Day 2	Area 3 – Developing or Managing Treatment Plans	
Day 3	Area 4 – Performing Calculations	
Day 4	Area 6 – Developing or Managing Practice or...	
Day 5	Practice Test #1	
Day 6	Practice Test #2	
Day 7	Take Your Exam!	

Two Week Study Schedule			
Day 1	Area 1 - Obtaining, Interpreting, or...	Day 8	Area 5 – Compounding, Dispensing, or...
Day 2	Evaluating Medical Records	Day 9	Area 6 â€" Developing or Managing Practice or...
Day 3	Area 2 - Identifying Drug Characteristics	Day 10	Practice Test #1
Day 4	Area 3 – Developing or Managing Treatment Plans	Day 11	Answer Explanations #1
Day 5	Drug Contraindications, Allergies, or Precautions	Day 12	Practice Test #2
Day 6	Lifestyle and Self-Care	Day 13	Answer Explanations #2
Day 7	Area 4 – Performing Calculations	Day 14	Take Your Exam!

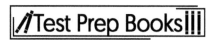
One Month Study Schedule						
Day 1	Area 1 - Obtaining, Interpreting, or...	Day 11	Drug Contraindications, Allergies, or Precautions	Day 21	Area 5 – Compounding, Dispensing, or...
Day 2	Evaluating Information from Patients	Day 12	Drug Interactions	Day 22	Equipment or Delivery Systems
Day 3	Evaluating Medical Records	Day 13	Therapeutic Monitoring	Day 23	Packaging, Storage, Handling, and Disposal of Medications
Day 4	Using Evidence-Based Literature and Studies	Day 14	Lifestyle and Self-Care	Day 24	Area 6 – Developing or Managing Practice or...
Day 5	Area 2 – Identifying Drug Characteristics	Day 15	Complementary and Alternative Medicine	Day 25	Vulnerable and Special Populations
Day 6	Brand, Generic, or Biosimilar Names and Physical Descriptions	Day 16	Medical Equipment	Day 26	Practice Test #1
Day 7	Boxed Warnings and REMS	Day 17	Area 4 – Performing Calculations	Day 27	Answer Explanations #1
Day 8	Area 3 – Developing or Managing Treatment Plans	Day 18	Dose Conversions	Day 28	Practice Test #2
Day 9	Medication Reconciliation and Indication of Uses	Day 19	Biostatistics and Epidemiological Measures	Day 29	Answer Explanations #2
Day 10	Duplication Therapy and Omissions	Day 20	Pharmacokinetic Parameters	Day 30	Take Your Exam!

Build your own prep plan by visiting:

testprepbooks.com/prep

10

Area 1 - Obtaining, Interpreting, or Assessing Data, Medical, or Patient Information

Evaluating Information from Instruments and Screening Tools

Health screenings are an essential part of determining medical risks for patients. **Screenings** determine the overall health of a patient, and they help the pharmacist and primary care provider select appropriate drug therapy and preventative strategies. Before performing or reviewing health screenings, pharmacists should review the patient's medical history. A review of systems is necessary to determine which screenings are required. During an initial assessment, a pharmacist should ask a few questions about each body system to determine the overall health of the patient. A health screen will be dependent on the patient's answers and medical history.

For example, a pharmacist may ask a patient if they frequently experience joint pain when assessing the musculoskeletal system. Should the patient report the presence of joint pain and issues with mobility, further studies may be required. Laboratory tests to measure calcium and vitamin D levels may be recommended. Additionally, if a primary care provider determines that a patient is at a high risk for osteoporosis, the patient may undergo a bone mineral density test to assess the quality and strength of the bones. The x-ray taken during a bone density test can help visualize how porous bones look. The more porous, the higher the risk of a fracture. Subsequently, medications such as alendronate (Fosamax) may be ordered to reverse the progression of osteoporosis.

Assessing a patient's dietary habits is an important component in determining their risk for conditions such as high cholesterol and diabetes. A patient who consistently eats a high-fat, high-carbohydrate diet may be at a higher risk of cardiovascular disease and diabetes. Laboratory tests such as a full cholesterol panel can help pharmacists and providers determine the need for cholesterol-lowering drugs. For example, if a patient's total cholesterol is above 200 mg/dL, triglyceride levels are above 150 mg/dL, and low-density lipoprotein (LDL) levels are above 100 mg/dL, the patient may require dyslipidemic drugs such as lovastatin (Altocor) to reduce the risk of atherosclerosis and heart disease. Lifestyle modifications such as a low-fat diet and an increase in physical activity should also be highly encouraged during patient education sessions.

Patients who are high risk for developing diabetes may require laboratory tests to determine glucose levels and hemoglobin A1C levels. The ideal fasting glucose levels should be below 100 mg/dL. Additionally, hemoglobin A1C measures the average level of glucose in the blood over a period of 60-90 days. Normal levels are below 5.7%. **Blood glucose testing** is another alternative that produces faster results and is less invasive. Blood is taken from a patient's fingertip and applied to a test strip. The test strip is analyzed by a glucometer that delivers results in seconds. Analysis from these screening tools allows the pharmacist and primary care provider to determine the best course of drug therapy.

Vital signs are an essential assessment for determining a patient's overall health status and usually include temperature, pulse rate, rate of breathing, and blood pressure. They can also be part of a cardiovascular risk assessment. Cardiovascular events such as heart attack and stroke are often caused by uncontrolled hypertension. In some cases, hypertension is not symptomatic, and patients are unaware they have high blood pressure. Measuring a patient's blood pressure can be a simple screening tool to determine their vascular health. Systolic blood pressures above 120 mmHg and diastolic blood

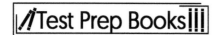
pressures above 80 mmHg place a patient at risk for cardiovascular events. High blood pressure can signal a primary care provider and pharmacist to encourage lifestyle changes such as low-sodium diets and increased cardio exercise. Uncontrolled hypertension may require medications such as beta-blockers, calcium channel blockers, and diuretics. Other annual wellness exams such as weight and body fat percentage are useful in evaluating a patient's overall health status or the effectiveness of drug therapy.

Evaluating Laboratory and Diagnostic Findings

Laboratory and diagnostic clinical parameters are important for the assessment of drug therapy efficacy. Labs and diagnostics are also essential before beginning a new drug regimen. Labs can provide an overview of the patient's health status and help determine the best course of treatment. Laboratory orders are based on the patient's disease process. A primary care provider will order labs that correlate with the patient's suspected or current medical condition. It is important for pharmacists to be familiar with the normal ranges of lab values to evaluate whether a patient's medication regimen is producing the intended results.

For example, a patient who reports fatigue, dizziness, and discoloration of mucous membranes may be diagnosed with anemia. Anemia will be diagnosed by a complete blood count (CBC) test that evaluates the number of red blood cells (RBCs), the amount of hemoglobin, and percentage of hematocrit in a patient's blood serum. Low levels of RBCs, hemoglobin, and hematocrit can assist in securing a diagnosis of anemia. Subsequently, the patient's provider may order iron supplements such as ferrous sulfate or erythropoietin stimulants such as epoetin (Epogen) to increase and maintain the production of red blood cells. Pharmacists need to evaluate the progression of increased lab values while the patient is receiving these treatments.

Patients may also report signs and symptoms of an infection. Infections can affect several body systems. Respiratory infections may display cough, sore throat, or exudates at the back of the throat. Skin infections may be accompanied by redness to the site, purulent drainage, and pain. Gastrointestinal infections may present with diarrhea, vomiting, and nausea. White blood cells (WBC) in a complete blood count laboratory test will signal the presence of an infection in the body. At times, further studies such as blood cultures, nasal swabs, stool cultures, and wound cultures may need to be obtained to determine the causative organism. Interpretation of these results will aid in the selection of the appropriate antibiotic or antiviral medication. For example, a patient diagnosed with a staphylococcus infection on a throat culture may be placed on Nafcillin to treat the respiratory illness. **Nafcillin** is an anti-infective used in the treatment of respiratory tract infections due to staphylococci.

Pharmacists should also be aware of the link between medical illnesses and the potential complications if drug therapy is not initiated. For example, a patient diagnosed with atrial fibrillation is at risk for blood clots. **Atrial fibrillation** is a condition in which the heart does not beat regularly and there is a disconnect between the pumping action of the atria and the ventricles of the heart. This can lead to blood pooling in the heart and formation of blood clots. Patients with a diagnosis such as atrial fibrillation may be placed on anticoagulation therapy. Blood thinners used for treatment include warfarin (Coumadin). Patients taking Coumadin require routine monitoring of the prothrombin time and international normalized ratio (INR). Careful monitoring of these lab values determines efficacy of treatment and safe levels of medication. Ideal INR levels should be between 2.0 and 3.0.

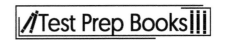

Evaluating Information from Patients

Before beginning drug therapy, a pharmacist is required to perform a **patient interview** and accurately assess important information that will aid in the management of proper treatment. There are several standards of care that should be met when selecting an appropriate drug therapy. The first standard of care involves collecting patient-specific information during an interview that will help a pharmacist understand the patient's health status and drug-related needs. Demographic information is important in understanding the patient's individuality and determining any barriers present that will interfere with adherence of therapy and completion of medication goals. Age is an important piece of demographic data that is necessary for appropriate dosing and selection of medication. For example, if a patient has a lower respiratory tract infection, the dosage of the anti-infective will vary based on age. Children's dosages are usually based on weight while adult dosages may be more standardized. Patients in the geriatric stage may also require smaller dosages to account for declining organ function. Height and weight are important for dosing medications such as enoxaparin (Lovenox). **Lovenox** is an anticoagulant medication and its dose needs to be accurately calculated based on the patient's weight in kilograms.

The patient's living situation is another important element to assess during the interview. Assessment of the living situation can include asking about family members, dependents, and caregivers. If a patient has small children, safety should be taken into consideration when selecting the type of container used to secure medication. If an elderly patient lives alone, a pharmacist must ask about caregivers or family members who will assist with medication administration.

The patient's socioeconomic status and work situation should also be assessed. This will help determine if the patient will be able to afford their medication. Patients who are not insured and have high-cost medications will often prioritize basic needs over their healthcare. The patient's occupation can help determine any risk factors for existing medical conditions and drug therapy. For example, if a patient takes a bronchodilator such as montelukast (Singulair) for asthma and works in a factory where smoke, dust, and strong fumes are prevalent, further education and safety precautions may be required.

Another important piece of information to obtain during an interview is the patient's medication experience. The medication experience includes the patient's attitude towards drug therapy, their understanding of the intended effects, expectations of the desired outcome, and medication administration behaviors. A patient's initial impression of a medication will help determine their decision-making process. For example, a patient may hesitate to take a chemotherapy medication that may cause vomiting and loss of hair during the course of treatment. Prompt education on the benefits of a medication despite possible side effects should be delivered to the patient. The overall goal is to improve a patient's medication management experience.

There are other components to the patient interview. Pharmacists should review the patient's immunization record and encourage them to receive appropriate vaccinations for their age group and geographical area. Social drug use can have many adverse effects when mixed with medications. Nicotine, caffeine, street drugs, and alcohol can alter the way medications are metabolized and cause potential side effects. Pharmacists should ask about amount, frequency, and type of substances used. For example, if a patient drinks a considerable amount of caffeine daily or smokes several cigarettes a day, this can cause vasoconstriction and lessen the therapeutic effects of antihypertensive medications.

In order to identify potential adverse drug reactions, a pharmacist should ask the patient if they have any allergies or have experienced any complications due to medications in the past. Allergic reactions

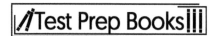

should be documented accordingly, including the severity of the allergy. Health aids, special needs, and health alerts should be assessed during the interview for safety purposes. Physical limitations, cognitive impairment, and language barriers can potentially lead to medication errors. For example, if a patient is hard of hearing, they may not interpret instructions correctly if given over the phone. The pharmacist may need to recommend that the patient is educated in a face-to-face format.

Evaluating Information from Practitioners

Therapeutic records serve to effectively communicate the patient's treatment plan with other health care providers. Communication with physicians should include the identification of problems and recommendations to improve the patient's medication regimen. **Physician reports** for medication management services should be comprehensive, organized, and to the point. The report should clearly identify the patient, their date of birth, age, gender, and medical record number. The patient's history of allergies is an important component that should be presented early in the report to prevent serious harm to the patient. It is useful to include the patient's caffeine, tobacco, and alcohol use. Usage of these substances may influence the care decisions made by practitioners. For example, if a patient has a history of drinking large amounts of alcohol on a daily basis, liver function and proper metabolization of medications may be inhibited. Medication dosages may need to be adjusted based on the patient's liver function tests. Smoking can narrow the blood vessels and decrease circulation. Additionally, it can decrease the effectiveness of medications such as antidepressants, hypnotics, antipsychotics, and anxiolytics. Patient education on smoking cessation may be warranted to avoid inappropriate dosage adjustments.

Adverse reactions to medications are important components of the physician report that alert the practitioner to the harmful effects experienced by the patient. This helps the physician avoid prescribing medications in the same category that may cause the same adverse effects. A medication management report is crucial when the patient is being treated for multiple conditions by multiple doctors. The physician report can summarize all of the patient's interactions so all practitioners are aware of the current treatment. The report should address the disease the medication is treating and the evaluation status of the drug. For example, a patient who has a history of renal impairment, a cardiac dysrhythmia, diabetes, and hypertension may be treated by a nephrologist, cardiologist, and internal medicine physician. All of the practitioners would have to be informed of the patient's medications in order to coordinate a safe and effective plan of care. The number of conditions, active medications, and daily doses are important pieces of information to evaluate drug therapies. It is also useful to include the estimated monthly cost of medications. The patient's ability to pay for their medications can influence their compliance with treatment.

Physician reports should also include any drug therapy problems, including dosages that are too low to be effective, nonadherence, dosages that are too high to be safe, and adverse drug reactions. A clear distinction should be made regarding which disease process the drug therapy problem is affecting. For example, if a diabetic patient is unable to afford their insulin, they would most likely not purchase the medication and discontinue its use. Nonadherence to this medication can cause complications of their diabetes and possible disruption of other disease processes. Pharmacists would have to communicate this to physicians and collaborate on possible cost-effective alternatives.

The final component of the physician report for medication management should include a pharmacist evaluation and recommendation. In this section, pharmacists have the opportunity to communicate their judgment on the drug treatment and its effect on the patient's goals and overall outcome of

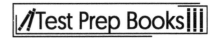

therapy. Often, pharmacists will be required to provide physicians with alternatives. It is important to clearly state the drug therapy problem and reason for presenting different options.

Alternative options should be safe, effective, and cost-efficient to the patient. Concise information and a strong reason for the preferred drug should be outlined to help decrease the chance of physicians having to question the alternatives. For example, if a patient with a history of hypertension and a second-degree heart block has stopped taking captopril (Capoten) because it caused a persistent, dry cough, the pharmacist should be prepared to provide recommendations for alternative treatment. Given the patient's history of a second-degree heart block, pharmacists would have to be cautious recommending a beta-blocker such as atenolol (Tenormin), which may cause a significant decrease in the heart rate. The overall goal of alternative therapy is to facilitate the care of the patient and provide guidance to physicians when drug therapy problems exist. Continuous feedback between the physician and the pharmacist is crucial to help achieve the goals of therapy.

Evaluating Medical Records

A patient's **medical record** includes any recent and relevant prescribed, non-prescribed, and herbal medications as well as any acute and chronic medical conditions. During an assessment, a pharmacist must evaluate the patient's history of medication use. Medications taken within a six-month period are important to note. The primary reason is to assess whether a present medical condition has been treated in the past. If a condition is recurring and has been treated effectively in the past with a certain medication, it is likely that the same medication will have the same outcome. Alternatively, if a patient has been treated ineffectively with a medication in the past, changes in drug therapy should be considered. A list of current medications is necessary to make an informed decision about drug therapy. The medication record should include:

- The indication for the medications
- The number of medications being taken to treat the same medical condition
- How the patient is taking the medications
- The patient's response to their current drug therapy

It is important to make it known that herbal and over-the-counter medications are considered drug therapies. Pharmacists should carefully evaluate the type, amount, and frequency of non-prescribed medications being taken. These medications can cause drug interactions and unwanted side effects. For example, if a patient is prescribed an anticoagulant such as warfarin (Coumadin) for the treatment of blood clots and is currently taking gingko biloba for its antioxidant properties, pharmacists should be aware that combining both of these medications may cause increased bleeding.

The medication's **"indication"** refers to all the clinical reasons why a patient might take that specific medication. Medications can be used to cure or prevent a disease, slow the progression of an illness, supplement nutritional deficiencies, correct abnormal lab results, provide relief from symptoms of a disease, and assist in diagnostic procedures. It is important for a pharmacist to interpret why a patient is taking a medication.

The **Food and Drug Administration (FDA)** approves the indication of a medication for labeling and marketing based on the information submitted by the pharmaceutical industry. However, patients may be prescribed a drug for purposes other than the labeled use. For example, **chlorpromazine** (Thorazine) is an antipsychotic medication used primarily in the treatment of mood disorders. Thorazine may also be prescribed in patients with gastroparesis who have uncontrolled hiccups. The indication of a medication

15

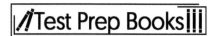

is important for the establishment of goals in therapy. The patient's medical conditions are a crucial part of the medical record for determining the appropriateness of drug therapy. Information such as illnesses, surgical procedures, pregnancies, and injuries can assist a pharmacist in creating an effective medication plan with the patient.

Pharmacists should also avoid over-collection of data that will not prove beneficial to the current drug therapy. For example, if a patient lists multiple surgeries in the past but none of them have caused physical or cognitive limitations, they may not be a priority in the selection of medications. However, if a patient has history of a renal transplant, the pharmacist must consider dosage adjustments to maintain the integrity of organ function.

Pharmacists should also be vigilant about unclear or conflicting information in the patient's medical record. Many healthcare providers contribute to the patient's medical record and reconciliation of the patient's medication history and medical conditions should be performed to ensure that the record reflects the patient's accurate history. For example, a patient's medical record may state history of hypertension. If no medications are noted, the pharmacist should clarify when the diagnosis was made and what type of follow up treatment was given.

A patient's medical record should also include any recent laboratory or diagnostic data. In order to evaluate the patient's current health status, a recent laboratory panel and diagnostic screenings may be required. Pharmacists should be mindful of the economic impact repetitive testing may have on the patient. For example, a patient prescribed a statin medication such as lipitor (Atorvastatin) will require a cholesterol panel to evaluate baseline labs. If the medical record reflects that the patient had laboratory work performed in the past couple of weeks or month, repetitive testing may not be required. However, if labs are not present or are significantly outdated, communication with a medical provider may be warranted to obtain baseline data. Diagnostic imaging is equally important in the patient's medical record. Diagnostic tests such as x-rays, ultrasounds, CT scans, and MRIs are required to evaluate the progress of drug therapy. For example, if a patient is taking an antibiotic medication to treat an abdominal abscess, an ultrasound or CT scan may be required to assess the dimensions and progression of the abscess after drug therapy is initiated.

Evaluating Signs and Symptoms

One of the goals of drug therapy is to alleviate the symptoms of a disease. Each disease process has characteristic signs and physical symptoms. It is important for a pharmacist to recognize the physical manifestations of various medical conditions to determine if the goals of drug therapy are being met. Upon an initial assessment of a patient's health status, a focused review of systems can help select the appropriate treatment. For example, if a patient says that they wake up at night to urinate, feel thirsty, and have excessive hunger, these may be signs of diabetes. Additional questions should be asked to obtain more information on accompanying signs and symptoms of diabetes such as poor wound healing, decreased vision, and peripheral extremity pain. These symptoms reported by a patient should be documented and promptly reported to the provider for treatment. Medications such as insulin, biguanides, and sulfonylureas may be ordered. The overall goal of therapy would be to see a decrease in the polydipsia, polyphagia, and polyuria in combination with normal serum glucose levels.

Endocrine disorders can have various signs and symptoms throughout the different body systems. **Hypothyroidism** is a condition in which there is an underproduction of hormones essential for metabolic functions. Patients will report loss of energy, weight gain, constipation, muscle cramping, weakness, and

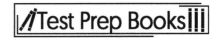

intolerance to cold temperatures. It is important to link these physical manifestations with a laboratory test to confirm a diagnosis. Primary care providers may order labs such as thyroxine (T4), triiodothyronine (T3), and thyroid stimulating hormone (TSH) to determine whether a patient has this condition. Once confirmed, patients may be started on medications to replace T4 levels such as levothyroxine (Synthroid). Another example is a patient with a medical diagnosis of asthma.

Asthma is a condition in which the respiratory airways become inflamed due to an allergen. The narrowing of these airways can lead to respiratory distress if not appropriately treated. Patients may report chest tightness, trouble breathing, cough, and wheezing when exposed to allergens or strenuous physical activity. Pharmacists should recognize these as signs of an acute asthma attack. Patients may be prescribed inhaled bronchodilators such as albuterol (Proventil) to help widen the respiratory airways. Expected goals of therapy include the prevention of asthma attacks and decrease in respiratory symptoms.

Upon review and assessment of the gastrointestinal system, patients may report heartburn, regurgitation of food, and excessive burping. All these symptoms combined indicate gastroesophageal reflux disease. These patients may be placed on proton pump inhibitors such as protonix (Pantoprazole) to decrease the amount of acid production in the stomach. Evaluation of therapy will include a decrease in the presenting gastrointestinal symptoms and greater toleration of food.

A patient's mental status and behavior should be an important topic of discussion during the patient interview and throughout drug therapy. Patients with depressive mood disorders may report a reduction in appetite, concentration, and attention span. Patients may also appear fatigued and unkempt. Antidepressants such as paroxetine (Paxil), sertraline (Zoloft), and citalopram (Celexa) may be prescribed. The overall goal of these medications is for the patient to return to a normal level of functioning. Pharmacists should also be aware that it may be weeks before behavioral symptoms improve.

Health and Wellness

The overall goal of healthcare is to keep people healthy and prevent the development of chronic illnesses. One of the main duties of healthcare providers is to encourage healthy lifestyles and seek primary care for early detection of illness. Pharmacists have a duty to identify patients who need to be educated about harmful practices and correct their modifiable risk factors. Many chronic conditions are preventable. Several risk factors that contribute to the development of a disease or exacerbate complications of current illnesses include:

- Unhealthy diets
- Sedentary lifestyles
- Smoking
- Alcohol
- Drug use

When performing an assessment on a patient, pharmacists should inquire about **dietary habits**. Patients should be asked about their daily intake of nutrients, eating patterns, and any challenges contributing to an unhealthy diet. Patients who report eating high-fat, high-calorie meals should be educated on the complications of these dietary patterns. The development of atherosclerosis is one of the leading causes of heart disease. **Atherosclerosis** is an accumulation of fat within the vessel walls. Prolonged elevated

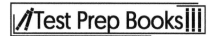

levels of cholesterol and triglycerides can potentially lead to heart disease, heart attacks, and heart failure. Additionally, patients who report eating high-carbohydrate, high-sugar diets may be at risk for the development of diabetes. Education on the effects of simple carbohydrates on the body should be discussed with patients. Chronically elevated glucose levels can lead to insulin resistance and organ dysfunction as a result of diabetes. Similarly, high-sodium diets can cause the body to retain fluid. Patients should be educated on the correlation between excess fluid and high blood pressure. Patients with other risk factors such as stress, smoking, and obesity can develop uncontrolled hypertension. Elimination of unhealthy dietary patterns can maintain wellness and prevent complications of diseases.

Exercise is an important topic of discussion with patients who report sedentary lifestyles. Lack of exercise can lead to obesity, osteoporosis, mood disorders, and back pain. The Centers for Disease Control and Prevention recommends aerobic and muscle strengthening activities for at least 150 minutes a week.

Smoking is a modifiable risk factor that can affect various body systems. Smoking can lead to tooth decay, erectile dysfunction, bronchitis, atherosclerosis, and lung cancer. In combination with other harmful risk factors, smoking can lead to the development of many chronic illnesses such as coronary artery disease, hypertension, emphysema, and peripheral arterial disease. Pharmacists should encourage cessation of smoking and be prepared to discuss the harmful effects of tobacco with the patient.

Abuse of substances such as alcohol and other drugs can also contribute to the development of disease. Alcohol is primarily metabolized in the liver. Excessive alcohol intake can lead to the destruction of liver cells and cause inflammation, cirrhosis, and liver failure. Most medications are also metabolized by the liver. Decreased liver function may lead to toxicity and harmful side effects.

Pharmacists should also be aware of **hereditary risk factors** that may contribute to the development of disease. For example, a patient who has family history of breast cancer should be encouraged to schedule annual wellness exams for possible mammograms at an earlier age. Mammograms are a screening tool that can detect early signs of breast cancer. **Maintenance of health** is a collaborative effort that can help prevent the development of disease and progression of chronic illnesses.

Using Evidence-Based Literature and Studies

Application of pharmaceutical care practice helps to maintain the health and safety of patients and overall communities. It is essential for pharmacists to become familiar with the integration of knowledge in care practice. Understanding the patient, the disease process, and the corresponding drug therapy are the three basic concepts in establishing a safe and effective plan of care. A prudent pharmacist will obtain knowledge on the most commonly encountered concepts in practice. Establishing a learning agenda on the best practices for the given conditions will allow the pharmacist to establish safe and effective drug therapies.

In addition to knowing the pharmacology and pharmacotherapy of medications, pharmacists should know the clinical appropriateness of drugs. The patient's physical signs and symptoms act as parameters to establish goals of therapy. Best practices are established from well-known disease processes and a vast number of pharmaceutical care encounters. For example, some of the most common disease indications for drug therapy in the nation include hypertension, diabetes, hyperlipidemia, vitamin deficiencies, depression, and pain. As a result, pharmacists can focus on understanding the

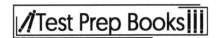
characteristics of the disease, the intent of the drug treatment, and the overall goals of therapy. Documented clinical indications serve as a guideline for treatment options.

Clinical pharmacology knowledge is developed and based on four key areas, including indication, efficacy, safety, and adherence. In treatment, **effectiveness** refers to the benefit obtained by an individual, whereas efficacy describes the benefits obtained by an entire population. Pharmaceutical care practitioners should always question whether a medication is appropriately indicated at the present time. For example, a patient's chronic asthma may be the indication for corticosteroids. **Corticosteroids** suppress the inflammatory response in the respiratory airways and aid in bronchodilation. To evaluate the effectiveness of treatment, practitioners should question whether the drug product and dosage regimen is producing the desired outcome for each medical condition. A patient with chronic pain, for instance, may be taking an opioid such as hydromorphone (Dilaudid). If the patient's pain persists after weeks of therapy, the dosage should be reevaluated. Pharmacists should be knowledgeable of the side effects of the medication, tendency of drug dependence, and safe ranges for dosing. Opioids are considered non-ceiling drugs with few limits on their doses but can cause respiratory depression and coma if not monitored appropriately.

Safety considerations include the likelihood of adverse reactions and toxic side effects. Proper dosage recommendations, patient education, and laboratory values can minimize the risk of this occurring. For example, a patient taking aspirin should be educated on the signs and symptoms of salicylate poisoning, such as ringing in the ears, nausea, vomiting, and severe abdominal pain. Additionally, serum salicylate values greater than 40 mg/dL can signal an overdose. **National consensus guidelines**, such as the Adult Treatment Panel and Joint National Committee, recommend the best evidence-based approach to treat or prevent a disease process.

These guidelines are created based on published clinical trials and extensive clinical expert experience. National guidelines serve as an outline for the approach to drug treatment. Textbooks are a common resource pharmacists use to produce a therapeutic framework and can help educate the practitioner on a patient's medical condition, associated symptoms, and current best practices. Textbooks used to help pharmacists better understand drug therapies include Lexicomp's *Drug Information Handbook, Handbook of Clinical Drug Data, Pharmacotherapy Handbook,* and *Pharmacotherapy: A Pathophysiologic Approach.* Knowledge of the patient's disease process can help influence the selection of drug therapy. A downside of printed textbooks is the limited scope of practice or outdated information.

Published clinical trials can also serve as the primary resource for up-to-date information on treatment modalities. Clinical trials are outlined in journals such as the *Journal of the American Pharmacists Association* and the *New England Journal of Medicine.* Randomized clinical trials provide measures that describe the benefit of a new treatment. One of these measures is the **number needed to treat (NNT)**. NNT expresses the benefit of the new treatment compared to a control group. For example, a trial administers omeprazole to 100 patients with erosive reflux esophagitis and a placebo to 100 patients with the same condition. If all 100 patients who took omeprazole see an improvement in their condition and none of the patients who received a placebo see an improvement in theirs, this would indicate that the treatment is effective and necessary. It is important for the pharmacist to interpret clinical trial results before applying them to drug therapy plans.

Practice Quiz

1. To determine the average glucose level of a patient over a period of 2 to 3 months, which laboratory result should the pharmacist evaluate?
   a. Hemoglobin A1C
   b. Fasting blood glucose
   c. Glucose tolerance test
   d. Capillary blood glucose

2. A patient is taking levetiracetam (Keppra) for the management of seizures. Which of the following labs should a pharmacist evaluate? (Select ALL that apply.)
   a. White blood cell count
   b. Platelet count
   c. Red blood cell count
   d. Liver function tests
   e. Creatinine test
   f. Blood urea nitrogen (BUN) test

3. Which signs and symptoms are expected for a patient taking chlorpromazine (Thorazine)? (Select ALL that apply.)
   a. Increased ability to perform activities of daily living
   b. Decreased heart rate
   c. Decreased appetite
   d. Increased ability to sleep
   e. Decreased hallucinations

4. Rank the following foods based on their sodium content (lowest to highest milligrams per portion):
   I. 3.5 oz of cooked asparagus
   II. 3.5 oz of avocado
   III. 3.5 oz of cheddar cheese
   IV. 3.5 oz of canned corn
   a. I, II, IV, III
   b. I, II, III, IV
   c. II, I, IV, III
   d. I, III, II, IV

5. Which manifestation is expected for a patient taking propylthiouracil (PTU)?
   a. Weight gain
   b. Decreased dyspnea
   c. Increased T4 levels
   d. Increased appetite

See answers on next page.

Answer Explanations

1. A: The hemoglobin A1C level provides an estimate of the average level of glucose in the body over the past 2 to 3 months. Hemoglobin A1C is a blood component that carries oxygen and binds to glucose. Normal values should be below 5.7%. Choice *B* is not correct. A fasting blood glucose measures the basal sugar levels when a patient has not had a meal overnight. This does not provide an insight into the history of glucose levels. Choice *C* is performed to measure the body's ability to absorb glucose after sugar is ingested. Blood glucose levels are taken before the test and 2 hours after ingestion of sugar. Normal glucose levels 2 hours after ingestion should be below 100 mg/dl. Choice *D* does not provide an average of glucose over a period of time. Blood samples are taken from blood vessels near the surface of the skin, and they provide the current glucose level.

2. A, C, and D: Levetiracetam (Keppra) is an anticonvulsant medication that decreases the incidence of seizure activity. Keppra may cause hematologic effects resulting in decreased erythrocytes and leukocytes. Erythrocytes are red blood cells used for oxygen transport throughout the body. Leukocytes are white blood cells used to fight off infections. Keppra may also cause hepatic abnormalities resulting in abnormal liver function tests. Choice *B* is not correct. Platelets are blood components that aid in blood clotting. Keppra does not directly affect platelets. Choices *E* and *F* assess kidney function. Keppra is not known to directly affect kidney function.

3. A, D, and E: Chlorpromazine (Thorazine) is an antipsychotic medication used in the treatment of chronic and acute psychosis. It treats conditions such as bipolar disorder, schizophrenia, and schizoaffective disorder. Patients with psychotic symptoms experience hallucinations, anxiety, hostility, and delusions. Physical symptoms include insomnia, loss of appetite, and decreased energy to perform activities of daily living. Thorazine is intended to increase the ability to perform independent activities, improve sleep patterns, and decrease or eliminate hallucinations. Choice *B* is not correct. Thorazine does not have a cardiovascular indication. Choice *C* is incorrect. Thorazine is intended to improve appetite.

4. A: It is important for pharmacists to encourage patients to follow a low-sodium diet to avoid the development of medical conditions such as hypertension and heart disease. A list of food groups is beneficial when educating patients about sodium content. Cooked asparagus contains the lowest amount, with 1 mg of sodium per portion. Avocado contains 4 mg of sodium per portion. Canned food contains more sodium than fresh food. Canned corn contains 236 mg of sodium per portion. Cheddar cheese contains the highest amount of sodium, with 620 mg per portion.

5. A: Propylthiouracil (PTU) is an antithyroid medication used in the treatment of hyperthyroidism. Patients with hyperthyroidism have an increased metabolism and exhibit signs such as elevated heart rate, increased appetite with weight loss, and heat intolerance. The goal of PTU is to inhibit weight loss associated with rapid metabolism. Choice *B* is incorrect. Difficulty breathing is not a characteristic sign of hyperthyroidism. Choice *C* is incorrect. Hyperthyroidism causes an increase in T4, the thyroid hormone responsible for metabolism. The goal is to decrease these levels. Choice *D* is incorrect. Hyperthyroidism causes an increase in appetite with excessive weight loss. The goal is to retain weight.

Area 2 - Identifying Drug Characteristics

Pharmacology, Mechanism of Action, or Therapeutic Class

Pharmacology refers to how medicine is used, including its possible effects and the way it acts on the human body. When filling a prescription, it is important to understand how a drug works. Not only does knowledge about the pharmacology of a medicine help to identify possible drug interactions, but it also helps to facilitate patients' understanding of why medications are prescribed for them. It is important to recognize that drugs with a similar therapeutic effect might have different mechanisms/modes of action.

Once absorbed into the body, medications are transported to target cells in several different ways. The most common mechanism for transport is **passive diffusion**. **Diffusion** occurs when a substance travels from an area of high concentration to an area of low concentration. Medications that act by passive diffusion are pushed into the bloodstream where they exert their action. For example, medications ingested orally will initially have a higher concentration in the stomach. The lower concentration in the bloodstream will cause the medication to diffuse from the stomach into the bloodstream.

Facilitated diffusion is a process in which the medication binds to a carrier such as an enzyme or protein before it can diffuse from an area of high concentration to an area of low concentration.

Medications that are moved from an area of low concentration towards an area of high concentration use the **active transport mechanism**. A carrier substance and cellular energy is required for medications to be transported to target cells using the active transport mechanism.

The mechanism of action varies among the different class of medications. The following chart describes the different classes.

Class I medications	Sodium channel blockers	Block the movement of sodium into the cardiac cells
Class II medications	Beta-adrenergic blockers	Block the sympathetic nervous system from stimulating beta receptors in the heart
Class III medications	Potassium channel blockers	Prolong the refractory period in both ventricles and atria, prolong the action potential, and slow repolarization
Class IV medications	Calcium channel blockers	Block the movement of calcium into conductile and contractile cells in the myocardium

For example, opioid medications such as morphine, fentanyl (Sublimaze), and hydromorphone (Dilaudid) act via a gate control action. These medications bind to opioid receptors in the brain and block transmission of pain impulses from one nerve cell to another. Opioid analgesics can bind to different types of pain receptors and the degree to which they block pain impulses will determine the level of

22

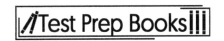

analgesia a patient will experience. The mechanism of action for antiseizure medications such as phenytoin (Dilantin), fosphenytoin (Cerebyx), and diazepam (Valium) functions primarily by decreasing the movement of ions into the nerve cells.

Antiseizure medications also alter the activity of neurotransmitters such as gamma-aminobutyric acid (GABA) which decrease the excitability of nerve cells. These mechanisms of action decrease the possibility of seizure activity. Adrenergic drugs such as epinephrine (Adrenalin), pseudoephedrine (Sudafed), and isoproterenol (Isuprel) have several different mechanisms of action. Adrenergic drugs directly interact with postsynaptic receptors on the membrane surface of target organs and tissues. This interaction causes an alteration in the permeability of the cell membrane and allows molecules such as enzymes and ions to enter the cell and aid in its reproduction. Stimulation of these receptors results in sympathetic effects in the body such as increased blood flow, heart rate, and oxygen consumption.

Corticosteroid medications such as hydrocortisone, fluticasone (Flovent), and cortisone (Cortone) are lipid-soluble drugs that enable simple diffusion through cell membranes into the target cells. Once inside the target cells, corticosteroids bind to receptors and travel to the cell nucleus where they interact with deoxyribonucleic acid (DNA) and either stimulate or suppress gene transcription. This action can help inhibit tissue repair, prevent the increase of lymphocytes, and impair phagocytosis. Due to their immunosuppressive mechanism, corticosteroids are primarily used to treat inflammatory and immune response disorders such as allergies, ulcerative colitis, and cerebral edema.

Additionally, medications have a specific peak and duration. The **peak** is the timeframe when there is maximum concentration of the medication in the circulatory system. How long the medication exerts its effects is known as the **duration**. The **mechanism of action** is the way a substance exerts its effect on target tissues. Active ingredients have several ways of producing their pharmacological effects such as binding to an enzyme, blocking a receptor, interrupting cell growth, or stimulating hormone production. In order for a generic medication to be considered bioequivalent, its active ingredient must produce the same mechanism of action and have a near equal peak as the branded medication. The same bioequivalence rule applies when prescribing alternative medications within a drug class.

Patients who develop allergies, experience adverse effects, or do not tolerate a medication well will require a different medication that has a similar mechanism of action and can produce the same therapeutic effect. Pharmacists should become familiar with equivalency tables so that they can suggest alternatives when needed. For example, if a patient needs to substitute clonazepam (Klonopin) for flurazepam (Dalmane), a benzodiazepine equivalency table can be used to determine the appropriate dosage. 0.25-1 mg of clonazepam (Klonopin) is approximately equivalent to 15-30 mg of flurazepam (Dalmane). Likewise, if a patient requires an alternative to carvedilol (Coreg), a beta blocker equivalency table can be used to determine the dosage of the substitute drug. 12.5 mg of carvedilol (Coreg) is equivalent to 50 mg of atenolol (Tenormin), 100 mg of labetolol (Normodyne), and 5 mg of timolol (Istalol).

Commercial Availability and Prescription or Non-Prescription Class

Before a medication can be marketed for use as a prescribed or an over-the-counter medication, it must go through an approval process. Safety is a high priority and medications must first be tested on animals before clinical trials on humans can occur. Efficacy of the medication is determined after three phases of clinical trials. During these trials, the medication is tested on healthy volunteers and patients who have a

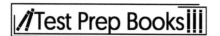

condition the medication is intended to treat. The medication then goes through an approval process by the Food and Drug Administration. Once a medication is determined to be safe and effective, it is marketed for patient use and providers are able to prescribe it. Post-marketing studies continue after its release to ensure side effects and long-term effectiveness are documented.

Each medication that is approved to be released has a unique identity. The physical characteristics must differ from other medications on the market. These characteristics will identify the medication and be useful for tracking purposes. A medication in pill form is required to have a unique design to include a shape, pattern, and color. Medications must also be imprinted with an identifier such as letters, numbers, the medication name, or a logo. Medication labels will identify the characteristics of the tablet. **Prescribed medications** are intended to be administered only to the patient for whom it was prescribed.

When providers write a prescription, they have taken into consideration the patient's allergies, past medical history, current symptoms, and intended therapeutic response. Medications that are not prescribed by a provider are available as **over-the-counter medications**. These medications can be purchased without a prescription and are intended to be used by anyone who is experiencing the symptoms listed on the medication label. When dispensed, prescribed medications will contain a leaflet with information about the medication. The leaflet will include instructions on administration, characteristics of the medication, and an ingredient list of the drug. Over-the-counter medications have this information on the label or the secondary packaging. Included on the label will be the active and inactive ingredients of the drug.

Patient Package Inserts (PPIs) are developed and submitted voluntarily to the FDA by the manufacturer. PPIs are approved by the FDA. For certain classes of medications, it is mandatory that PPIs be provided to patients—these include oral contraceptives and estrogen-containing products. The FDA warrants the safe and effective use of these products by requiring that patients be fully informed about the benefits and risks associated with the uses of these medications.

Manufacturers also voluntarily submit PPIs for other medications to the FDA for approval; however, distribution of these PPIs to patients is not mandatory.

Commercially-available pharmaceuticals carry an expiration date based on the stability data. The **expiration date** refers to the calculated timeframe within which a product retains its physical and chemical stability and therapeutic efficacy, based on a published monograph.

The active ingredients are typically listed at the top of the label and are ordered by their dosage concentration. The purpose of the ingredient is listed next to its name. For example, Aleve-D Sinus & Cold is a medication available over the counter. The medication label on the carton includes active and inactive ingredients, uses, warnings, directions, and miscellaneous information. The primary ingredient listed is 220 milligrams of Naproxen sodium, followed by 120 milligrams of extended-release pseudoephedrine hydrochloride. **Naproxen** is a non-steroidal anti-inflammatory medication with a listed purpose of pain relief and fever reduction. **Pseudoephedrine** is a nasal decongestant with the purpose of relieving a stuffy nose. In addition to the primary ingredients, labels must include a list of inactive ingredients. Inactive ingredients help the medication retain its shape and enhance its chemical stability. Patients taking over-the-counter medications may have an allergy or sensitivity to one or more of the inactive ingredients. Disclosure of inactive ingredients improves safety and minimizes the risk of allergic reactions.

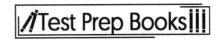

Brand, Generic, or Biosimilar Names and Physical Descriptions

Before a medication can be approved for use, initial animal studies and subsequent clinical trials in humans must be performed. When a medication is deemed safe, it is marketed as a brand. **Branded medications** contain an innovative chemical composition that is not currently on the market; they are initially exclusive to the company that develops them. Over time, these medications can be replicated in a generic form. **Generic medications** are more cost-effective and often become the first choice when dispensing a prescription. In order for a generic medication to be approved, it must be bioequivalent to the branded medication. **Bioequivalence** of a drug is determined by the pharmacokinetic action of the active ingredient. Each synthetic drug is absorbed, distributed, metabolized, and excreted in the body.

Each medication that is developed has a patent that prevents other companies from producing a medication that has the same molecular structure and the same active ingredient as the original drug. The Food and Drug Administration (FDA) prohibits generic drug companies from producing their version of a brand name drug until the patent expires. This exclusivity is placed as an effort to recoup the costs involved with developing and marketing a new medication. As a result, every medication has different physical attributes. Each medication that is developed must be unique in its color, shape, or form. **Pharmaceutical trade dress** is a trademark law that prevents generic drug companies from developing a medication that looks exactly like the brand name medication. This law is designed to prevent medications from being counterfeited.

Medications are developed in various forms, including capsules and tablets. Capsules and tablets are meant to be taken via the oral route. The drug must travel through the oral cavity and down the esophagus and be absorbed in the stomach or small intestine. Each tablet has a specific shape whether it's oval, round, flat, or capsular. Capsules travel easier through the esophagus, whereas flat tablets may adhere to the esophageal tissues.

The size of the medication is also important. Many patients have issues swallowing large pills. Dysphagia can lead to aspiration of medications into the lung and cause choking due to the blockage. Medications that are not passed properly through the pharynx into the esophagus have a risk of disintegration before they reach the stomach. This can lead to pain, ulceration of the esophagus, and possible perforation. The Food and Drug Administration and the U.S. Department of Health and Human Services suggest that tablets greater than 8 millimeters in diameter can cause issues with swallowing. For example, potassium chloride supplement tablets are typically large in size. An oval shaped extended-release tablet can range between 15–23 millimeters in diameter. Pharmacists should be cautious when dispensing these medications to ensure that patients have no problems swallowing. Additionally, if medications are enteric coated or extended release, they cannot be crushed, chewed, or split. Potassium supplements are also available in powder form and should be dispensed accordingly.

Tablets should be identified by their color, shape, and imprint. The imprint is a series of numbers and letters that are stamped on the capsule or tablet. This identifies the medication as being approved by the Food and Drug Administration for marketing and usage. The shape may vary and can be in the form of a circle, rectangle, or oval, or it can have 3–8 sides. Colors may be solid or have a combination of patterns. Medications that do not have these physical attributes are not approved by the FDA and may be classified as vitamins, diet pills, herbal supplements, foreign drugs, or illicit substances.

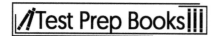

Boxed Warnings and REMS

The Institute of **Safe Medication Practices (ISMP)** provides impartial, timely, and accurate drug safety information. The ISMP provides pharmacy resources such as "do not crush" lists, black box warnings, error-prone abbreviations lists, confused drug names lists, high alert medications, and tall man letters. The ISMP also manages the **National Medication Errors Reporting Program (MERP)** and the **National Vaccine Errors Reporting Program (VERP).** Currently, the ISMP is the only national nonprofit body concentrating on the prevention of medication errors.

FDA Market Recalls are another type of warning issued for a drug, where minor violations need to be corrected or the drug needs to be removed from the market. Medical device recalls are part of FDA Medical Device Safety Alerts.

For medications with serious risks that may outweigh their benefits, the FDA may require a **Risk Evaluation and Mitigation Strategy (REMS).** The FDA's evaluation of a medication to determine whether an REMS is necessary considers several factors including serious risks, potential and known adverse effects of the drug within the afflicted population, and the seriousness of the condition being treated. The FDA also considers the size of the population expected to use the medication, the expected duration of treatment, the beneficial expectation of the drug, as well as other factors. It is the responsibility of the drug manufacturer to develop and implement the REMS for their drugs. The **iPledge program** is an example of an REMS for acne medications that contain Isotretinoin. Isotretinoin is contraindicated in pregnancy and can cause serious birth defects.

The REMS outline the requirements of the prescriber, patient, and pharmacy to ensure safe and effective use. To obtain a prescription for isotretinoin, females who can bear children must register with the iPledge program and verify they are not currently pregnant with a urine or blood test performed by a certified laboratory. The physician is required to counsel patients regarding the risks associated with the medication as well as document which two forms of contraception the patient is taking and enter the information into the iPledge system. Once the information is entered in iPledge, including the results of a second pregnancy test, the patient has seven days to obtain the medication from the pharmacy. The pharmacy must also register with iPledge to be able to verify that all patient requirements have been met. This requires entering the patient's iPledge ID and documenting the Risk Management Authorization (RMA) number on the prescription as well as the date it must be picked up by. If, however, the patient does not pick up the medication, then the RMA must be reversed in the iPledge system and the drug must be returned to stock.

Pregnancy or Lactation

It is important to assess a female patient's pregnancy status. Medications are assigned a **risk factor level** of A, B, C, D, or X. These different risk factor levels determine the probability that a medication will cause harm to an unborn fetus. Medications assigned an A risk factor level are the safest. Category A medications have been determined to be safe for administration in a pregnant female. Category B medications have been tested on animals, and no harm to the fetus has been shown. However, studies in pregnant women are not well controlled to determine its safety. Category C medications have been tested on animals, and adverse effects occurred in the unborn fetus. Studies are not well controlled in pregnant females to make a safety determination. Category D medications have demonstrated a risk to the fetus in well-controlled studies in pregnant women. However, the benefits that these medications provide in the treatment of a condition outweigh the possible risks identified in studies. If pregnant,

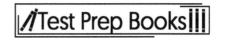

female patients should be asked to provide their estimated delivery date. The most damaging effects to a fetus usually occur during the first trimester of pregnancy.

During pregnancy, medications should be prescribed carefully to prevent harm to the developing fetus. For some medications, there might not be enough data available regarding safety during pregnancy, and therefore, they must be used cautiously after weighing the benefits versus the risks. Many medications are contraindicated during pregnancy, as they have teratogenic effects and can cause birth defects. If a patient is on a teratogenic medication prior to pregnancy, the medication should be stopped upon conception. A few examples of medications that are contraindicated in pregnancy include ACE inhibitors (e.g., ramipril, enalapril, lisinopril, etc.), ARBs (e.g., losartan, candesartan, irbesartan, etc.), isotretinoin, tetracycline antibiotics, hormonal therapies, and immunosuppressants (e.g., methotrexate).

Breastfeeding mothers have unique healthcare needs, including the administration of medications. Many substances pass through breastmilk or can otherwise affect the quantity or quality of a mother's milk supply. Nursing mothers can still take many medications safely, although the formulation and timing of the dosage may shift. Pharmacists are an important source of education and counseling for nursing mothers, as they can help these patients understand how to safely take medications to limit infant exposure to active pharmaceutical ingredients. This can include timing medications right after nursing sessions, so that enough time passes before the next nursing session so that any active pharmaceutical ingredients have metabolized.

Patients may also receive a different form of the medication. For example, topical anesthetics typically have poor oral absorption abilities. Therefore, a mother who requires pain relief may be able to use a topical ointment at the site of pain rather than taking an oral medication that would be more likely to enter her milk supply. Finally, pharmacists can help dispel misinformation about how medication affects lactation. Many patients may forego medications such as ibuprofen, believing it could affect their breastmilk, and needlessly suffer from pain and discomfort. However, research indicates that many routine medications do not affect infants adversely, even if small amounts enter the mother's milk supply. Other patients may believe that over-the-counter medications, such as aspirin, are harmless to nursing infants. However, this medication can adversely affect the baby. Pharmacists play an important role in ensuring that mothers receive the health care they need while also supporting the mother's breastfeeding goals and the health and safety of the nursing infant.

Practice Quiz

1. Rank the following antipsychotic medications based on their peak action (shortest to longest):
   - I. Haloperidol IM
   - II. Olanzapine PO
   - III. Chlorpromazine PO
   - IV. Trifluoperazine IM
   a. I, II, IV, III
   b. I, IV, III, II
   c. IV, III, II, I
   d. I, III, II, IV

2. Which of the following over-the-counter cold remedies has the highest concentration of pseudoephedrine per dose?
   a. Advil Cold and Sinus
   b. Dimetapp Cold and Allergy
   c. Actifed Cold and Allergy
   d. Robitussin Cold and Flu

3. Where does paroxetine (Paxil) exert its mechanism of action?
   a. Serotonin reuptake transporter
   b. Vesicle containing serotonin
   c. Serotonin receptors
   d. Receiving neuron

4. A pharmacist is dispensing adrenergic agonist medications. Which receptor, when activated, causes dilation of the renal blood vessels?
   a. Dopamine
   b. Alpha-1
   c. Beta -1
   d. Beta-2

5. A pharmacist is providing education to a patient taking oral morphine for chronic pain. The pharmacist tells the patient that maximum analgesia should be expected how long after the patient takes the dose?
   a. 10 to 20 minutes
   b. 30 minutes
   c. 60 minutes
   d. 60 to 90 minutes

See answers on next page.

Answer Explanations

1. B: The peak action of medications refers to the highest concentration of the active substance in the circulatory system. The onset of the intramuscular route is faster than the oral route. Therefore, the peak action will be reached quicker. The fastest peak action is for haloperidol IM at 30 to 45 minutes. The peak action for trifluoperazine IM is 1 to 2 hours. The peak action for chlorpromazine PO is 2 to 4 hours. The longest peak action is for olanzapine PO at 4 to 5 hours.

2. C: Multi-ingredient nonprescription cough, cold, and sinus remedies have a combination of drugs to alleviate a variety of symptoms. All the listed medications contain pseudoephedrine. Pseudoephedrine is a nasal decongestant that constricts blood vessels to relieve a runny nose. Actifed Cold and Allergy has the highest concentration of pseudoephedrine per tablet (60 mg). Advil Cold and Sinus has 30 mg of pseudoephedrine per tablet. Dimetapp Cold and Allergy has 15 mg of pseudoephedrine per 5 ml of solution. Robitussin Cold and Flu has the lowest concentration of pseudoephedrine per tablet (10 mg).

3. A: Paroxetine (Paxil) is a selective serotonin reuptake inhibitor (SSRI) used in the treatment of depression. Serotonin is a neurotransmitter responsible for regulating mood and assisting with the reward center in the brain. It is released from vesicles found in presynaptic cells. Then it travels to a receiving neuron where it transmits its effects. The reuptake of serotonin requires a transporter to recycle it back into the cell. Paxil competes for the binding site and inhibits the reuptake of serotonin. Paxil helps the body use the available serotonin more effectively to decrease the symptoms of depression.

4. A: Adrenergic agonist medications such as dopamine, dobutamine, and epinephrine stimulate receptors responsible for vasodilation, smooth muscle relaxation, and increased myocardial contractility. Dopamine receptors are specifically responsible for renal blood vessel dilation with low, moderate, and high doses of dopamine (Intropin). Choices *B*, *C*, and *D* do not have renal blood vessel dilation properties. Alpha-1 receptors are responsible for vasoconstriction to increase blood pressure and decreases nasal congestion. Beta-1 receptors are responsible for increased myocardial contractility, heart rate, and rate of conduction through the AV node of the heart. Beta-2 receptors are responsible for bronchodilation in the respiratory airways.

5. C: Oral administration of morphine has an expected peak activity 60 minutes after ingestion. Choice *A* is the expected time frame for morphine administered intravenously. Choice *B* is incorrect; 30 minutes is the expected peak when morphine is administered intramuscularly. Choice *D* is the most delayed effect and is expected when morphine is administered via the subcutaneous route.

Area 3 – Developing or Managing Treatment Plans

Triage or Medical Referral

Triage is the practice of prioritizing patient treatment from highest risk and need to lowest risk and need. Historically, triage is most commonly associated with mass casualty and catastrophic events, such as war or natural disasters. In these contexts, patients who require the most resources and have the highest chance of surviving if they receive those resources are treated first. Patients who are unlikely to survive even with treatment and patients who are not critically ill are seen later. Healthcare administrations have seen how the benefits of triaging care can help manage the ever-increasing demands on primary care, community health, public health, and geriatric health services.

Pharmacists have the necessary clinical background and knowledge to determine how best to manage a patient's care and can provide a multitude of non-emergency services such as medication dispensation, medication monitoring, immunizations, health coaching, and health education that can prevent an emergency situation or manage the patient's need until a specialty appointment becomes available. They can also partner with healthcare systems to determine a patient's health needs and refer critically ill patients immediately to necessary services, bypassing wait times associated with busy emergency department waiting rooms and intake paperwork. Pharmacies and pharmacists can often meet the needs of patients who need primary care support or chronic care management support, therefore reducing the burden on emergency services and physician offices.

Managing a patient's drug regimen is a collaborative effort between a pharmacist and other members of the healthcare team. Primary care providers are responsible for managing a patient's medical condition and prescribing appropriate drug therapy. Pharmacists are an additional resource to verify that the medications prescribed by providers are safe, appropriate, and effective for the selected patient. Providers may refer patients to specialists or other care providers to address the needs of the patient. Constant evaluation of the patient's response to drug therapy is needed for possible modification of the care plan.

Pharmacists are also responsible for recognizing signs and symptoms of adverse reactions to medications and worsening of a disease process. Medications have an array of possible side effects. Some are common while others are potentially dangerous. For example, loop diuretics such as furosemide (Lasix) can be ototoxic. Pharmacists should be aware of the possibility of hearing loss while taking this medication. Questions regarding the sense of hearing should be assessed during follow up appointments. Should a patient report that they are experiencing hearing loss, prompt discontinuation of the medication and referral to a medical provider is warranted if the condition does not improve.

One of the goals of therapy is the resolution of clinical signs and symptoms. Patients who do not show improvement or exhibit a decline in their health status should be referred to a medical provider for care. For example, a patient prescribed an antibiotic for an upper respiratory infection with manifestations of coughing, throat irritation, and runny nose would expect to see resolution of these symptoms a couple of days after starting drug therapy. Should the patient return and report increased cough and a new onset of shortness of breath or chest pain, the pharmacist should recognize that the patient is having complications of their disease process and requires further medical care. Pharmacists should also be able to identify when a patient requires primary, urgent, or emergency care.

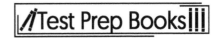

Patients who take over-the-counter medications may ask pharmacists for advice on selecting them. Pharmacists should be prepared to ask screening questions to ensure the patient's signs and symptoms do not require a higher level of care. For example, a patient reporting diarrhea may seek advice for over-the-counter treatments. Diarrhea can cause a large amount of fluid loss and lead to electrolyte imbalances. A pharmacist should be prepared to screen the patient for accompanying symptoms such as weakness, dry mouth, and dizziness. These symptoms can be a sign of dehydration. Significant dehydration can lead to hypotension, loss of consciousness, and kidney failure. Patients experiencing alarming symptoms should be referred to a medical provider for care.

Keeping track of laboratory results is an important aspect of drug therapy follow up. Lab values that are out of range can have significant adverse effects. For example, a patient taking spironolactone (Aldactone) for management of congestive heart failure may have an increase in potassium levels. **Aldactone** is a potassium-sparing diuretic that minimizes the excretion of potassium and may cause hyperkalemia. Hyperkalemia can lead to cardiac dysrhythmias and chest pain if not addressed. Symptomatic patients should be promptly referred to a medical provider for correction of the electrolyte imbalance.

Therapeutic Goals or Outcomes

Developing goals of therapy is a standard of care for pharmaceutical care practice. Goals should be patient centered and have several measurement criteria. Goals are mutually negotiated between health care providers and the patient to establish parameters used in evaluating the effectiveness and safety of drug therapy. Goals should also be realistic in relation to the patient's future and present capabilities. In pharmaceutical care, care plans are organized based on the indication for drug therapy. Some goals of therapy include reducing or eliminating symptoms of an illness, curing or preventing a disease, slowing the progression of an illness, normalizing laboratory values, and assisting with a diagnostic process. Modification of treatment plans will always be dependent on the patient's goal of therapy and clinical parameters. For example, the therapy goal for a patient with a local infection is to receive the correct medications based on antibiotic sensitivity to prevent systemic spread and subsequent complications. Patients with terminal illness may have pain management as their primary drug therapy goal.

Therapeutic goals allow the practitioner to safely manage each of the medications ordered. Strict organization of expected outcomes avoids mistakes, confusion, and errors of omission. For example, a patient with a couple of medical conditions may be taking several medications to effectively manage their comorbidities. Multiple drug therapies that are used for the same indication can be successfully grouped together within the same care plan. This allows for evaluation of the pharmacotherapeutic approach of each condition. A patient who has a history of hypertension and heart failure, for instance, may be taking multiple diuretics to decrease volume in addition to beta-blockers to control blood pressure. It is important to establish a therapeutic goal to maintain safe efficacy and adequate daily functioning.

Patient-centered therapy goals should always have a specific structure and include realistic, observable, and measurable time frames. Patients must always know what to anticipate from drug therapy and when results are expected to appear. For example, a patient with hypothyroidism may be started on levothyroxine. A therapy goal may be the achievement of normal thyroid function as indicated by a thyroid-stimulating hormone level of 4.5 mIU/L or less within 3 weeks of medication initiation. A patient with diabetes may be started on metformin with a goal of reducing the glycosylated hemoglobin (A1c) to less than 7% within 9 months. If the patient is unable to achieve this goal by the specified time frame,

31

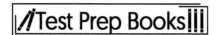

modification is required. Adjustments to the medication dosage and frequency or the addition of other antihyperglycemic agents may apply. Goals of therapy that aim to cure a disease apply to medical conditions such as urinary tract infections, pneumonia, or gastrointestinal concerns.

Therapeutic goals may include the resolution of infection or the complete suppression of symptoms within a specified time frame. For example, a patient taking loperamide (Imodium) for diarrhea would expect to see a decrease in the number and fluidity of stools and a reduction in abdominal cramping within 24 to 48 hours. Therapeutic goals that focus on reducing or eliminating symptoms of a disease aim to help the patient return to an acceptable level of functioning. An example of this would be major depression. Patients with depression experience symptoms such as fatigue, decreased appetite, disturbed sleep patterns, and reduced concentration. Drug therapy may include antidepressants such as sertraline (Zoloft), citalopram (Celexa), and fluoxetine (Prozac). Patients should be adequately informed that antidepressants typically require several weeks to begin their efficacy. Symptoms such as fatigue can improve within days, and follow-up evaluations every 6 to eight weeks are required for continued control.

Goals of therapy that aim to prevent a disease process include medical conditions such as stroke and diabetes and preventive drugs such as vaccines. A postmenopausal woman, for example, is at a high risk for development of osteoporosis. The goal of therapy would include adequate serum calcium levels to prevent weak bones and possible fractures. In addition to drug therapy such as alendronate (Fosamax), an elderly patient may be encouraged to maintain an adequate intake of vitamin D and perform weight-bearing exercises to strengthen bones. Medications administered before a diagnostic test have a goal of successful completion of the procedure. For example, a patient with anxiety who is unable to tolerate enclosed spaces necessary for an MRI (magnetic resonance imaging) may require alprazolam (Xanax) prior to the diagnostic procedure.

Medication Reconciliation and Indication of Uses

Personalized care plans are important when initiating and revising drug therapy. Patients should actively participate in the care process and be involved in modifications to their treatment. Effective communication and documentation of the personalized care plan is important because it provides the patient with a summary of their medications, disease process, and personal health information. Patients are able to take this summary with them to physician visits and have it available in case of emergencies. The care plan also provides the patient with an overview of their progress and allows them to record observations or questions that can later be discussed with their pharmacist or physician. Personalized care plans also empower the patient to be actively involved in the decision and modification of drug therapy.

A personal pharmaceutical care plan has several components. The plan should identify the patient with their name, address, and date of the current care plan. **Medication-related information**, such as allergies, adverse reactions, or special instructions should be included. A summary of all the patient's current medications is a major part of the care plan and focuses on the medication indication, name, directions for use, and prescriber information. Patients should be educated on why the medication is being taken and how often it should be administered. If patients are taking several medications that interact with one another, the care plan should clearly state directions for use. For example, a patient receiving interferon alfa-2b for leukemia may experience flu-like symptoms, such as fever, aches, and pains after its administration. Acetaminophen (Tylenol) is used to decrease the effects of the

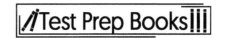

medication, but it must be taken prior to the interferon alfa-2b administration. This information would need to be communicated to patients and their caregivers.

Additionally, the care plan should include information for each of the medications prescribed, including the goals of therapy, how to take the medication, common side effects, and follow-up checkpoints. Effective communication regarding the treatment plan should be user-friendly and medical jargon should be avoided. For example, a diuretic for hypertension should be explained to the patient in lay terms. The patient should be able to recognize that this medication is used to lower blood pressure and can increase frequency of urination. A patient taking a proton-pump inhibitor for gastritis should be aware that this medication decreases stomach acid and relieves heartburn. Directions for use should also be translated into statements the patient can understand. For example, a prescriber may write a prescription for 600 mg of ibuprofen (Motrin) to be taken TID with meals. The patient would need to understand the medication should be taken 3 times a day (every 8 hours) with food to decrease stomach upset caused by nonsteroidal anti-inflammatory (NSAID) medications.

In addition to medication information, the personalized care plan should include health advice for the patient to assist them in reaching their treatment goals. Health advice can include **nonpharmacological approaches**, such as diet, exercise, and avoidance of harmful substances. For example, a patient taking a statin to lower cholesterol should be encouraged to eat a low-fat, low-cholesterol meal and exercise at least 150 minutes a week to decrease the risk of heart disease. The description of the medication is also valuable to the patient. Medications are dispensed in different shapes, sizes, and colors. Communicating these medication characteristics to the patient and their caregivers allows for better recognition of the drugs.

Follow-up checkpoints are key components of the care plan that monitor goal progress. Additionally, a follow-up checkpoint may be created to monitor side effects of medications after initiation of treatment. For example, a patient taking clindamycin (Cleocin) for a wound infection should expect to see a decrease in redness, inflammation, and purulent drainage. However, possible side effects of Cleocin include severe diarrhea and vaginal yeast infections due to the suppression of normal flora by antibiotics. The follow-up checkpoint can evaluate the decrease in primary symptoms and the appearance of adverse effects. Follow-up dates should be a mutual agreement between the patient and their pharmacist or physician. After a pharmacist has prepared the care plan for the patient and applicable caregivers, a pharmacist signature is required to ensure the care plan is legible and realistic for the patient.

Polypharmacy can be a barrier for patient compliance with drug therapy. A high percentage of patients take several medications a day to treat multiple comorbidities. Managing multiple drug therapies can cause confusion and the inability to follow instructions properly. For example, a patient who has diabetes, hypertension, and a cardiac arrhythmia may be taking multiple medications that target different body mechanisms. Additionally, the medications may need to be taken at different times of the day. Patients need to be educated thoroughly on the dosages, frequency, indication, and side effects of drugs before initiation of therapy.

Patient education also prevents misuse of drugs. Patients with polypharmacy may take the drug for the wrong reason. For example, a patient taking more than ten medications may confuse the shape, size, and color of the pills. If not cautious, patients can take multiple doses or a medication not intended for the current situation. Patients may also develop tolerance to a medication and self-prescribe higher doses to obtain the same effects. The most commonly misused medications include stimulants such as methylphenidate (Ritalin), opioids such as oxycodone (Oxycontin), and central nervous system

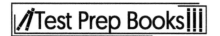

depressants such as phenobarbital (Luminal). When overuse no longer matches the goal of therapy, modification of treatment is necessary. Patients will need to be reevaluated for presenting symptoms and overall goals of drug therapy.

Duplication Therapy and Omissions

It is a pharmacist's responsibility to identify drug therapy problems. Drug therapy problems include:

- Unnecessary drug therapies
- Additional need for drug therapy
- Ineffective medication treatment
- Ineffective dosages

One of the causes for unnecessary drug therapy is duplication of medications. Patients may be prescribed multiple drug products to treat a condition that can ideally be treated with one medication.

Duplicate drug therapy increases the risk of additive side effects and extra costs for the patient. For example, a patient with chronic renal failure may require a variety of medications to manage the illness. The kidneys are responsible for maintaining fluid balance. Ineffective renal function may lead to fluid overload and subsequent hypertension. Patients with chronic renal failure often require antihypertensive medications such as ACE inhibitors, calcium channel blockers, and diuretics. Medications such as furosemide (Lasix) are loop diuretics that decrease excess volume but cause the excretion of electrolytes such as potassium. Patients with chronic renal failure retain large amounts of potassium. These patients may be prescribed medications such as Kayexalate to eliminate excess potassium. A patient prescribed both a loop diuretic and Kayexalate may experience excessive loss of potassium. Hypokalemia can cause muscle weakness, abnormal heart rhythms and paralysis. Pharmacists should promptly notify providers when duplicate drug therapy is noted to avoid adverse effects.

Another potential drug therapy problem category is the need for additional therapy. Upon review of a patient's medical record, pharmacists should note all medical conditions. Any untreated condition may require an initiation of drug therapy. In addition to reviewing illnesses, reviewing laboratory and assessment data will help determine if the condition is well controlled or requires provider intervention. It is important for pharmacists to collect comprehensive patient data when presenting omission of drug therapy to the provider. For example, if a pharmacist notes that the patient is a newly diagnosed diabetic but does not have any hypoglycemic medications, evaluation of the laboratory data should follow. Laboratory data such as serum glucose levels and hemoglobin A1C are useful in determining if the disease is well controlled. Normal serum glucose levels should be between 70-110 mg/dl. Normal hemoglobin A1C levels should be below 5.7%. Elevated results may indicate the progression of the disease.

Additionally, documentation of the review of systems may reveal signs and symptoms related to the illness. If a newly diagnosed diabetic reports having decreased sensation in the lower extremities, this may be peripheral neuropathy. **Peripheral neuropathy** means that nerve endings have been damaged as a result of sustained hyperglycemia. Non-healing wounds, excessive thirst, hunger, and increased urination are all additional symptoms of poorly controlled glucose. Laboratory and clinical parameters will aid the pharmacist in communicating drug therapy omission to the patient's provider.

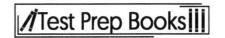

Drug Dosing and Duration of Therapy

Although medications are developed for the treatment of a medical condition, there are numerous variables for the dosages, frequencies, and indications of each individual drug. Furthermore, a number of medications have unlabeled uses that treat alternative conditions not listed as a primary indication. Patient assessment and evaluation of their medical conditions enable providers to establish individualized goals of therapy.

Most medications are metabolized in the liver, so liver function is important for dosing. Intact liver function is required for medications to be converted to water-soluble molecules that can later be excreted by the kidneys. Patients who do not have an intact liver may require smaller doses of medication. The inability to metabolize drugs in their entirety can lead to toxicity and cumulative adverse effects. Liver function can be assessed by laboratory data. Enzymes such as alanine transaminase (ALT), aspartate transaminase (AST), and alkaline phosphatase (ALP) help metabolize proteins. When the liver is damaged, these enzymes will be released into the bloodstream and result in high laboratory values. Subsequently, providers will adjust dosages of hepatotoxic medications. For example, antiretroviral drugs such as didanosine (Videx) and zidovudine (Retrovir) can cause increased AST, ALT, and ALP. Decreased hepatic function can lead to hepatic steatosis, an abnormal retention of fat within liver cells. Fatty liver can lead to scarring, decreased liver function, and increased acidity in the blood. The resulting lactic acidosis can be fatal if not corrected promptly. Prescribers may choose to order lower doses to maintain organ integrity.

Renal function is another assessment that must be conducted prior to prescribing medications. The kidneys are primarily responsible for excreting excess waste, including medication concentrations. Decreased kidney function may lead to cumulative effects and toxicity. Laboratory parameters such as creatinine clearance and blood, urea, and nitrogen (BUN) levels must be obtained and evaluated. Normal creatinine clearance time is approximately 95 ml/min. Patients with levels significantly below this value will require dosage adjustments. For example, **amantadine** (Symmetrel) is an antiparkinson agent which is entirely excreted via the urine. The medication is to be used cautiously in patients that have a creatinine clearance below 50 ml/min. Dosages need to be adjusted accordingly for patients with renal impairment.

A number of medications have multiple therapeutic uses. Although the pharmacologic effect is the same, the intended response will differ. For example, a patient with gastroparesis may suffer from intractable hiccups. This patient may be prescribed chlorpromazine (Thorazine) for the treatment of hiccups, nausea, and vomiting. **Thorazine** is more commonly used as an antipsychotic medication for the treatment of acute and chronic psychosis. Additionally, Thorazine has an unlabeled use for the treatment of vascular headaches. Another example of a medication with multiple therapeutic uses is sildenafil (Viagra/Revatio). **Sildenafil** is primarily used for the treatment of erectile dysfunction in men. As **Viagra**, it works by increasing blood flow to the corpus cavernosum and producing an erection. As **Revatio**, its function is to produce vasodilation of the pulmonary vascular bed. Revatio is used in the treatment of pulmonary hypertension. Dosages for this medication vary depending on their intended use. It is important for pharmacists to assess reports that identify which conditions are managed with individualized drug therapy. The medical record should reflect the medical condition that is being treated with the selected medication.

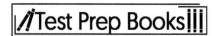
Route of Administration, Dosage Forms, and Delivery Systems

Medications can be administered via several routes. The route of administration affects how quickly a medication is absorbed into the bloodstream. Absorption determines how quickly the active substance will take effect. There are different routes of administration for medications, including the following:

- Orally or by mouth: oral tablets, capsules, liquid preparations (elixirs and suspensions)
- Nasally: sprays or drips
- Intravenously (IV): goes through the veins and must be liquid
- Intramuscularly (IM): goes into the muscle and must be liquid
- Subcutaneously: usually an injection under the skin
- Epidurally: may be infused into epidural space in the spinal cord
- Transdermal route: medication is absorbed through the skin via patches and creams
- Rectally: these are usually suppositories and some cream medications
- Sublingually: under the tongue
- Inhalation route: many sprays and nebulizer solutions are inhaled into the lungs
- Ocular route: into the eye, usually in the form of solutions and suspensions
- Aurally: into the ear, usually in the form of solutions and suspensions

One of the most common routes is the **oral route**. Once a medication is ingested, it travels to the stomach where enzymes will facilitate its absorption or delay the mechanism of action. For example, a medication like sucralfate (Carafate) is used to heal gastric ulcers. The medication is intended to be given on an empty stomach to exert its maximum effect. Conversely, medications like aspirin and other non-nonsteroidal anti-inflammatory drugs may cause gastric irritation and are recommended to be taken with food.

Drugs administered via the **intramuscular route** are injected into major muscles of the body including the deltoid, vastus lateralis, and ventrogluteal. Medications that require a target effect and quick onset may be administered intramuscularly. Alternatively, patients who are unable to ingest oral medications may require the intramuscular route instead. For example, a person who develops a sudden allergic reaction and develops anaphylaxis may lose consciousness or have swelling of their airway. A medication like epinephrine (Epipen) can be self-administered into the muscle at the first sign of an allergic reaction. Patients with known allergies should be instructed on the use of an Epipen and the importance of having it with them at all times for emergency purposes.

One of the routes that has the fastest onset is the **intravenous route**. Venous access provides a direct entry into the bloodstream. Medications administered via the intravenous route will have a rapid onset and are used widely to treat conditions such as nausea, pain, and hypertensive crisis. For example, one of the priorities for post-surgical patients is pain management. In an acute care setting, administering medications such morphine, hydromorphone, and fentanyl via the intravenous route will enable faster pain relief and better surgical outcomes.

Drug Contraindications, Allergies, or Precautions

Medications are intended to produce effects that alleviate physical symptoms, cure illnesses, and prevent long-term complications of disease. They do this by working to replace or supplement a chemical function in the body. Due to their synthetic makeup, medications can also cause unintended effects. There are thousands of medications that have been approved for use by the United States Food

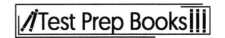

and Drug Administration. Each medication has a unique chemistry that produces a mechanism of action when it is absorbed, distributed, and metabolized. Medications are then primarily excreted from the body via the kidneys as liquid waste. It is important for pharmacists to recognize contraindications, special precautions, and warning labels when dispensing medications for patients.

The following are symptoms that indicate an **allergy** to a medication:

- Hives
- Skin redness and rashes or other types of reactions
- Swelling in the face, throat, tongue or other area of the body
- Difficulty breathing, wheezing, or chest tightness
- Irregular or rapid heartbeat

Severe forms of these reactions can indicate an **anaphylactic reaction**, which is life-threatening and requires immediate emergency treatment. Emergency Medical Services (9-11) should be contacted right away in cases of suspected anaphylactic reactions to any substance. It is common for patients to confuse allergic reactions and adverse effects. Therefore, it is important for the pharmacy staff to ask about the symptoms a patient experiences so the reaction can be categorized correctly.

There are some medications and supplements that contain food-based ingredients, and therefore, precautions need to be taken when prescribing such substances to a patient with food allergies. The coatings of medications, for example, can have excipients such as lactose, maltodextrin, and other starches that can cause allergic reactions in patients who are susceptible to those ingredients. Other medications, including Prometrium (a hormone medication), contain peanut oil so patients with peanut allergies should avoid such formulations. Some calcium products and omega-3 supplements are derived from shellfish; hence, a person with a seafood allergy may need to avoid these supplements. Patients with dietary restrictions, such as celiac disease or gluten intolerance, should avoid capsules made with gluten fillers or gelatin. If there are any questions about the ingredients, it is best to contact the manufacturer.

Although each medication is distinctive, all medications are part of a classification of drugs. In general, medications belonging to the same class will produce similar effects and provide a common therapeutic response. Likewise, drugs under the same classification will have similar contraindications, warnings, and precautions. For example, antineoplastic medications such as tamoxifen, mitomycin, and cisplatin are contraindicated in patients with previous bone marrow depression. Antineoplastics disrupt the DNA synthesis and function of tumor cells. Patients with bone marrow suppression may have an additive immunosuppressive response. Most antineoplastic medications are pregnancy category D. Category D medications can produce teratogenic effects to the unborn fetus and are therefore contraindicated in pregnancy.

Antipsychotic medications such as clozapine, haloperidol, and risperidone are all contraindicated in patients who have central nervous system depression. These types of medications often produce a sedative effect. In combination with central nervous system depression, they can induce a comatose state and/or cause death. Antipsychotic medications should also be used cautiously in patients with symptomatic cardiac disease. Antipsychotics have anticholinergic properties that can potentially cause an increase in the rate of the heart. Patients with cardiac disease may experience cardiac overload and potentially lead to heart failure.

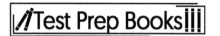

Individual medications may have unique warning labels that should be emphasized to the patients whenever a prescription is dispensed. For example, transdermal fentanyl (Duragesic) patches are meant to dispense medication over time. Due to fentanyl's prolonged peak and duration, dosages tend to be higher than opioids administered orally, intravenously, or intramuscularly. The risk of overdosing is increased with transdermal patches and the patches should be handled carefully by the person applying this medication. Improper handling of transdermal opioid patches can lead to fatalities, especially in children who have easy access to these medications.

Antitubercular medications such as isoniazid (INH) can induce hepatitis. When isoniazid is metabolized in the liver, it produces a liver toxin known as acetylhydrazine. Special precautions should be taken in patients with liver disorders. Prompt assessment of laboratory data such as alanine aminotransferase (ALT), aspartate aminotransferase (AST), and serum bilirubin levels should be performed before and during therapy. Elevated laboratory values indicate liver damage or drug-induced hepatitis.

The Beers List is a collection of medications that are more likely to cause adverse effects in the geriatric population. As people age, the risk of drug toxicity, disease development, and polypharmacy increases. Medications that cause an increase of adverse effects in the elderly can have a significant impact on their quality of life and lead to hospitalizations or permanent injury. Some of the medications found on the Beers List include alprazolam (Xanax), fluoxetine (Prozac), and barbiturates. Pharmacists should also be aware of fall safety among the elderly. Medications that cause sedative effects or sensory disturbances are more likely to cause falls in the geriatric population. Careful assessment of caregiver availability and home safety strategies should be performed when providing instructions for home use. Some of the medication categories that increase the risk for falls include antidepressants, narcotics, and vasodilators.

Adverse Drug Effects, Toxicology, or Overdose

Medication management includes establishing the safety of the drug regimen and supervising adverse effects of therapy. The usual cause of safety concerns are medication dosages that are too high or too frequently taken. **Adverse effects** result in either an unintended response to the pharmacology of the drug product or idiopathic effects. Patients may develop symptoms that were not present at the start of therapy. Medications often have several mechanisms of action and can affect multiple body systems, resulting in both beneficial and adverse side effects. For example, **aspirin** is an analgesic-antipyretic-anti-inflammatory drug that reduces pain, fever, and swelling. In addition to these beneficial effects, aspirin inhibits cyclooxygenase 1 (COX -1), which can decrease the protective mucous lining of the stomach and inhibit platelet aggregation. Patients taking aspirin for pain relief may exhibit signs of gastric irritation and bleeding.

The intended outcome will determine which of the effects are beneficial and which are adverse. For example, a patient who requires a decrease in viscosity of the blood to prevent a stroke or heart attack may be prescribed 81 mg of aspirin daily. The intended effect is blood thinning and not analgesia or fever reduction. Gastric irritation would be considered a secondary adverse effect. Adverse effects manifest themselves as clinical signs and symptoms or abnormal laboratory results. **Drug toxicity** occurs when the dosage of a medication is too high. Prompt identification of drug toxicity can prevent permanent organ dysfunction. An excessive dose of a drug or drugs can lead to an overdose which can be fatal.

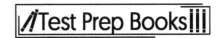

Laboratory tests should be evaluated on a scheduled basis to monitor drug therapy. For example, patients with high cholesterol may be prescribed a statin such as atorvastatin (Lipitor), simvastatin (Zocor), or rosuvastatin (Crestor). These medications inhibit an enzyme required for liver synthesis of cholesterol and can cause liver damage if not monitored properly. Laboratory values such as alanine aminotransferase (ALT) and aspartate aminotransferase (AST) can help determine the extent of liver toxicity. Laboratory values for statins should be ordered upon initiation of therapy and 6 to 12 weeks after starting the medication. **Digoxin** (Lanoxin) is a cardiac glycoside that improves cardiac output. Digoxin is used to treat heart failure and improve a patient's quality of life. Digoxin toxicity is precipitated by electrolyte imbalances, such as hypokalemia, hypomagnesemia, and hypercalcemia. Therefore, laboratory tests for potassium, magnesium, and calcium allow for prompt treatment of any imbalances.

Serum digoxin levels are important to monitor before and during the initiation of therapy to avoid toxic serum levels of 2 ng/mL or greater. Early manifestations of digoxin toxicity include nausea, confusion, and decreased appetite. Cardiac dysrhythmias, such as premature ventricular contractions (PVCs) and sustained atrial fibrillation (AFib), may result from inadequate doses. Clinical parameters are the patient's signs and symptoms that result from drug safety concerns. Physical symptoms are dependent on the medication's mechanism of action. The majority of medications are orally ingested, and therefore the effects are primarily gastrointestinal related, such as nausea, vomiting, and diarrhea. Medications that act on the central nervous system, such as opioids, may cause drowsiness, somnolence, agitation, and confusion when toxicity exists.

Alternatively, patient education on self-monitoring of vital signs may increase the safety of therapy for medications that lower blood pressure and pulse rates. For example, a patient taking a beta-blocker such as atenolol (Tenormin) for hypertension should be educated on the secondary effect of bradycardia. Patients should be instructed to take their pulse rate daily to ensure the heart rate does not drop below 50 beats per minute (bpm). Dangerously low heart rates can cause cardiac dysrhythmias, fainting, and possible cardiac arrest. The dosage may need to be tapered before discontinuation of the drug.

Practitioners should also be vigilant of polypharmacy, a term used to describe the simultaneous use of multiple drugs to treat a single condition. Patients who take various medications may not be fully informed on the mechanisms of action or possible side effects of each drug. Establishing an administration schedule and providing patient education is important to avoid overlapping therapeutic effects. For example, a diabetic patient who takes insulin aspart (NovoLog) and glipizide (Glucotrol) should be educated on eating shortly after administration. Both drugs lower glucose levels and can lead to hypoglycemia. Severe hypoglycemia (blood glucose level less than 40 mg/dL) can cause permanent brain damage and cardiac dysrhythmias.

Drug Interactions

Drug interaction refers to the alteration in pharmacology (absorption, distribution, metabolism, elimination, efficacy, side effects, etc.) of a medication by various factors including disease conditions, prescription and OTC medications, and foods or nutritional supplements. These interactions may result in either an augmentation or decrease in the efficacy and/or toxicity of the respective medication. Drug interaction should be carefully reviewed in order to avoid serious life-threatening conditions.

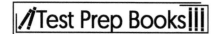

Incompatibility is defined as a change in medication components, such as the pH level, moisture, temperature, and color, that results in an undesirable product. The result can affect efficacy, safety, appearance, and stability of the medication. Incompatibilities can occur during dispensing, compounding, packaging, storage, and administration. The types of incompatibilities include physical, chemical, and therapeutic. Incompatibility occurs when two or more substances are mixed and form an unstable product. Two medications compounded together or administered at the same time may have varying pH levels and affect the mechanism of absorption.

For example, aspirin is an acidic medication with a pH level of 3.5. Aspirin is absorbed primarily in the stomach where the pH level is between 1.5–3.5. Other medications that have a low pH level include doxycycline (2–3) and ibuprofen (4). Due to their acidic nature, these medications can often cause stomach irritation. Enteric coating is a barrier made of plastic polymer that covers the medication and prevents its disintegration within the gastric environment. Medications that are alkaline are absorbed further in the gastrointestinal tract. The pH level of the small intestine is between 7–8.5. Alkaline medications, such as erythromycin, methotrexate, and penicillin G, are affected by the pH level in the stomach and are best absorbed in the small intestine.

Manipulation of the pH levels can lead to insolubility and instability of a medication. When compounding medications, pharmacists can add acidifying agents, such as phosphoric, nitric, or acetic acid, to lower the pH level of medications and increase their absorption. Alternatively, alkalizing agents, such as sodium carbonate, trolamine, and potassium hydroxide, increase the pH level and neutralize acidic substances. These chemical reactions increase the stability of the ingredients and allow compounded medications to function therapeutically. Chemical incompatibility may lead to precipitation of a medication. Precipitation results in turbidity, haziness, or the formation of crystals within the diluted drug solutions and can cause the inactivity or toxicity of active ingredients. Precipitates can occlude the catheter and form an embolus.

Emboli can travel through the bloodstream and cause ischemic organ failure. One of the main reasons for chemical incompatibility is a difference in pH levels of solutions. For example, **intravenous ertapenem** is an antibiotic medication with a pH level of approximately 7.5. **Lactated Ringer's** is an intravenous solution that contains electrolytes and has a pH level of 6.5. When mixed with ertapenem, it produces a stable solution that can be infused intravenously. Mixing ertapenem with dextrose solutions can cause instability and result in the formation of precipitates. Dextrose has a pH level of approximately 4.3. The acidic fluid does not react well with the alkaline medication and forms precipitates. Other alkaline drugs that are not compatible with acidic fluids include phenytoin, diazepam, and blood products.

Therapeutic incompatibility results when two or more medications exert opposing mechanisms of action. This results in antagonistic effects or interference with drug absorption. For example, quinidine is an antiarrhythmic medication that decreases myocardial excitability and slows the conduction velocity of the heart. **Epinephrine** is an antagonistic medication that increases the excitability of the heart in patients with cardiac arrest. These medications have opposite properties that would interfere with their mechanisms of action. It is important for pharmacists to reconcile all medications to ensure that interactions do not exist or interfere with their therapeutic purposes. For example, if a patient is taking levothyroxine for hypothyroidism, pharmacists should ensure that the patient is not taking bile acid sequestrants, such as cholestyramine. **Cholestyramine** is a cholesterol-lowering agent that decreases the absorption of oral levothyroxine. Incompatible medications should be administered at different timeframes to avoid mixing.

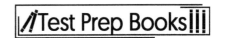

Medications that are synergistic produce actions in the same direction or enhance the action of each other when given simultaneously. **Synergism** can be additive or supra-additive. **Additive** refers to a combination of drugs that produces the same effect and results in an elevated therapeutic response. When the combination of medications produces a greater effect than individual drugs, it is known as **supra-additive synergism**.

Therapeutic Monitoring

Therapeutic monitoring is measuring the amount of drugs present in the blood. The efficacy and safety of a drug are determined quantitatively by comparing the amount of the drug needed to achieve a specific therapeutic goal and the amount at which toxicity occurs. The **therapeutic index**, or TI, compares the concentration of a drug in the blood at levels considered to be effective and at levels that are toxic. The therapeutic index is equal to the ratio of the toxic dose, or TD, for fifty percent of subjects and the effective dose, or ED, for fifty percent of subjects.

$$TI = \frac{Toxic\ dose}{Effective\ dose} = \frac{TD_{50}}{ED_{50}}$$

Generally, a medication with a high therapeutic index has a broader margin of safety and does not require close monitoring by a physician. For example, **Simvastatin**, a statin medication, is used to reduce cholesterol and is available in strengths ranging from 5 mg to 80 mg. Statins require minimal monitoring, such as annual bloodwork for cholesterol screening. Like many medications, Simvastatin can have adverse effects, but overall it is considered safe because of its broad therapeutic range.

Medications with a low therapeutic index are referred to as narrow therapeutic index drugs**. Narrow therapeutic index**, or NTI, medications have a small window between being effective and lethal. Some NTIs can have significant drug and dietary interactions that can complicate dosing. Examples of narrow therapeutic index medications include the anticoagulant Warfarin, thyroid medications such as Levothyroxine, transplant rejection medications like Cyclosporine, and the anticonvulsant Phenytoin, to name a few. Narrow therapeutic index medications require close monitoring of a patient by the physician to ensure their use does not result in therapeutic failure, serious injury, or death. **Vancomycin** is a narrow therapeutic index antibiotic medication that is used to treat serious bacterial infections like Methicillin-resistant Staphylococcus aureus (MRSA).

The antibiotic Vancomycin is typically delivered via intravenous infusions when treating these types of bacterial infections and requires extensive monitoring to ensure efficacy. To effectively inhibit bacterial growth, Vancomycin must hit a peak blood concentration followed by a low concentration called a trough. Dosing is repeated until a steady state, or the balance between infusion and elimination of the medication in the body, is achieved. A trough level is usually drawn before the fourth dose in the course is administered, as this is when the drug is at its lowest concentration in the bloodstream. Vancomycin is cleared from the body by the kidneys; therefore, kidney function must also be monitored to ensure adequate elimination from the body. Renal impairment may allow for the buildup of the medication in the body, possibly leading to irreversible nephrotoxicity. Vancomycin is most effective at a specific and steady concentration in the bloodstream, so it is vital to monitor the patient's level to determine adjustments in dosing.

The blood thinner Warfarin is another example of a narrow therapeutic index medication. **Warfarin** is an anticoagulant used to prevent the formation of blood clots in the body. Achieving the correct dose can be challenging in Warfarin patients because of its narrow therapeutic range. Warfarin dosing is further

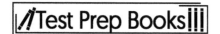

complicated by the fact that it interacts with other medications, dietary supplements, and some foods. A patient taking a blood thinner should avoid taking nonsteroidal anti-inflammatory drugs (NSAIDs) like aspirin or ibuprofen or dietary supplements such as garlic, as these can increase bleeding. In some foods like leafy greens, which are rich in Vitamin K, Warfarin acts to slow down the process of clotting factor production by blocking Vitamin K.

Vitamin K is a fat-soluble vitamin which is necessary to produce clotting factors like the protein Prothrombin. A dose too low can allow for clot formation and result in stroke, embolism, or heart attack. A dose too high can cause uncontrolled bleeding in the body. Warfarin patients require close monitoring by performing a PT/INR test to determine how quickly the blood is clotting. **Development of the International Normalized Ratio (INR)** helped to standardize these test results and account for any laboratory variations that may affect test results. The INR values range from zero to five, with the standard therapeutic target INR for a patient taking Warfarin being between two and three. A low INR value can put the patient at risk of clot formation, whereas a higher INR value can put the patient at risk for excessive bleeding.

Anticonvulsants are considered narrow therapeutic index medications and are used to minimize seizure activity in patients with seizure disorders such as epilepsy. Determining the correct therapeutic dose requires the patient to self-monitor any medication side effects and seizure activity, such as how frequently seizures occur or duration of the seizure. In addition, bloodwork must be monitored to ensure organ function is within range and blood concentration of medication is at a steady state.

Drug Pharmacokinetics or Pharmacodynamics

Pharmacokinetics is the study of the fate of a medication in the body. The knowledge of a medication's pharmacokinetics helps to determine dosing. Pharmacokinetics of a medication includes four parameters: absorption, distribution, metabolism, and elimination. **Absorption** refers to the process of the medication entering blood circulation. **Distribution** is the process of dispersion of the medication throughout the body, including the site of action. **Metabolism** is the process of degradation of the parent molecule into different metabolites. **Elimination** refers to the process of removal of the parent molecule and the metabolites from the body.

The pharmacokinetic of a medication can be affected by various factors including:

- Age
- Race
- Gender
- Genetic factors
- Dosage form
- Disease conditions
- Foods
- Concurrent administration of other conditions

Pharmacodynamics refers to the study of the effects of a medication at the site of action. This helps to ascertain the mechanism of action of a medication and to determine the dose-response relationship by analyzing the interaction of a drug with its receptors at the target organ or site.

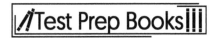

Evidence-Based Practice

Evidence-based practice (EBP) is a health care delivery framework that uses findings from rigorously performed research, relevant practitioner expertise, and patient preferences to develop and implement a medical treatment. EBP is a systematic approach that aligns closely with the scientific method to plan and test a medical intervention. The approach begins with a clinical question, which is generally focused on the patient's health concern and how to resolve it. In EBP, clinical questions are best formed using the PICO method, which stands for Patient/Population/Problem, Intervention, Comparison, and Outcome. This helps the practitioner develop their question by considering the following aspects: the patient they want to serve OR the target population they want to serve OR the health problem they are trying to address; the category of treatment they are considering; what they will compare the treatment results to in order to determine whether or not it was effective; and what outcome they are hoping to achieve.

Once the clinical approach has been developed, the provider should review high quality literature to find information. High-quality literature sources include manuscripts published in peer-reviewed journals, textbooks, case studies from reputable sources (e.g., a university or health care system), and some journalistic publishing. In general, good, relevant research in EBP should be current, pertain to the same demographic as the patient, and have reliable and externally valid results. Anecdotes from the general population or from non-expert sources, opinion pieces, editorial pieces, and crowd-sourced encyclopedia sites are low-quality information sources and should not be used in EBP. Once this literature review is complete, consulting with field experts adds more information to the evidence pool. Field experts should be reputable, respected, and seasoned in their field; ideally, they have worked with large numbers of patients whose conditions and treatments are relevant to the clinical question that has been formed.

Finally, this evidence base should be presented as transparently and simply as possible to the patient who will receive the intervention. It is important that the patient understands the evidence and treatment recommendations so that they can make an informed decision about their health plan. If a patient is distrustful of their provider, does not understand the treatment recommendation, or otherwise has a personal barrier to treatment, a successful intervention is unlikely. The patient may experience harm and the medical facility may have wasted organizational resources. When presenting information to the patient, the provider should be mindful of any possible biases or bedside manner that could sway the patient. Once the patient and provider have collaborated on the treatment plan, the intervention can begin. The patient should be monitored and evaluated with respect to the intervention, and findings should be documented and disseminated as appropriate. If the intervention is not successful, the practitioner should plan to go through this process again and design another intervention to test.

Lifestyle and Self-Care

Many medical conditions can be prevented by following a healthy lifestyle and adequate diet. Drug therapy is often the last resort when lifestyle changes do not correct a condition or complications are present. Patient education on lifestyle choices and self-care is a crucial element in preventing disease and managing comorbidities. In collaboration with other members of the healthcare team, pharmacists have a duty to encourage patients to adapt healthier lifestyles. Diseases such as hyperlipidemia, diabetes type II, some forms of hypertension, and heart disease are preventable by initiating healthier

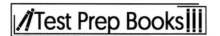
diets and active lifestyles. Patients who are prescribed medications to manage these diseases should still receive education on healthy foods and recommended timeframes for physical activity.

For example, a patient with hyperlipidemia has an excess of low-density lipoprotein (LDL) cholesterol and possibly elevated triglycerides. One factor that can increase cholesterol levels is a diet high in saturated fat. An excess amount of cholesterol can lead to atherosclerosis, or fatty plaques that attach themselves to the walls of arteries within the circulatory system. An accumulation of atherosclerosis can lead to heart disease and eventually heart attacks and heart failure. Pharmacists have the ability to counsel patients on diets that can eliminate or reduce the risk of heart disease development. Foods that are rich in protein such as egg whites, fish, chicken, lean beef, and legumes should be encouraged as an alternative to high trans-fat foods such as sweets, desserts, fried foods, and full-fat dairy products. High-density lipoprotein (HDL) cholesterol helps to eliminate bad cholesterol and prevent the progression of heart disease. Foods rich in omega-3 fatty acid, such as salmon, tuna, and sardines, help to increase HDL levels and lower LDL levels.

In addition to healthy diets, patients should be encouraged to perform cardiovascular exercise. According to the American Heart Association, adults should exercise at least 150 minutes per week. In addition to aerobic activity, moderate to high intensity muscle strengthening is recommended twice a week to support muscular and bone health.

Patients who are at risk for developing diabetes type II should also be encouraged to modify their diets and increase their physical activity. Diabetes develops when glucose levels are consistently high within the body. Foods that increase glucose levels include high-sugar items such as sweets, breads, pasta, and certain fruits. Patients should be encouraged to eat complex carbohydrate foods such as brown rice, whole wheat bread, and peas to maintain better control of their glucose levels. Physical activity can also decrease insulin resistance and increase the use of glucose as energy.

Hypertension is a disorder in which there is increased vascular resistance leading to an increase in blood pressure. Hypertension can be caused by unmodifiable risk factors such as age, family history, and race. However, there are risk factors that can be modified such as smoking, stress, and high-sodium diets. Patients who smoke should be encouraged to stop. Tobacco damages the lining in the arterial walls and causes narrowing of the vessels. In combination with smoking, stress can increase blood pressure and lead to a chronic condition. Pharmacists should encourage patients to perform stress-relieving activities such as meditation, yoga, and deep breathing. Mindfulness techniques help patients refocus and alleviate stress associated with work, life, or family challenges. Patients should also be encouraged to do activities they enjoy outside of their normal work routine to increase their sense of well-being. Diets that are high in sodium cause an accumulation of fluid in the body. Excess fluid leads to increased vascular resistance and subsequent high blood pressure. Patients should be encouraged to eat foods low in sodium such as vegetables, fruits, and grains to regulate fluid within the body.

First-Aid

First aid refers to the initial care a person can receive if they find themselves in a critical health situation. First aid may come from a bystander or a trained first responder. It may consist of providing treatment for a minor concern, or it could include interim support until a person is able to receive comprehensive emergency care. For example, providing chest compressions to a person experiencing a heart attack until they can be transported to a hospital is a form of first aid. Cleaning a cut, applying antiseptic ointment, and bandaging the wound is also considered first aid. If a person appears to be in

44

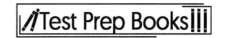

medical distress, the first-aid provider should immediately note if there are any sources of danger that could also compromise their safety.

If the scene is clear, the first-aid provider should assess the patient and determine what materials are needed, or if additional help is needed. If emergency care is needed, the first responder should ideally ask for another bystander to call emergency services, so they do not have to leave the distressed person unattended. However, this is not always possible; in that case, the first aid provider may need to make the call themselves. First-aid certification courses can help bystanders learn how to best assess the condition of a person and how to aid in various health contexts. These include lacerations, burns, overdose, falls, cardiac arrest, allergic reactions, heat or cold events, and pediatric support. Since pharmacists regularly see patients and customers who are ill or injured, they may be more likely to offer first-aid assistance. Additionally, patients and customers may ask pharmacists for advice about first-aid techniques or products to keep in their personal first aid kits.

Complementary and Alternative Medicine

Dietary supplements, herbal medications, and alternative medicine are the primary drug therapy for many patients. There is a misconception that herbal supplements are not harmful to the body. However, non-prescribed supplements can lead to disease complications and interact with pharmaceutical medications. Dietary supplements and herbal medications are marketed by various companies claiming that they are all natural and will often replace the effects of prescribed medications. Although most supplements contain naturally occurring ingredients, their concentration may greatly exceed daily nutritional needs.

Additionally, dietary and herbal supplements are not approved by the FDA and control studies are not widely performed. Dietary supplements, unlike OTC medications, are not regulated by the FDA. The Dietary Health and Supplement Act of 1994 defines the guidelines that dietary supplements must meet, including those that:

- Contain a vitamin, mineral, herb, botanical, and/or amino acid
- Are sold as a capsule, tablet, powder or liquid
- Are not purposefully marked to be the sole source of nutrition
- Has the labeling "dietary supplement"

The safety of herbal supplements cannot be established without a sufficient number of controlled studies. Like prescription medications, herbal supplements can also lead to toxicity. For example, some of the top selling herbal supplements are Ginkgo, St. John's Wort, and ginseng. Each of these supplements are said to have a positive effect on the body. **Ginkgo** is a leaf extract taken to improve memory and cognitive function. It is commonly used by patients with Alzheimer's to improve cognition. Its mechanism of action is to increase blood flow to the brain and peripheral extremities. Additionally, it inhibits platelet aggregation. Patients taking gingko as treatment for cognitive disorders or peripheral arterial disease need to be evaluated for concurrent use of antiplatelet medications such as aspirin to avoid excessive bleeding.

St. John's Wort is an herb that is said to increase serotonin in the brain. This herb is used to treat mild to moderate forms of depression. St. John's Wort causes interactions with a large number of medications and can decrease the therapeutic effects of birth control pills, antivirals, and organ transplantation drugs. Ginseng is a plant root with multiple uses. **Ginseng** is often used to increase strength, stamina, and endurance. It is also used to promote sleep and help relieve symptoms of depression. Depending on

45

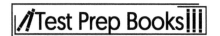
the dose, ginseng can inhibit platelet aggregation and can stimulate or depress the central nervous system. Ginseng can interact with medications having antiplatelet properties such as Plavix. In diabetic patients, ginseng may increase the risk of hypoglycemia if taken concurrently with glucose lowering medications.

Pharmacists should be prepared to educate patients on the characteristics of herbal supplements, their intended use, adverse effects, and contraindications with other medications or medical conditions. Pharmacists should also inform patients that products manufactured by reputable companies with standardized ingredients are generally safer to use. Standardized ingredients indicate that there is a specific dosage in each tablet or capsule as opposed to a variety of ingredients with unknown potency.

Similar to herbal supplements, vitamin supplementation is often self-prescribed. Some patients believe that taking excessive amounts of vitamins will benefit their bodies and improve organ function. However, large doses of all types of minerals can be toxic. In combination with dietary intake, supplements can lead to vitamin levels that exceed daily recommended limits. Each vitamin has a **tolerable upper intake level (UL)**. This term refers to the maximum amount of intake that is considered safe and not likely to pose a health risk. Exceeding the ULs may lead to toxicity. For example, the UL for vitamin D is 400 international units (IU). If a patient is taking vitamin D supplements, a multivitamin containing additional vitamin D, and eating a diet rich in fortified milk, cumulative quantities can lead to toxicity. Below is a table of some of the most common supplements with their primary use and contraindications.

Supplement	Primary Uses	Contraindications/Safety
Saw palmetto	Relieves urinary symptoms and retention in men who have benign prostatic hypertrophy (BPH)	Side effects include diarrhea, stomach upset, and headache. It may reduce levels of the prostate-specific antigen (PSA) and cause a false-negative. PSA is a screening test for prostate cancer.
Ginkgo biloba	Improves cognition, memory, and blood flow to the peripheral extremities	Increased risk of bleeding with medications that inhibit platelet aggregation such as Plavix and aspirin.
Melatonin	Improves sleep in patients with insomnia and used in the treatment of jet lag	Contraindicated in patients with history of depression, liver disease, and stroke. Patients with kidney impairment should use caution as it can cause cumulative effects and toxicity.
Black cohosh	Relieves menopause symptoms such as hot flashes, vaginal dryness, and mood swings by decreasing the release of the luteinizing hormone (LH).	Side effects include nausea, vomiting, bradycardia, and visual disturbances.

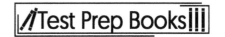

Supplement	Primary Uses	Contraindications/Safety
Echinacea	Stimulates the immune system and relieves symptoms of a common cold	It is not to be used in patients with immune system suppression and liver disease as it can cause toxicity.
Valerian	Used as a muscle relaxant and anxiety reducer	Patients taking sedative medications should not take this supplement as it can depress the central nervous system.
Ginger	Treats nausea and morning sickness	Can increase blood clotting time and cause miscarriages in early pregnancy.

Medical Equipment

Pharmacies should have appropriate equipment and supplies in order to formulate pharmaceutical admixtures per the specified standards. Equipment should be routinely cleaned and kept dry to minimize contamination with the formulation ingredients and extraneous materials. Pharmaceutical compounding generally requires the following equipment and auxiliary supplies in addition to therapeutic ingredients to formulate a compound:

- Class A prescription balance or analytical balance to weigh the ingredients
- Weighing papers, wax papers, or measuring boats
- Spatula to transfer ingredients
- Mortar and pestle for grinding and mixing
- Graduated cylinders (10 ml and 100 ml)
- Ointment slab
- Cream or ointment base
- Wetting or levigating agent to reduce particle size
- Personal protective equipment (PPE)

The following considerations should be considered when selecting tools and equipment for compounding practice:

- Equipment and utensils used in pharmaceutical compounding should have a suitable design and capacity that will allow for effective admixing. The type and size of the equipment to be utilized depends on the intended purpose of compounding, the dosage form, and the volume/amount to be compounded.

- The surface of the equipment should be chemically-inert and should not alter the admixture through chemical reaction, addition, or absorption.

- Tools and equipment should be properly stored to avoid contamination and routinely cleaned.

- All electronic, automated, mechanical, and other instruments used in preparing or testing admixtures should be routinely calibrated and inspected.

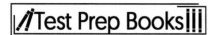
- The cleaning of equipment should include extra care and caution when the preparation includes cytotoxic agents, antibiotics, and hazardous materials.

- When possible, equipment can be dedicated for a specific job that involves hazardous chemicals or requires high precision. Disposable equipment should be used to reduce the bio-burden and cross-contamination.

Practice Quiz

1. Which of the following outcomes can be expected for a patient taking tranylcypromine (Parnate)? (Select ALL that apply.)
    a. Improved energy level
    b. Increased appetite
    c. Decreased anxiety
    d. Decreased weight
    e. Increased sleep

2. What is the best route for the absorption of nelfinavir (Viracept)?
    a. IV
    b. IM
    c. PO
    d. Sub-Q

3. What is a therapeutic use of sodium polystyrene sulfonate (Kayexalate)?
    a. To treat hypernatremia
    b. To treat hyperkalemia
    c. To treat hypomagnesemia
    d. To treat hypocalcemia

4. A patient is prescribed metformin (Glucophage) to help regulate their serum glucose levels. In combination with drug therapy, which food the pharmacist should encourage the patient to ingest to manage their disease?
    a. Orange juice
    b. White rice
    c. Kidney beans
    d. Crackers

5. A pharmacist is reviewing the home medication list for a patient taking clopidogrel (Plavix). Which herbal supplement would cause the pharmacist concern?
    a. Echinacea
    b. Chondroitin
    c. Capsaicin
    d. Ginkgo biloba

See answers on next page.

49

Answer Explanations

1. A, B, C, and E: Tranylcypromine (Parnate) is a monoamine oxidase (MAO) inhibitor used in the treatment of depression. Patients who have a diagnosis of depression commonly experience anxiety, insomnia, lack of enjoyment in daily activities, and the inability to carry out activities of daily living (ADLs). The expected outcomes of a medication like Parnate include an improvement in energy, appetite, and rest. Decreased anxiety is also expected. Choice *D* is not an expected response for this type of mood stabilizing medication.

2. C: Nelfinavir (Viracept) is an antiretroviral medication used in the treatment of the human immunodeficiency virus (HIV). Viracept is mostly excreted through feces and metabolized in the gastrointestinal system. Viracept is manufactured as a tablet or powder. Oral administration is the intended route of administration. Choice *A* is the intravenous route. Choice *B* is the intramuscular route. Choice *D* is the subcutaneous route. Choices *A*, *B*, and *D* require the medication to be manufactured in liquid form.

3. B: Sodium polystyrene sulfonate (Kayexalate) is an electrolyte modifier/hypokalemic medication used in the treatment of hyperkalemia. Potassium levels above 5.0 mEq/L can have adverse effects such as cardiac dysrhythmias, hypotension, and muscle weakness. Kayexalate promotes the excretion of potassium and absorption of sodium in the large intestine. Choice *A* is sodium levels above normal. Choice *C* is lower than normal magnesium levels. Choice *D* is lower than normal calcium levels. Kayexalate does not treat Choices *A*, *C*, or *D*.

4. C: Glucophage (Metformin) regulates glucose levels in patients with pre-diabetes or diabetes. The goal of diabetes management is to control sugar levels. Diabetic patients should focus on eating foods that are low in sugar and include complex carbohydrates. Kidney beans are plant based and include protein, fiber, and antioxidants that help manage diabetes. Choice *A* is not correct. Simple sugars raise the blood glucose rapidly, and fruit juices are not recommended for diabetic patients. Choices *B* and *D* are refined carbohydrates that raise blood sugar quickly. Alternatives such as brown rice and whole wheat pasta are recommended.

5. D: Ginkgo biloba is a leaf extract used by patients with declining cognitive function. Ginkgo inhibits platelet aggregation and may increase the risk of bleeding. Antiplatelet medications such as Plavix may cause additive effects and increase the risk of bleeding. Choice *A* is incorrect. Echinacea is used to stimulate the immune response. It does not have a direct effect on blood clotting. Choice *B* is incorrect. Chondroitin is used to manage arthritis. It is derived from cartilage and does not affect blood clotting. Choice *C* is not correct. Capsaicin is derived from cayenne pepper and is used topically to relieve pain. It does not have an effect on blood clotting.

Area 4 – Performing Calculations

Patient Parameters and Laboratory Measures

Drug therapy requires an evaluation of the effectiveness of treatment. The two most common parameters to evaluate the efficacy of treatment include clinical and laboratory data. **Clinical parameters** include the manifestation of the patient's physical signs and symptoms. The goal of drug therapy is to see an improvement of the initial presenting symptoms. At the start of therapy, the patient's clinical symptoms should be documented and compared throughout the therapy and at the finalization of medication management. The pharmacotherapy workup examines the indication of therapy, the drug product, the dosage regimen, and the outcome. Modifications are dependent on the patient's response and achievement of therapy goals. For example, a patient who presents with excruciating pain in the lower back due to an injury will require analgesics to minimize the pain and improve joint movement. If the patient is prescribed ibuprofen (Motrin) 800 mg 3 times a day for the next week, the goal of treatment would be for the patient to have decreased back pain and increased physical functionality. If the patient's pain is decreased, collaborative efforts by practitioners should be made to change the dosage, frequency, or type of drug therapy to provide the patient with adequate pain relief.

A thorough patient assessment should be made at the start of therapy to effectively establish clinical parameters at the time of evaluation. For example, a patient who presents with cough will need to be assessed for the severity, frequency, and alteration in daily activities as a result of the cough. Should the patient be prescribed a non-narcotic antitussive such as Delsym 60 mg PO (by mouth) every 12 hours, evaluation of the patient's cough is required as directed. A decrease in the severity of the cough and effective sleep patterns would be expected. When physical manifestations are not present, practitioners must rely on laboratory data to evaluate the effectiveness of drug therapy. Certain medical conditions, such as hyperlipidemia, silent hypertension, diabetes, and anemia, often do not display physical symptoms. Therefore, practitioners must examine laboratory parameters to modify medication management. For example, a patient with a cholesterol level of 250 mg/dL and low-density lipoprotein (LDL) level of 160 mg/dL would likely not have initial physical manifestations of dyslipidemia. Therefore, a practitioner would have to rely on blood cholesterol and lipid levels to assess the effectiveness of treatment.

It is also important to note that the maximum desired effect resulting from drug therapy will vary between medications. The timing of the laboratory data is important in determining the efficacy of the drug treatment. For example, a statin drug such as lovastatin (Mevacor) begins to take effect within 5 to 14 days. However, the full extent of its intended purpose does not occur until several weeks after initiation. Patients who are taking medications to lower their blood pressure will require laboratory parameters in the form of vital signs. In order to assess the efficacy of antihypertensives, a systolic and diastolic pressure would be required.

Additionally, patients taking beta-blockers such as metoprolol (Lopressor) or atenolol (Ternormin) that cause bradycardia may require a pulse rate check. Patients taking medication for cardiac dysrhythmias such as adenosine will require a diagnostic electrocardiogram as a laboratory parameter. Modification of medications will be dependent on the rate of goal completion or decrease in clinical and laboratory parameters. For example, if a patient had an initial blood glucose level of 350 mg/dL at the start of

51

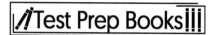

insulin therapy, the expectation would be to lower the glucose levels to less than 120 mg/dL. Should this patient have a glucose level of 250 mg/dL at the first follow-up, this would indicate insulin therapy is working but may require modifications.

Additionally, it is important to assess all contributing lifestyle factors, such as diet, exercise, timing and administration of the medication, and management of comorbidities, that can have an impact on drug efficacy. Alternatively, if a patient is displaying a rapid drop in parameters accompanied by physical manifestations, safe discontinuation of the drug is required. For instance, if a patient taking metoprolol (Lopressor) for high blood pressure presents with a follow-up blood pressure of 110/59 but a pulse rate of 39, modifications to the dosage or prompt discontinuation of the drug would be applicable. Bradycardia can lead to syncope, decreased cardiac output, and cardiac arrest.

Quantities of Drugs to be Dispensed or Administered

A medication dose is the total quantity of medication that is administered to a patient. Also called the **absolute dose**, the drug dose is determined by the patient's provider. Relative doses are those that need to be calculated based on a patient's weight. For example, **Lovenox** is an anticoagulant medication that is prescribed based on weight when used for therapeutic purposes. The usual dose is 1 mg/kg of weight. If a patient weighs 60 kilograms, the absolute dose would be 60 mg: $60 \times 1 = 60$. Kilograms is the preferred unit of measurement when calculating medication dosages. If the patient's weight is available in pounds, it must be translated into kilograms. For example, if the patient weighs 176 pounds, the weight needs to be divided by 2.2 since 1 kg = 2.2 lbs:

$$176 \text{ lbs} \div 2.2 \text{ lbs} = 80 \text{ kg}$$

The patient weighs 80 kilograms. The patient's Lovenox dose would be 80 milligrams: $80 \times 1 = 80$.

Most medications administered to adult patients are a standard dose. However, there are certain instances in which the dose of the medication needs to be calculated. For example, geriatric patients are at a higher risk of toxicity due to alterations in absorption, metabolism, distribution, and excretion. Older adults have decreased plasma proteins necessary for drug transport, as well as diminished gastrointestinal motility and blood flow, which are required for absorption. The same concept applies to patients with liver disease, renal dysfunction, and heart failure. The lowest dose available should be prescribed for these patient populations.

Body size determines the availability of fatty tissue. Medications that penetrate through fatty tissue do not require standard dosage adjustments. However, medications such as heparin, vasopressors, and aminoglycosides are distributed based on body composition, and their dose should be based on body weight. Similarly, patients who are underweight have an alteration in body mass, and dosages will need to be based on individual weight. Body size is the main reason why medication dosages need to be calculated for the pediatric population. Dosages are prescribed as milligrams for every kilogram of weight. Furthermore, neonates and premature infants require further dosage adjustments due to the immature function of various body systems.

Rates of Administration

Medications and nutritional support that are administered via an intravenous route or through an enteral tube require a specific **rate of administration**. Although the medications and supplementation will be administered by healthcare providers working at the bedside, pharmacists are responsible for

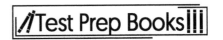

dispensing the medication and, in many instances, calculating the rate of administration. A common route of administration that requires an infusion rate is via the venous system. **Intravenous (IV) medications** that are combined with a diluent require controlled administration. IV fluids that are prepared in 250 milliliter, 500 milliliter, or 1 liter bags are usually administered via an infusion pump. Infusion pumps regulate the rate at which medications enter the body. However, the rate of administration must be manually programmed by a healthcare provider.

Infusion pumps are set to deliver volume in milliliters per hour. When performing calculations, the units of measurement are converted to milliliters and hours to obtain an accurate rate of administration. For example, if a provider orders 50 milligrams of medication to be administered every hour via a continuous infusion, the first step is to verify the available stock. If the medication is supplied as 250 milligrams in a 500 milliliter bag, the next step is to find out how many milligrams are available in each milliliter of solution. To find this, the dose needs to be divided by the volume: $250 \div 500 = 0.5$. There is 0.5 milligram in each milliliter of solution. The ordered dose is 50 milligrams per hour. To find the rate per hour, the ordered dose needs to be divided by the supplied dose: $50 \div 0.5 = 100$. The infusion pump would need to be set at 100 mL/hr to deliver 50 milligrams of medication every hour.

Similarly, patients who have an **enteral tube,** such as a percutaneous endoscopic gastrostomy, nasogastric, or nasojejunal tube, require nutrition via liquid supplementation. Based on the patient's caloric and nutritional needs, providers will order a certain volume of nutritional supplementation. For example, a 250 milliliter carton of Peptamen feeding supplement provides 250 calories per serving. Should a patient require a daily 1750 calorie diet, the order will likely read to administer 7 cartons daily. If the order is to administer a continuous infusion, a rate of administration is calculated. Each carton contains 250 milliliters. $250 \text{ mL} \times 7 \text{ cartons} = 1,750 \text{ mL}$. In a 24-hour period, the patient would receive 1,750 milliliters of supplemental volume. To find the hourly rate, the total volume is divided by 24: $1750 \text{ mL} \div 24 \text{ hrs} = 72.9 \frac{\text{mL}}{\text{hr}}$. Depending on the infusion pump capabilities, the rate would be entered as 72.9 milliliters per hour or 73 milliliters per hour if rounded to the nearest whole number.

Dose Conversions

Conversions should take place if needed prior to calculating ratio and strength percentages. For example, if the active ingredient is supplied as milligrams but the base is in grams, one of the two values must be converted before calculation. Using solids as an example, if 2 grams of the active ingredient is mixed into a base of 98 grams, the total quantity needs to be determined prior to providing the final concentration. The weight of the active ingredient needs to be added to the base. In this case, the total quantity is 100 grams. The active ingredient (2 grams) is divided by the total quantity to determine the final concentration in decimal form: $2 \div 100 = 0.02$.

To determine the percentage, the decimal is multiplied by 100: $100 \times 0.02 = 2$. The final weight/weight concentration is 2%. The same formula applies when calculating the concentration of solid/liquid preparations. For example, if 150 grams of an active ingredient is added to 500 milliliters of normal saline base, the total quantity is 500 milliliters. Active ingredients in solid form dissolve into the base and are not included in the total volume. To find the concentration, the active ingredient is divided by the base: $150 \text{ grams} \div 500 \text{ milliliters} = 0.3$. The decimal is multiplied by 100 to find the percentage: $100 \times 0.3 = 30$. The final weight/volume concentration is 30%.

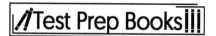

Drug Concentrations

Medication dosages are defined by their concentration. The **concentration of a medication** is determined by how much of the active ingredient is found in its supplied form. The ingredients of a medication can be mixed into either a liquid or solid base and expressed as a ratio strength. Based on the formulation, **ratio strengths** are displayed as a fraction. For example, if a solid ingredient is mixed into a liquid base, the ratio is expressed as weight/volume. If the ingredient is in liquid form and is turned into a solid, such as a cream or ointment, the ratio is volume/weight. If both the ingredient and the base are liquids, the ratio is expressed as volume/volume. Similarly, if both the ingredient and the base are solids, the ratio is weight/weight. With liquid formulations, the percentage represents how many grams of the active ingredient are present in 100 milliliters of solution. In solid formulations, the percent strength is represented by how many grams of the active ingredient are found in 100 grams of solid. It is also important to note that the supplied units should match.

Quantities of Drugs or Ingredients to be Compounded

Compounding is a term used to describe the mixing, combining, or altering of medication ingredients to suit the needs of individual patients. Pharmacists who are licensed can compound medications to provide the patient with a tailored medication. Compounding may be necessary when a patient is allergic to dyes or when the formulation, such as a capsule, cannot be swallowed. These medications are then compounded to a different form or altered to provide the absence of the allergen. Compounded medications are not approved by the Food and Drug Administration but do require oversight to ensure safety. Mixing and preparing medication dosages is dependent on various factors, such as tonicity and pH levels of solutions, dilution, concentration, and osmolarity of prepared medications.

One of the most common types of compounding occurs with intravenous (IV) solutions. Medications are supplied as stock doses, and pharmacists dilute these into compatible IV fluids. Calculation of dose and volume are performed using dimensional analysis. When using dimensional analysis, all units should cancel each other out to arrive at the desired unit. If the units do not match, they must be converted prior to calculating dosages. For example, if the stock volume is in liters but the base solution is in milliliters, the volume needs to be the same unit (milliliters and milliliters) prior to diluting medications.

For example, if a pharmacist needs to prepare a syringe that contains 2 grams of medication mixed with 40 milliliters of diluent and the stock medication is 400 mg/mL, all units need to match before proceeding to the next step. The 2 grams of medication need to be converted to milligrams. 1 gm = 1,000 mg. The syringe must contain 2,000 milligrams of medication. To find the milliliters needed, the medication dose is divided by the stock medication: 2,000 mg ÷ 400 mg = 5 mL. The pharmacist would need to add 5 milliliters of the stock medication into the 35 remaining milliliters of diluent to supply a syringe that contains 2 grams of medication.

Providers often order a medication dose that is not available as ordered. Pharmacists need to compound medications to dispense the appropriate drug dose to the patient. When combining medications, pharmacists must ensure that all dose units match before performing calculations. Diluting and concentrating are common compounding practices when a prescriber orders a dose that differs from an already prepared medication. To equal the ordered dose, pharmacists can use the algebraic method to determine the volume of medication that is needed from the already prepared formulations. When using the algebraic method, it is important to note that the intended result is the volume of the most concentrated already-prepared medication. For example, if a provider orders 30 milliliters of 2%

54

[]

[]

 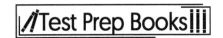

solution, but the stock doses are 30 milliliters of 1% and 30 milliliters of 2.5%, the formula should be set up to solve for the volume of the 2.5% solution that is needed. The formula to be used is as follows:

$$Desired\ final\ volume \times (smallest\ concentration\ available - final\ desired\ concentration)$$
$$\div (smallest\ concentration\ available - highest\ concentration\ available)$$

Using the example provided, the formula would be set up as follows: $30\ mL \times (1\% - 2\%) \div (1\% - 2.5\%)$. The answer to this equation is 20 milliliters. The pharmacist would need to mix 20 milliliters of the 2.5% solution and 10 milliliters of the 1.5% solution to dispense 30 milliliters of 2%.

It is important to note that when medications are compounded, the chemical properties should not change, and the only varying factor is the volume of the active ingredient. For example, a patient who is unable to take an oral tablet may require the medication to be changed to a liquid form. The pharmacist will need to calculate how many tablets are required to formulate a specific volume. For example, a patient has an order for 150 milligrams of a medication daily. The only available form of the medication is a tablet. The available compounding formulation is 25 mg/mL in a 30 milliliter suspension.

To find the total dose of medication needed, dimensional analysis will be used. The formula will be as follows: $(25\ mg/1\ mL) \times 30\ mL$. The total milligrams needed from the tablets is 750. The tablets are 150 milligrams each. In order to make a 30 milliliter suspension, the pharmacist will have to incorporate 5 tablets when compounding the medication: $750\ mg \div 150\ mg = 5$ tablets. To find the new dose in liquid form, the ordered dose is divided by the supplied dose: $150\ mg \div 25\ mg = 6\ mL$. To receive the appropriate dosage, the patient would need to take 6 milliliters of solution to equal the ordered dose.

Nutritional Needs and Nutrient Sources

Nutritional intake for patients is attained through various sources. A patient who has no deficits can tolerate oral intake of nutrients. It is important to collect a patient's medical history to determine specialized diets and caloric needs. In collaboration with primary care physicians and dieticians, a pharmacist can help educate a patient on proper nutritional needs. For example, a patient with a history of diabetes may benefit from the 1,800 calorie ADA diet. An **ADA diet** is a nutritional plan established by the American Diabetes Association. This diet helps patients with diabetes control their daily blood sugar levels by incorporating whole grains, lean meat, poultry, and foods rich in fiber. Foods that are rich in Omega-3 fatty acids, such as salmon, walnuts, and shellfish, can decrease the level of triglycerides in the blood. Elevated triglycerides are a risk factor for heart disease in diabetic patients. Multiple studies have found that 4 grams of Omega-3 fat improve insulin sensitivity and decrease the hemoglobin A1C levels in diabetics. As a reference, a 3-ounce salmon fillet has approximately 1.8 grams of Omega-3 fat while 1 ounce of walnuts contains approximately 2.5 grams.

Patients who are unable to ingest food orally may obtain their nutrition through enteral tubes. The most common type of enteral feeding tube is a **nasogastric tube (NGT)**. NGTs are inserted through the nose and end internally at the stomach. A **nasojejunal tube** begins at the nose and ends internally in the small intestine. A nasojejunal tube allows for precise nutritional absorption, as 95% of nutrients are absorbed in the first part of the small intestine. **Enteral tubes** are used in acute care settings. Chronic enteral nutrition may require a percutaneously placed gastrostomy tube. This method is invasive and requires an endoscopic procedure. Food that is administered through these enteral tubes is in the form of a liquid that contains carbohydrate, fat, protein, electrolyte, vitamin, fiber, and water content.

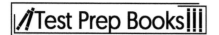

Providers will calculate nutritional needs using the **basal metabolic rate (BMR)**. The BMR is the amount of calories that are burned in a 24 hour period. For women, the standard formula is:

$$655 + (4.35 \times \text{weight in pounds}) + (4.7 \times \text{height in inches}) - (4.7 \times \text{age in years})$$

In men, the standard formula is:

$$66 + (6.23 \times \text{weight in pounds}) + (12.7 \times \text{height in inches}) - (6.8 \times \text{age in years})$$

The BMR is then multiplied by the activity factor. The pharmacist will need to know a patient's activity level, ranging from sedentary to very active. For sedentary patients, the standard factor of 1.2 is used. The standard factor for lightly active is 1.375, moderately active is 1.55, and very active is 1.725. The BMR is multiplied by the activity factor to find the total daily caloric needs of the patient.

Selection of the enteral formulas will be dependent on the patient's disease process and individual nutritional needs. Patients who are unable to receive their nutrients orally or enterally may require **total parenteral nutrition (TPN)**. Parenteral nutrition is administered via an intravenous line and contains elements such as amino acids, glucose, fat, micronutrients, and electrolytes. When TPN formulas are calculated, the patient's age, sex, height, weight, stress factors, lipid need, and protein intake are considered. Due to the possibility of complications, such as catheter-related infections, electrolyte imbalances, and allergic reactions, parenteral nutrition is often a last resort for the intake of nutrients.

Biostatistics and Epidemiological Measures

Biostatistics focuses on statistics that pertain to human health and medicine. It is a critical part of clinical research trials and helps to evaluate whether results are significant and useful to a target population. Important biostatistical measures are summary measures, which provide information about a sample data set. Summary measures include the sample mean, variance, and standard deviation. The sample mean is the average of all values in the data set. Variance looks at the difference between an individual data point and the sample mean. Standard deviation looks at the data points as a whole to see if they are collectively closer to or farther away from the sample mean.

If most data points are near the sample mean, the sample has a low standard deviation. Samples with high standard deviations indicate that there is high variability in the sample. Variation can help a researcher hypothesize why differences exist or do not exist. For example, a researcher may look at a sample of lung cancer rates in a community and calculate the mean age for the sample. If individual data points are clustered around a specific age, the researcher may hypothesize a reason as to why lung cancer cases are higher in this age group. The findings can then be extrapolated to the larger population.

Epidemiology examines biostatistical findings to determine health and disease patterns in communities and make recommendations for population-level health interventions. For example, if the researcher from the lung cancer data set noted that a high concentration of cases existed in older men who were previously employed at the local coal plant, a recommendation could be made to implement practices that protect current workers' respiratory health. Common measures in epidemiology include ratio, proportion, incidence rate, prevalence, and mortality rate.

Ratios describe one measure relative to another measure (e.g., rate of coal workers who develop lung cancer versus non-coal-workers who develop lung cancer). **Proportion** is defined as the comparison of one part to a whole (e.g., seventy-year-old coal workers with lung cancer versus all ages of coal workers with lung cancer). **Incidence rate** refers to how quickly disease occurs in a specific population (e.g., the

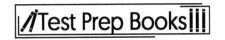

age at which each coal worker developed lung cancer). **Prevalence** refers to the total number of cases in an entire population (e.g., the total number of lung cancer cases in coal workers over total number of coal workers). **Mortality rate** refers to the number of deaths that occur due to a specific factor or disease over the entire population (e.g., the total number of lung cancer deaths in coal workers over the total number of all lung cancer deaths).

Pharmacoeconomic Measures

Cost can be a factor in compliance with drug therapy. If a patient cannot afford their medication, the likelihood of noncompliance increases. Patients are more likely to prioritize basic needs such as groceries, utilities, and housing over medical treatment. If a prescribed medication is out of the patient's economic capability, the risk of disease development is great. Noncompliance with drug therapy leads to worsening physical signs and symptoms, disease progression, and hospitalization. The added costs of emergent medical attention will further add to the economic burden and cause a strain on the healthcare system. **Pharmacoeconomics** refers to understanding how the costs of medicines affects the pharmaceutical industry and its patients.

Part of a patient interview requires assessment and evaluation of their ability to pay for their medical care. Patients should be asked about their medical insurance status, occupation, and financial means. Pharmacists should also be knowledgeable about the prices of medications.

Medical insurances group and price medications based on five tiers. The higher the tier, the more expensive a medication will be.

- Tier 1 medications are the most commonly prescribed due to their generic form and low cost.

- Tier 2 medications are usually branded medications or generic medications that are more expensive than tier 1 drugs.

- Tier 3 medications are branded medications for which no generic form is yet available.

- Tier 4 medications include primarily branded drugs that are higher in cost.

- Tier 5 medications are specialty drugs that treat complex conditions such as cancer.

Tier 1 medications can be as low as a few dollars for a 30-day supply whereas a tier 5 medication can cost thousands for one individual dose.

Although cost is an important aspect of medication management, healthcare providers must prioritize efficacy and safety of medications. Drug therapy that is chosen solely based on cost can be ineffective and produce adverse effects, toxicity, and chronic impairments. The cost to treat complications from drug therapy will greatly outweigh the cost of the medication.

Generic medications are close replicas of branded medications. Their chemical composition closely resembles the original drug and they are determined safe to use by the U.S. Food and Drug Administration. If the pharmacokinetic difference between a branded medication and a generic medication is not significant, the generic medication should be chosen when there are socioeconomic challenges.

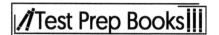

Collaboration with case managers and social workers should take place when patients require financial assistance. Resources can be made available that will help patients receive adequate drug therapy. For example, Medicare Part D provides drug coverage for patients over the age of sixty-five who have Medicare insurance. For a reasonable premium, the insurance carrier will network with pharmacies to provide medications to patients at a lower cost.

Pharmacists should also be familiar with **pharmacy assistance programs**. Patients who disclose their inability to pay for medications should be referred to programs such as GoodRx, Prescription Care, and Rx Outreach. These types of programs evaluate the patient's ability to pay for their medication based on their income, state of residence, and household size. Eligible patients can obtain their medications at a discounted price through these assistance programs.

Pharmacokinetic Parameters

Half-life is a pharmacokinetic parameter that represents the unit of time over which the concentration of a medication in circulation drops to half of its initial concentration. For example, if a medication has a half-life of 15 hours, blood concentration of the drug decreases 50% every 15 hours. The longer a medication's half-life, the longer the effects persist; therefore, lower therapeutic doses or longer dosing intervals should be used. Medications in the same therapeutic class might have different half-lives, resulting in varying durations of action. Knowledge of a medication's half-life helps to determine the necessary dosage and the frequency of administration.

A medication's half-life depends on the elimination rate kinetics of the respective medication. There are two common types of elimination rate kinetics that are studied in pharmacology: first order kinetics and zero order kinetics.

When a medication follows **first order elimination kinetics**, the medication undergoes a linear rate of elimination in proportion to its concentration. However, the elimination half-life remains constant independent of the initial concentration of the reactant. The metabolism and elimination of most of the drugs follow first order kinetics.

Zero order kinetics refers to a reaction that proceeds at a rate independent of the concentrations of the reactants. For example, alcohol metabolism in the liver follows zero order kinetics.

Practice Quiz

1. A patient is prescribed levetiracetam (Keppra) suspension 500 mg PO BID. The available medication is 100 mg/ml. How many teaspoons should the pharmacist tell the patient to administer at home with every dose? (Round the final answer to the nearest WHOLE number.)

2. A patient is prescribed thyroid (Thyrar) PO 2gr/day. How many milligrams need to be dispensed daily for this patient? (Round the answer to the nearest WHOLE number.)

3. A patient is prescribed bismuth subsalicylate (Pepto-Bismol) PO 15 ml QID for the treatment of diarrhea. How many ounces of liquid should the pharmacist recommend as a daily dose? (Round the final answer to the nearest WHOLE number.)

4. A patient is prescribed guaifenesin (Robitussin) PO 200 mg q4hr for the management of cough. The medication is available as a syrup 100 mg/5 ml. How many teaspoons should the pharmacist instruct the patient to take per dose? (Round the final answer to the nearest WHOLE number.)

5. A patient weighing 175 pounds has an order for linezolid (Zyvox) IV 10 mg/kg BID. The medication is supplied as a 200 mg/10 ml. How many milliliters should be dispensed per dose? (Round the final answer to the nearest WHOLE number.)

See answers on next page.

Answer Explanations

1. 1 teaspoon: To determine the volume of medication required for each dose, the available medication needs to be divided into the ordered dose. Each milliliter contains 100 mg of medication. The patient needs to take 5 ml of volume with each dose (500 mg/100 mg = 5 ml). For home use, the volume needs to be converted to teaspoons, and 1 teaspoon = 5 ml. The patient needs to take 1 teaspoon of medication per dose. The frequency of the medication is not relevant when determining the volume per dose.

2. 130 milligrams: The ordered dose is for 2 grains of medication a day. Grains need to be converted to milligrams to obtain the answer, and 1 grain = 65 milligrams. The total dose per day is 130 milligrams (65 mg × 2 grains = 130 mg).

3. 2 ounces: To determine how many ounces the patient will require every day, the ordered dose needs to be converted to ounces, and 1 ounce = 30 milliliters. The ordered dose is 15 ml. The total ounces per dose are 0.5 ounces (15 milliliters ÷ 30 milliliters = 0.5 ounces). The patient needs to take this medication four times a day. QID = every 6 hours or four times a day. The patient will take a total of 2 ounces per day (0.5 oz × 4 = 2 oz).

4. 2 teaspoons: To find the total number of teaspoons, the ordered dose needs to be converted to milliliters. The medication available provides 100 mg for every 5 milliliters. The ordered dose is 200 mg, and the required volume per dose is 10 milliliters. (100 mg/5 ml = 200 mg/10 ml). One teaspoon is equal to 5 milliliters. The ordered dose requires 10 milliliters. The number of teaspoons required per dose is 2 (10 ml/5 ml = 2 teaspoons).

5. 40 ml: To find the total number of milliliters required per dose, the patient's weight needs to be converted to kilograms first: 1 kilogram = 2.2 pounds. The patient weighs 79.5 kilograms (175 lbs/2.2 kg = 79.5 kg). To find how many milligrams are required per dose, the weight needs to be multiplied by the ordered dose (10 mg). The patient will require 795 milligrams of medication per dose (10 mg × 79.5 kg = 795 mg). For every 10 milliliters, the supplied dose is 200 mg. Using dimensional analysis, the total ordered dose should be multiplied by 10 milliliters and divided by 200 to obtain the total volume. The required volume is 39.7 milliliters (795 mg × 10 ml = 7,950 mg), (7,950 mg/200 mg = 39.7ml). The question asks to round to the nearest whole number, and 39.7 ml rounds to 40 ml.

Area 5 – Compounding, Dispensing, or Administering Drugs, or Managing Delivery Systems

Physicochemical Properties of Drug Products

Every medication that is approved for use has a unique therapeutic effect based on physical and chemical properties. **Physicochemical properties** refer to the specific structure, solubility, and chemical reactions that define a medication. The **solubility** of a medication refers to its ability to dissolve in a solid, gaseous, or liquid solvent. Medications that are highly soluble in fat can cross cell membranes faster than those that are more soluble in water. Fat-soluble medications concentrate heavily in fat tissues, whereas water-soluble medications remain in the bloodstream and interstitial spaces. Cholesterol-lowering medications such as atorvastatin, fluvastatin, and simvastatin are all lipid-soluble drugs that can cross the blood-brain barrier and reduce the presence of atherosclerotic plaques within the cranial arteries.

Excess fatty plaques can block circulation and lead to strokes and neurovascular deficits. Another fat-soluble medication is digoxin. **Digoxin** is an antiarrhythmic medication used to treat atrial fibrillation. Digoxin is stored in the tissues and released slowly into the bloodstream to maintain a stable serum level. Other lipid-soluble medications that readily cross the blood-brain barrier include rifampin—an antibiotic used primarily in the treatment of tuberculosis—and most psychotropic medications used in the treatment of psychiatric and mood disorders. Vitamins are also classified as either water-soluble or fat-soluble. Water-soluble vitamins, such as vitamins B and C, are excreted in the urine when excess amounts are ingested. Fat-soluble vitamins, such as vitamins A, D, E, and K, are stored in the tissues and can cause toxicity if there is an excessive amount ingested.

Other properties include the **protein binding capability** of the drug. Medications that are minimally bound to proteins will travel more efficiently across cell membranes. This action produces a higher concentration of the drug within the bloodstream. Only the free-flowing portion of a medication will exert its mechanism of action on body cells. The rest of the percentage is stored in muscle, fat, and various body tissues for later use. Storage of the medication decreases the concentration of the drug in the bloodstream and minimizes the risk of toxicity. For example, warfarin is an anticoagulant medication that is 99% protein bound. This means that only 1% of the medication is available in the bloodstream. If compounding altered the percentage of unbound medication, this would increase the availability in the bloodstream and increase the risk of bleeding.

Medications are made up of active and inactive ingredients. The **active ingredient** of a medication is the component that produces the therapeutic effect, as well as the unwanted side effects and adverse reactions. The **inactive ingredients** are those that have no effect on the medication's absorption or metabolism. Inactive ingredients aid in the ease of use and can include preservatives, coloring, and substances to hold the shape of the medication. For example, the active ingredient in aspirin is acetylsalicylic acid. This active ingredient inhibits the activity of enzymes that cause inflammation, fever, and pain. This same ingredient also interferes with blood clotting and the production of substances that protect the stomach lining, causing bleeding and gastrointestinal irritation. The inactive ingredients such as triacetin, corn starch, and hypromellose act as binding agents and fillers to hold the tablet together. Patients who are unable to digest inactive ingredients or are allergic to them may require a

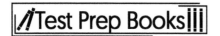

compounded medication. Pharmacists can remove or manipulate inactive ingredients to personalize medications for patients.

Various factors affect the solubility of medications. **Solubility** is defined as the ability of solutes to be dissolved in liquid, solid, or gaseous solvents. A **solvent** is a substance that can dissolve a solute, such as a medication. For example, when a medication is administered orally, the drug must dissolve within the gastrointestinal system in order to be absorbed into the bloodstream. Medications are classified based on their solubility and permeability. **Permeability** refers to how readily a medication crosses between cell membranes. Medications that are highly soluble and highly permeable include acetaminophen, metoprolol, and verapamil. These medications do not require enhancements, such as salt formation, surfactant use, or particle size reduction, to produce solubility. Medications that have a low solubility and permeability and are poorly absorbed in their oral form are best administered via the intravenous route. **Taxol**, an antineoplastic medication used in the treatment of metastatic cancers, is an example of a poorly-absorbed medication not typically given via the oral route.

Some of the factors that affect solubility include temperature, pH level, contact area, and dosage form. Each medication has a distinctive molecular structure that functions positively with the molecular structure of body cells. High temperatures can break the bonds that hold these molecules together. Without the original molecular structure, medications can lose their potency, be degraded, or become toxic. Medications can withstand temperatures of approximately 77 degrees Fahrenheit or lower. This corresponds with the instructions to store medications at room temperature. Medications stored above 86 degrees Fahrenheit can degrade and lose their potency. Patients should be advised not to self-administer medications that have been exposed to extreme temperatures.

The **pH level** is another physicochemical drug property that can affect solubility. Medications are formulated as either an acid or a base. Medications given orally interact with degrading enzymes in the stomach. The stomach has an acidic pH level of approximately 1.5–3.5. Medications such as insulin that can be degraded by acid are not given orally. These medications are given parenterally so they are not affected by digestive processes. Alternatively, medications that are easily degraded in the stomach can be protected by an enteric coat. Enteric coating is made from plastics, waxes, or fatty acids and serves as a protectant to ensure the medication does not dissolve within the stomach. Some medications that are enteric coated include nonsteroidal medications such as naproxen, diclofenac, and sulfasalazine, and antibiotics such as erythromycin, amoxicillin, and cephalexin.

Solubility is also affected by the contact area with the solvent. Drugs that are ground have greater contact surface area with solvents and are more soluble than those that are left intact. Oral medications may be ground into a powder to allow for easier administration. Patients who have feeding tubes or who suffer from dysphagia and are unable to swallow intact medications may require medications in powder form. It is important to note that not all tablets can be crushed or ground. Medications that are enteric coated, such as nonsteroidal anti-inflammatory drugs and antibiotics, have a protective covering to prevent them from being dissolved in the stomach and causing irritation. Crushing or grinding these types of medications can cause stomach irritability and improper absorption. Sustained-release medications, such as codeine, morphine, and oxycodone, are meant to deliver medications over a prolonged period of time. Grinding them may lead to a large initial dose and insufficient therapeutic effects.

Liquid forms do not require binders and lubricants to produce a tablet or capsule shape. Oral suspensions have a faster absorption time than solids. However, liquid forms may have a lower stability and a shorter half-life than solid forms and may require dosage adjustments. The **half-life of a**

62

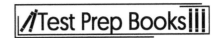
medication refers to the amount of time it takes for a medication's serum concentration to reduce by 50%. The **dosage form** determines how readily molecules disperse within a solvent. **Gaseous medications** such as inhalers or nebulizers are more soluble than liquid medications. Due to this property, the dosages vary significantly with each medication. For example, corticosteroids can be administered by inhalation, orally, topically, and parenterally. At different dosages, they exert different effects. **Budesonide** is a corticosteroid that treats asthma by producing bronchodilation when inhaled. The dosage is prescribed in micrograms. When used systemically, it treats ulcerative colitis and Crohn's disease by decreasing inflammation in the gastrointestinal tract. When given orally, the dosage is prescribed in milligrams.

Handling Hazardous or Non-Hazardous Sterile Products

Medications that are administered directly into the blood stream such as intravenous (IV) fluids and injections must be prepared in a sterile fashion. **Sterile preparations** are done in an environment where there are no microorganisms, such as bacteria and viruses, that can cause infections. Contamination of sterile products poses a high risk of infection to the patient if the contaminated products are not disposed of and exchanged promptly. During preparation and compounding of sterile medications, there are certain materials and equipment needed to successfully maintain a sterile environment. Medications are supplied in various forms, including liquids, powders, inhalants, and creams. Some of the common pieces of equipment used for mixture of medications include a mortar and pestle for grinding, flasks and graduated cylinders for measuring, and spatulas for mixing. Containers used to hold medications include vials, syringes, and bags for intravenous fluids. Equipment for medication administration includes needles, IV tubing, and catheters for medication transport throughout the body.

Producing sterile products requires an **autoclave**—a heated container that works under high temperatures and pressures to sterilize reusable products such as flasks and spatulas. The autoclave removes hazardous waste from the surface of the equipment being used. Airborne particles that can cause contamination of workspaces are controlled by a compounding hood. The flow of air is filtered by the hood to ensure no cross-contamination with the environment occurs. Any surfaces used to perform the preparation and compounding of medications should be disinfected with a germicidal solution to eliminate any bacteria, viruses, and fungal spores.

Pharmacists performing sterile preparations are also required to follow strict hand hygiene and application of personal protective equipment. Shoe, hair, and beard covers should be applied to ensure all organism-harboring surfaces are not visible. Masks and goggles are also applied to prevent transmission of organisms via saliva and tears. Hands are the primary source of organism exchange and require a systematic washing process. Before donning sterile gloves, hands must be scrubbed for at least 30 seconds to include all surfaces, fingernails, wrists, and forearms. Sterile gloves should be inspected for any tears or holes once applied. Sterile gloves should only touch sterile items. If contaminated, proper disposal should occur, and new sterile gloves should be applied. Pharmacists should refer to specific facility policies for the use of alcohol-based disinfecting solutions on gloves and work surfaces should contamination occur.

Handling Hazardous or Non-Hazardous Non-Sterile Products

Nonsterile preparation and compounding of medications require a clean environment. Unlike sterile processes, **nonsterile protocols** are used for medications that are ingested orally or applied topically to the skin. **Oral medications** travel through the esophagus into the stomach. The stomach's environment

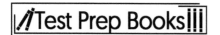

is equipped to eliminate most pathogenic bacteria with the acidic nature of hydrochloric acid. Similarly, the skin is the first layer of defense against organisms. Medications that are administered orally or topically still require a clean environment during preparation to reduce the risk of infection. The facility where compounding is taking place should be away from routine dispensing stations and high traffic areas and isolated from potential chemical contaminants. The workstation should be free of previous drug product and chemicals.

Workstations should be cleaned with an approved cleaner or solvent before and after use. Pharmacists should also follow hand hygiene practices prior to handling equipment and medications. The equipment being used, such as flasks, graduated cylinders, spatulas, beakers, refrigerators, and freezers, should all be properly maintained and sanitized according to facility protocol. Attire should be based on the type of medication being compounded. Hazardous materials require safety goggles, gloves, mask, gown, and foot and hair covers. Should a pharmacist have an open lesion or an illness, appropriate precautions should be taken to avoid microbial contamination. For example, if a pharmacist preparing a medication has a cough, a mask that fully seals the nose and mouth should be applied to avoid airborne transmission of organisms.

Nonsterile preparation allows pharmacists to customize medications. Medications that require a custom dose, addition of flavoring, or removal of inactive ingredients can be compounded using a clean environment. Medications produced via this method include oral suspensions; medicated shampoos; dissolving oral products; and topical creams, lotions, or ointments. For example, **ketoconazole** (Nizoral) is an antifungal medication usually prescribed as an oral tablet for the treatment of candidiasis. Ketoconazole can also be compounded into a topical cream to be used locally or as a shampoo for the treatment of dandruff.

Equipment or Delivery Systems

Automated systems and technology used in pharmaceutical practice assist with increasing efficiency and productivity and improving patient care. There are various forms of technology that function to perform tasks autonomously. **Automated delivery systems** are used to measure, fill, label, and dispense medications. Automated systems improve workflow and can multiply the number of prescriptions that are filled electronically as opposed to physical transcription. In some cases, dispensing systems can process hundreds of prescriptions per hour, providing pharmacists with extra time to do other tasks such as patient counseling, education, screening, and vaccinations.

Automated systems also improve patient adherence by creating innovative "smart" pill bottles that alert a patient when a dose has been missed, computer software that sends reminders for refills and pickups, and electronic calendars that remind patients when to take their next dose of medication. For example, a patient who picks up a prescription at their local pharmacy may be offered the opportunity to enroll in a text messaging system or instructed to download a pharmacy application on their phone. The text messaging system will send reminders to the patient when their medication supply is likely running low. If a patient is on a 90-day prescription medication, the system will alert the patient a few days before the refill is due. Phone applications also allow patients to place their electronic refill order for faster service.

Automated systems used for adherence improve communication with patients, provide tools that help patients stay on track with their drug therapy, and remind patients to refill their medications to improve compliance. Digital prescription technology is a popular form of ordering and refilling prescriptions. This

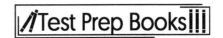

technology allows patients to order their prescriptions through an electronic device. Prescription technology is connected to a pharmacy management system and alerts pharmacy staff when an order is ready to be filled. This reduces paper trails and minimizes time spent on faxing orders and receiving phone prescriptions. Studies have shown that digital prescriptions improve patient adherence, perception of care, and satisfaction. Prescription technology is convenient and allows patients to be in control of their drug therapy.

An effective way to interact with patients and pharmacy technicians is through telepharmacy. **Telepharmacy** involves videoconferencing or telephone conferencing from a remote location and allows pharmacists to interact with patients who are unable to physically visit a pharmacy. Pharmacists can verify photo identification through telepharmacy and provide education and counseling to patients regarding their drug therapy. Telepharmacy expands access to care for patients who live in rural or medically underserved areas. For example, a patient who has begun therapy on a new medication may live 50 miles away from the nearest pharmacy. The patient may have questions regarding its use, safety precautions, food interactions, or specific instructions of when to take the medication. Telepharmacy allows the patient to contact their pharmacist via video or teleconferencing to clarify any concerns. This method improves patient knowledge about their drug therapy and increases drug administration safety. In addition, it is cost-effective. One pharmacist can provide remote services to multiple pharmacy locations and necessary consultation to pharmacy technicians who are performing the hands-on dispensing process.

Self-service kiosks allow the patient to pick up their medications with no contact, but may require a video chat with a pharmacist prior to the machine dispensing their medication. In the acute care setting, automated pharmacy systems are used by health care professionals such as nurses and respiratory therapists. Drug dispensing systems have customizable, high-capacity drawers that can be configured to meet the needs of the facility. Most drug dispensing systems are able to allocate a refrigerated drawer, a cabinet tower for common medications, and a narcotics dispenser for controlled substances.

In an **open-matrix configuration**, a health care worker will have access to all of the drawers in the dispensing system. Newer designs lock all of the drawers and only allow access to the medication that is required. Locked systems improve medication safety and security. Drug dispensing systems include a technology-based managing system in the form of a virtual console. Virtual consoles allow pharmacists to track errors, view inventory, and report usage to health care managers. Dispensing systems that include bar-code technology also improve charge-capture accuracy. **Charge-capture** is a process in which the medication cost is added to the patient's hospital bill. Inaccuracy during the dispensing process may cause an error in billing and decrease revenue for the facility.

Instructions and Techniques for Drug Administration

When dispensing medications to patients, pharmacists should be prepared to explain proper technique for self-administration of the drug. Medications are supplied in various forms, including oral tablets and suspensions. Patients taking tablets or capsules should be assessed for dysphagia. If there is any indication that the patient has trouble swallowing, a different form of medication should be provided. Alternatively, if the medication can be crushed, patients should be instructed to mix it with a liquid before ingestion. To help the medication pass properly through the esophagus, pharmacists should instruct patients to drink the medication with a full glass, or 8 ounces, of water. If medications are supplied as a liquid, the pharmacist must provide the patient with a medication cup with properly marked units of measurement. Syringes and medication spoons are alternatives. Oral liquids should be

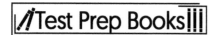
measured on a flat surface at eye level to ensure accuracy. Household utensils should not be used, as they can vary in size and provide inaccurate measurements.

Ear and eye drops are also common, and proper technique should be discussed. Eye drops should not be administered directly on the eyeball. The drops should be administered into the lower lid of the eye. Additionally, to avoid systemic effects, light pressure should be applied to the corner of the eye to cover the tear duct. When administering ear drops, the head should be slightly tilted to the opposite side, the top of the ear pulled up and back, and the drops inserted into the ear canal. If ear drops are being administered to a child, the top of the ear should be pulled straight back to accommodate the immature anatomy of the ear.

Metered dose inhalers (MDIs) with medications such as albuterol (Ventolin), fluticasone (Flovent), and budesonide (Pulmicort) have specific instructions that should be outlined when providing the patient with the medication. An MDI is a device that delivers medication directly into the lungs. Proper technique includes shaking the inhaler before use, forming a seal around the spacer with the lips, and breathing in slowly over a period of 3–5 seconds as the release button on the inhaler is being pressed. It is also important to educate patients on holding their breath for 10 seconds after inhalation to allow the medication to reach the lungs.

Patients who are prescribed subcutaneous medication, such as insulin and low molecular weight heparin, should be instructed on proper technique and body sites where injections can be given. Needles for subcutaneous injections should be approximately 5/8 inch in length. Needle length can be dependent on the patient's body composition and may require a shorter or longer needle depending on body mass and amount of subcutaneous fat. Injections should be administered at a 45 degree or 90 degree angle. Body sites where subcutaneous injections can be administered include the abdomen, thighs, shoulder blades, lower back, and back of the arm. It is important to educate patients on rotating sites if injection is administered daily or more frequently. Injecting the same site can lead to lipohypertrophy—a condition in which there is hardening of the tissues beneath the surface of the skin.

Packaging, Storage, Handling, and Disposal of Medications

Medications are packaged to protect the integrity of the substances. Packages prevent medications from being damaged or contaminated with environmental organisms. The packaging must have a surface where medication information can identify the substance found inside. There are different types of packaging that protect medications. **Primary packaging** is in direct contact with the medication and is supplied in the form of vials, blister packs, and bottles. The size of the primary packaging is dependent on the shape and form of the medication. Intravenous medications will likely be packaged in IV bags or vials requiring a syringe and needle for aspiration. Ampules are also used to store liquid medications. Ampules are made of glass. It is important to use the appropriate filter needle to ensure no glass particles enter the bloodstream upon intravenous administration.

Bottles are commonly used to store oral medications. The bottle is typically made of plastic and is orange or white in color. The orange color is translucent and prevents ultraviolet light from potentially harming photosensitive medications. The white bottles are not translucent and prevent light from penetrating though. Blister packs are used to store single dose medications that can be opened by puncturing the pre-formed plastic, paper, or foil lining. **Secondary packaging** is packaging that does not come into direct contact with the medication but helps add a second layer of protection. Secondary packaging can be in the form of a box, plastic bag, or carton. These surfaces can contain information

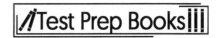

such as active and inactive ingredients, the manufacturer name, type of medication, side effects, and special warnings.

Medication labeling is required and mandated by the Food and Drug Administration (FDA). The medication label should include enough information to inform the patient of its use and any special precautions. Outpatient labels should include the following information:

- Name of the patient
- Name of the dispensing pharmacy
- Name of the prescriber
- Serial number of the prescription
- Name and strength of the medication
- Drug quantity
- Directions for use
- Date when medication was dispensed
- Refill availability
- Expiration date
- Physical drug description
- Special instructions for administration

All this information is necessary to ensure the patient safely takes the medication and is well informed about its attributes.

All medications should be closed and safely stored away from extreme temperatures or unclean environments. Medications that require controlled temperatures should include specific information when dispensing the medication to patients. When handling medications, pharmacists should always wear gloves. Gloves prevent the absorption of drug contents through the skin. Bare hands can potentially absorb some of the medication. For example, topical nitroglycerine exerts its therapeutic effect once absorbed into the skin. **Nitroglycerine** is a potent vasodilator used in the treatment of chest pain. If handled without gloves, it can cause hypotension and syncope. Nondisposable equipment used to prepare medications needs to be properly sanitized between each medication. Cross contamination can lead to improper dosages and presence of unwanted substances.

Medications that are expired or no longer being administered should be disposed of properly. Medication labels or inserts will instruct the patient on proper disposal of the medication. Some medications will need to be flushed down the sink or toilet when expired or no longer being used. However, medications that are flushed down the sink or toilet can contaminate sewer systems. The Food and Drug Administration has compiled a list of medications that are safe to flush due to their potential to be misused or accidentally ingested, which could result in toxicity and death. These medications include narcotics such as morphine, meperidine, oxymorphone, and Demerol. Other non-opioid medications include diazepam and sodium oxybate. Only medications found on the flush list should be discarded into the sink or toilet.

All other medications should be disposed of by other means. If thrown in the trash, the Food and Drug Administration recommends that medications be disposed of in a bag or container that can be sealed. All personal information should be removed or crossed out prior to disposal. The best way to dispose of unwanted or unused medication is to utilize the drug take back programs offered nationwide via pharmacies, mail-back methods, and drop-off boxes. The drug take back program is coordinated by the

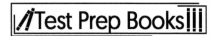

Drug Enforcement Administration and was created as an initiative to decrease drug abuse and misuse. Various sites will collect dispensed medications no longer being used by the patients and recycle or re-manufacture these drugs. This program ensures that medications are safely disposed of and decreases the risk of accidental ingestion by the patient or other members of the household.

Practice Quiz

1. Which statement indicates that a patient taking zolpidem (Ambien) ER understands how to self-administer the medication?
   a. "I will split the tablet when I need to take a smaller dose."
   b. "I will take the medication approximately one hour before bed."
   c. "I will crush the medication and mix with water for easier administration."
   d. "I will take the medication on an empty stomach."

2. A patient is prescribed carbamazepine (Tegretol) suspension 200 mg PO BID. The available suspension has a concentration of 100 mg/5 ml. How many teaspoons will the pharmacist dispense for a 24-hour period? (Round the final answer to the nearest WHOLE number.)

3. Which layer of the skin should the Mantoux tuberculin test be administered to?
   a. Epidermis
   b. Dermis
   c. Subcutaneous tissue
   d. Muscle

4. A provider has prescribed acetaminophen (Tylenol) 650 mg PO Q4H PRN for fever. Tylenol tablets are dispensed in 325 mg/tablet. How many tablets should be available in the dispensing system for the following 24 hours? (Answer must be numeric; round the final answer to the nearest WHOLE number.)

5. A hospitalized patient has an order for haloperidol (Haldol) 3 mg IM q2 hours PRN for agitation. The multidose vial concentration is 5 mg/mL with a total volume of 2 mL. How many vials would need to be available in the unit dispensing system for this patient in a 12-hour shift? (Answer must be numeric; round the final answer to the nearest WHOLE number.)

See answers on next page.

Answer Explanations

1. D: Zolpidem (Ambien) is a sedative/hypnotic used in the treatment of insomnia. Medication tablets should be swallowed whole preferably on an empty stomach for faster absorption and rapid onset of sleep. Choices A and C are incorrect. The patient is taking an extended release (ER) form of the medication. ER medications are meant to be released into the bloodstream over a longer period of time to avoid peaks in their action. Extended release medications should not be crushed, broken, or chewed in order to maintain the integrity of its mechanism of action. Choice B is not correct because patients should be encouraged to take the medication 15 to 20 minutes before bed. Sedatives have a quick onset, and the patient should be prepared to sleep shortly after ingestion.

2. 4 teaspoons: The ordered dose is 200 mg. For every 5 ml, the available dose is 100 mg. The patient will require 10 ml per dose (100 mg/5 ml = 200 mg/10 ml). The order reads to administer the medication BID, which means every 12 hours or twice a day. The total dose in a 24-hour period will be 400 mg (200 mg × 2 = 400 mg). To find the total milliliters per day, the milliliters per dose need to be multiplied by 2 (10 ml × 2 = 20 ml). Each teaspoon is equal to 5 ml. To find the total number of teaspoons, the total milliliters need to be divided by 5 (20 ml/5 ml = 4 tsp).

3. B: The Mantoux tuberculin test is a skin test administered to identify whether a patient has been infected with the bacteria that causes tuberculosis. The tuberculin liquid should be administered into the dermis layer of the skin. Intradermal injections will produce a wheal 6 to 10 mm in diameter. A wheal is a raised bump of skin; it can occur when liquid is introduced. If the test is negative, the wheal will flatten. If positive, 48 to 72 hours after the liquid is introduced the skin will harden and cause an induration. An induration greater than 5 mm is considered a positive TB test. The epidermis is the outermost layer of the skin.

Skin tests such as the tuberculin test need to be administered under the surface of the skin to produce the necessary induration if positive. The subcutaneous layer is used for medications such as insulin and heparin. The subcutaneous layer enables better control of medication release into the bloodstream. Metered flow prevents instantaneous effects that can be harmful to the patient. The muscle is a deep layer used for medications such as vaccines. The muscular layer has a strong supply of blood and enables quick absorption of medications into the circulation. Vaccines contain weakened viruses so the body can build immunity against them. Rapid recognition of these antigens is necessary for antibody production.

4. 12 tablets: The patient can potentially receive a dose every 4 hours (Q4H). In a day, the patient may receive up to 6 doses. The total dosage the patient may receive in a 24-hour period is 3900 g (650 mg × 6 = 3900 mg). The availability is 325 mg/tablet. The patient would require 2 tablets per dose (325 mg × 2 = 650 mg). A total of 12 tablets would need to be available to fulfill this order (325 mg × 12 = 3900 mg).

5. 2 vials: The patient may potentially receive up to 6 doses in a 12-hour shift (12 ÷ 2 = 6). In a 12-hour shift, the patient may receive up to 18 mg of the medication (6 doses × 3 mg = 18 mg). Each vial contains a total of 10 mg of medication (5 mg ÷ 1 mL = 10 mg ÷ 2 mL). The total number of vials needed is 1.8. The question asks to round to the nearest whole number (1.8 rounds to 2).

Area 6 – Developing or Managing Practice or Medication-Use Systems to Ensure Safety and Quality

Interdisciplinary and Collaborative Practice

Pharmacists are the central knowledge repository for drug therapy. Every other healthcare provider also has an important role in the management of patient care. Physicians, physician assistants, and advanced practice nurses work to prescribe medications and manage the patient's comorbidities. Nurses are responsible for administering drug therapy in the acute care and community setting. Other healthcare providers such as respiratory therapists and physical therapists are trained in administering specialized medications for their practice. Collaboration with these providers is an important part of patient-centered care. Pharmacists need to communicate to other providers about changes and assess documentation that may provide an insight into the patient's health status and efficacy of drug therapy.

Centralized electronic patient records enable multiple providers to document their findings. For example, physician documentation may include the medical conditions that are being managed by a specific drug. Progress notes may include whether the illness is acute or chronic, the intended therapy, and the overall goal of treatment. Pharmacists need to review these progress notes to accurately document the goals of drug therapy and communicate any information obtained from patient interviews.

Nurses who care for patients in the acute care setting are primarily responsible for administering most medications. Nurses also document the patient's toleration of a medication, and they are among the first to identify allergic reactions, side effects, and therapeutic responses to medications. Valuable information can be obtained from nursing flowsheets and progress notes. For example, if a patient taking Vancomycin develops a rash 15 minutes into the infusion, nursing documentation will reveal that this patient has developed an allergy. The patient's medical record will be updated to reflect the patient's allergy for future reference. If the patient is taking Lactulose for constipation and the nurse records a bowel movement several hours after administration, the medical record will reflect that the medication has provided its intended effect. In the community setting, nurses are also responsible for recording the management of drug therapy. For example, home health nurses commonly reconcile medications during a visit. Documentation regarding patient compliance will provide information regarding barriers to treatment.

Similarly, **respiratory therapists** are responsible for administering medications that help patients maintain their airway and breathing. Respiratory therapists may work with patients who receive aerosolized medications. Important information regarding the patient's toleration of the medication and physical condition may be recorded. Additionally, patients who are discharged home with nebulizers require patient education. Respiratory therapists often will teach patients how to use this medication delivery method. Documentation will reflect the patient's ability to use medication dispensing equipment which can have an impact on compliance.

Physical therapists have many duties, including wound care. Complex wounds may require topical medications. Licensed therapists are responsible for applying these medications during the procedure. The primary goals of wound care are to prevent infection and promote healing. Pharmacists can obtain

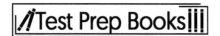

information on the efficacy of drug therapy by evaluating information found in the physical therapy notes.

Continuity and Transitions of Care

The patient is at the center of the **continuity of care model**. The patient is the object of the health care processes at work, it is the patient's case that is being managed, and they use the health care resources to reach their goal of wellness. In continuity of care, the whole patient is treated, not just an organ or an illness. Ideally, the community surrounding the patient is also involved in promoting good health and high quality of life.

The roots of continuity of care lie in a meaningful, long-term relationship between the patient and the health care providers. This relationship ensures that the patient is known. Their needs are anticipated through regular check-ups and follow-ups after the illness has run its course. The goal is to form a firm bond of trust between the health care provider and the patient. This trusting relationship and deep knowledge of the patient's case allow the provider to better advocate for the patient.

The main idea behind continuity of care is to avoid what happens all too often in health care: fragmentation of care. The responsibility of the patient's case is often shifted from one entity to another over the course of an illness. Initially, the patient's case is handled in a primary care setting or perhaps an emergent care setting, depending on the illness. Then the patient may become hospitalized, at which point the hospitalist and various specialists step in and take over. At discharge, the patient's case is then handed over to their primary care physician and community centers. Due to this shifting of care, it becomes ambiguous just who is overseeing the patient's care. The patient has a fragmented experience rather than continuity of care.

Transition of care refers to how patients receive medical care if they need to move to a different setting, facility, or care provider. This is a critical period, as it is a vulnerable time for patients and a high-risk period for medical errors that can compromise patient health and safety. Errors that occur during transitions of care include poor communication between providers, overlooked information, failure to schedule necessary follow-ups, failure to identify patient-specific barriers to health, and limited patient counseling. These errors are linked with poor patient outcomes and increased rates of hospital readmission (including for secondary diagnoses that result from poor management of the primary condition). Transitions of care should include standardized processes that focus on medication reconciliation, patient education regarding their medication and recovery, and shared decision-making for follow-up care between the patient and each healthcare provider.

Transitions of care should also include standard operating procedures for hand-offs between medical staff. These actions have been shown to improve outcomes when transitioning medical care. In this regard, pharmacists play a unique and valuable role in supporting transitions of care, as they are able to provide these specific services as well as additional bedside support, such as noting the patient's attitudes and preferences toward their care and potential barriers to recovery (e.g., low health literacy or caregiver support). Pharmacists are also well-equipped to identify gaps in general clinical service processes and aid other health care providers in closing these gaps, monitor patient discharge protocols, and recommend lifestyle changes that can help the patient with their recovery goals.

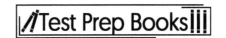

Disease Prevention, Screening Programs, and Stewardship

Disease prevention is integral to ensuring the physical and psychological well-being of individuals, groups, and the community at large. **Primary prevention** consists of the strategies implemented to prevent the onset of a particular disease process. **Secondary prevention** focuses on the early detection of disease and prevention of considerable damage from the disease process. Interventions to promote disease prevention also incorporate the utilization of the patient's support network, stress-management techniques, building effective coping skills, and encouraging healthy lifestyle choices.

Every biological system within the human body should be screened periodically to ensure that it is operating at optimal levels. At the start of every developmental stage, it is recommended that patients be screened and, if found deficient, treated and monitored for progress. Health screenings are suggested based on chronological age to guide both individual treatment and trends for developing community outreach. Armed with the data, providers collaborate to formulate an effective treatment plan.

Screening programs can also guide disease-prevention efforts on a larger scale. Screening data can be used to aide in the creation of medications and advertisement campaigns to target those individuals on the borderlines of a particular disease process. Health screenings also serve to identify gaps in access to healthcare, barriers to care, and disease maintenance. More engagement with health fairs, educational seminars, and print and social media campaigns may also result from health screenings.

Overall, health screenings are an integral piece of the healthcare puzzle. Pharmacists and other healthcare providers should discuss the importance of annual health-screening recommendations upon each patient encounter. If patients reject or accept the recommended testing, they become aware of any present risk factors.

In the context of pharmacies, **stewardship** primarily focuses on the responsible management of controlling diseases through managing chains of infection and implementing responsible antimicrobial practices. Infection control stewardship includes educating both the public and other health care professionals on processes that stop microbial infection transmission or eliminate infection from presenting in the first place. These can include practices such as sanitizing surfaces, implementing proper hand-washing techniques, promoting immunization schedules, encouraging the use of personal protective equipment, and isolating infectious patients.

The need for this area of stewardship arose from an increase in patient infections when in clinical settings, such as post-surgery. Pharmacists also focus heavily on antimicrobial stewardship, which promotes optimal antibiotic use in cases where infection occurs. This need arose from an increased prevalence in antibiotic-resistant pathogens due to antibiotic overuse and misuse. Under the practice of antimicrobial stewardship, pharmacists educate providers on limiting antibiotic prescription orders unless absolutely necessary for the patient's prognosis. Pharmacists also educate patients on correct antibiotic use, such as completing a prescription regimen. Many people who are prescribed antibiotics stop taking the medication when they begin to feel better but before all microbes are killed, leading to the survival of the fittest microbes that can resist available medications.

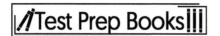
Vulnerable and Special Populations

In healthcare, vulnerable populations are those that face social and economic factors which increase their risk for experiencing poor health outcomes. These include low-income and rural communities, historically underserved minority groups, homeless populations, mentally ill populations, and the LGBTQ+ community. Special populations are those that may not have socioeconomic risk factors but require additional health support. Without this support, they can easily become vulnerable to poor health outcomes. Examples include pediatric patients, the elderly, and disabled people. In general, vulnerable and special populations are more susceptible to poor health and disease for myriad reasons. They often cannot access or afford high-quality health services, or they may feel discriminated against and are therefore less inclined to seek out medical services. Historically, some of these groups have been exploited by the medical community and consequently hold a strong distrust in providers.

Pediatric patients are more susceptible to some diseases, such as infectious illnesses, due to weaker immune systems. Elderly patients are also more vulnerable due to weakened immune systems and may suffer from chronic diseases that correlate with aging, such as cancer and arthritis. Collaborating with patients who fall within a vulnerable and/or special population requires policy support (e.g., increased funding), provider compassion and lack of judgment, and health approaches that support a sense of safety and build trust within the population. Pharmacists can support patients from vulnerable and special populations by encouraging shared decision-making, being honest and transparent with patients about their health care and medication plans, and developing working partnerships with trusted members in the community (e.g., a church, a social service agency, or a community non-profit that works with the target population).

Pharmacists can play a valuable role in risk-prevention programs, which are designed to reduce the incident and burden of chronic disease and injury. These topics are becoming more important as people live longer and become more susceptible to age-related diseases or injury. Many of these issues can be managed or prevented entirely through health-promotion techniques and education that pharmacists are trained to provide. **Risk-prevention programs** generally focus on supporting people to engage more frequently in healthy behaviors, educating people on dangerous or unhealthy behaviors to avoid, and improving access to health care and information. Successful risk-prevention programs that have become more common as pharmacist-led initiatives include self-management for chronic diseases (especially diabetes, hypertension, and asthma), fall prevention for older adults, and medication adherence.

When designing a successful risk-prevention program, pharmacists should consider the needs of their target patient population, survey the support and participation interest of other community health providers, and potential reimbursement mechanisms. For example, a location that primarily serves an elderly population may offer different risk-prevention programs than a pharmacist that works primarily with a cardiovascular health center. Locations that partner with colleges of pharmacy may be able to offer a wider range of programs due to the support and presence offered by pharmacy students. Finally, patients may not participate in programs that they are unable to afford; however, several self-management risk-prevention programs (such as diabetes self-management) are reimbursed through private insurance or Medicare, which tends to encourage higher participation rates.

Pharmacy Informatics

Pharmacy informatics is the combining of technology and information in the pharmaceutical field to provide an integrated approach to patient care. **Medication use** is a process that encompasses

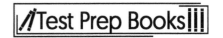

medication prescribing, order processing, administration, dispensing, and effects monitoring. There are various key elements within the medication-use system that affect the overall safety, morbidity, and mortality of drug therapy. One of the elements is **patient information**, which includes demographic and monitoring information. Included in this information is the patient's name, allergies, weight, age, vital signs, and lab values. This information aids in preventing adverse drug effects (ADEs). For example, patients with the same name and similar dates of birth would require other identifying information, such as current disease process, lists of medications, and pharmacy warnings. Quality improvement for patient information can be in the form of a second patient identifier and frequent updating of the medical record.

In addition to their name, patients should be identified using their date of birth or home address. Flagging patients in electronic medical systems alerts the pharmacist of possible patients with similar information. The second key element is drug information. Lack of knowledge about drug therapy is one of the most common causes of medication errors during prescribing and administration. Dosage errors are among the most frequent types of practitioner errors. For example, the medication order may read morphine sulfate IR 30 mg q4 hours (every 4 hours) as needed to manage pain. If the pharmacist misinterprets IR (immediate release) and enters ER (extended release), this can cause a significant accumulation of medication in the patient's system over time. An overdose is possible, and the patient may experience severe respiratory depression and coma.

Quality improvement would involve double-checking orders, verifying inconsistencies, and requesting practitioners use Food and Drug Administration (FDA)-approved drug names. Another key element of medication-use systems is miscommunication of drug orders and drug information among health care workers. Telephone orders increase the risk of misinterpretation of dosages, names, or frequencies. Having a second person listen to spoken orders on the integrated voice response (IVR) system can decrease the chance of medication errors. Abbreviations are another common cause of medication errors. For example, the abbreviation QD and QID can easily be misinterpreted if the medication order is ineligible. **QD** is a daily dose, whereas **QID** is to be administered 4 times a day. This error can have detrimental effects if misunderstood. Electronic prescriptions are becoming increasingly common and can minimize the effects of ineligible handwriting.

Drug labeling, packaging, and nomenclature is another key element of medication-use systems. Look-alike/sound-alike (LASA) drugs, absent drug labels, and vague drug labels result in incorrect dispensing and subsequent medication errors. LASA errors can be minimized by creating mixed-case lettering, in which a combination of capital and lowercase letters calls attention to the drug name. For example, hydroxyzine and hydralazine may look similar on a medication label. A combination of tall man (uppercase) and lowercase letters can help distinguish the medications. Hydroxyzine would be displayed as *hydrOXYzine,* and hydralazine would be displayed as *hydrALAzine*. Electronic images of medication with narrative descriptions of the tablet's color, shape, and lettering can also minimize the risk of incorrect dispensing.

A key element that focuses on accessibility and safe dispensing includes drug standardization, storage, and distribution. Medications should be stored in an organized, clutter-free environment. Expired, recalled, or returned medications should be stored separately from regular stock. Quality improvement techniques include stocking medications alphabetically, distinguishing and separating LASA medications, and ensuring proper labeling. Medication device acquisition, use, and monitoring is an additional key element that is precipitated by human error. Drug delivery devices such as pen injectors require comprehensive patient education to avoid misuse and medication errors. Health care professionals who

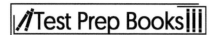

are unfamiliar with the use of devices should follow training protocols to ensure proper education to patients. Teaching patients how to measure and successfully administer medication using devices should be evaluated using the "teach back" method. With this method, the practitioner shows the patient how to use the device and requests a return demonstration to evaluate understanding. Key elements that are difficult to control involve environmental factors, workflow, and staffing patterns.

Medications should be prepared and dispensed in an environment where the practitioner can focus without distractions. For example, if a pharmacist's workstation is in a busy unit's medication room, the possibility of distractions is great. Nurses may enter the room constantly, the phones may be ringing, and background conversations may be present. This type of environment increases the risk of the pharmacist entering an incorrect order and dispensing the wrong medication for the patient. Short staffing and fast-paced environments may drive a practitioner to overlook orders and rapidly perform medication checks. Annual evaluation of knowledge supports the key element of staff competency and education. Educating the staff can supplement other error prevention strategies. Training should focus on new medications being used in the pharmacy, high-alert medications, protocols, policies, procedures, and medication errors currently affecting the facility. The final element in the clinical medication-use system is patient education. The patient's knowledge of a medication is the last line of defense for preventing medication errors. An informed patient may be able to distinguish incorrect dosages, characteristics of medications, and drug interactions.

Practice Quiz

1. A patient is taking phenazopyridine (Pyridium) for the relief of painful urination. Which of the following statements indicates patient understanding of the medication?
   a. "I should crush the medication and mix with water"
   b. "I should take this medication until I finish my antibiotic treatment"
   c. "My urine might turn a reddish-orange color"
   d. "I should take this medication once a day at bedtime"

2. Which statement made by a patient indicates that they understand the education provided for acetylcysteine (Mucomyst)?
   a. "I will flush unused medication down the toilet."
   b. "This medication will thicken my secretions."
   c. "I should dilute the medication in fruit juice."
   d. "This medication is odorless."

3. A pharmacist is following up on a patient's understanding regarding her new prescription of liquid penicillin V 500 mg PO TID. Which of the following statements would indicate that the patient requires further teaching?
   a. "It is best to take this medication on an empty stomach."
   b. "I will take this medication every 8 hours."
   c. "I will take this medication with a glass of orange juice."
   d. "If I keep this medication refrigerated, I must throw it away after 2 weeks."

4. Which of the following implementations improves the quality of medication-use systems? (Select ALL that apply.)
   a. Using the IVR system for telephone orders
   b. Using a workspace close to the drive-thru window and medication pickup line in a pharmacy
   c. Using mixed lettering for LASA medications
   d. Placing expired medications behind usable medications
   e. Practicing the teach back method with patients

5. A pharmacist is following up with a patient who is taking gentamicin for a complicated urinary tract infection. Which of the following statements made by the patient would concern the pharmacist?
   a. "I haven't had much appetite lately."
   b. "I have to raise the volume on the television higher than usual."
   c. "I have felt tired for the past week."
   d. "I have to get up multiple times a night to use the restroom."

See answers on next page.

Answer Explanations

1. C: Phenazopyridine (Pyridium) is a non-opioid analgesic medication used in the treatment of urinary tract symptoms such as itching, burning, frequency, urgency, and pain. One of the secondary effects of the medication is orange staining of the urine. Patients should be advised to wear liners to protect undergarments. Choice *A* is incorrect. Pyridium should not be crushed, chewed, or broken as it can cause increased gastric irritation. Choice *B* is not correct. Pyridium is an analgesic and should only be used until the urinary tract symptoms are relieved; it has nothing to do with finishing a course of antibiotics. Choice *D* is incorrect. Analgesic medications such as Pyridium should be taken as needed when discomfort is present.

2. C: Acetylcysteine (Mucomyst) is a mucolytic medication used to enhance the flow of respiratory secretions. Mucomyst is also the antidote for acetaminophen (Tylenol) poisoning. Patient education includes mixing it with fruit juices or other beverages to help mask the strong taste. Choice *A* is incorrect. Because of the risk of environmental contamination, unused medication should not be flushed down the toilet. Choice *B* is incorrect. Mucomyst is given to help loosen and liquify secretions. Choice *D* is incorrect. Mucomyst has a strong taste and an odor that is comparable to rotten eggs.

3. C: Penicillins should be taken with a full glass of water. Acidic fluids such as orange juice can destroy the medication before it is absorbed into the system. Choice *A* is a correct statement. Most penicillins should be taken on an empty stomach to avoid an excessively acidic environment, which can break down the medication. Ingesting food causes a release of gastric acid. Choice *B* is also a correct statement. The order indicates for the medication to be taken TID. TID stands for every 8 hours. Choice *D* is also a correct statement. Liquid forms of medications deteriorate and expire sooner, so they must be discarded after 2 weeks if refrigerated.

4. A, C, and E: Quality improvement strategies in medication-use systems should focus on safety. Telephone orders increase the risk of misinterpretation of medication names, dosages, and frequencies. The integrated voice response (IVR) system is a speech-recognition method to verify verbal orders. Look-alike/sound-alike (LASA) medications can easily be confused when dispensing. A combination of uppercase and lowercase letters in the name of the medication assists with differentiation. Patient education is key to preventing medication errors and adverse side effects. Patients should be educated on the use of medication dispensing tools. They should also be evaluated on their understanding of the instructions by asking them to demonstrate the skill. Choice *B* is not correct. When dispensing and preparing medications, working environments should be free of all types of distractions. Choice *D* is not correct because expired medications should be kept in a different drawer to prevent unsafe dispensing.

5. B: Gentamicin is an aminoglycoside used in the treatment of bacterial infections. Aminoglycosides have a risk of causing ototoxicity. Ototoxicity results in ringing of the ears, loss of balance, and decreased hearing. Hearing loss should alert the pharmacist of potential toxicity. Choices *A, C, & D* are not exclusive to aminoglycosides. Loss of appetite and fatigue are uncommon side effects of gentamicin. Polyuria is not a known side effect of gentamicin and may reflect another disease process.

Obtaining, Interpreting, or Assessing Data, Medical, or Patient Information

1. In an initial interview, the patient reveals a history of human papillomavirus (HPV). Which screening test will the patient require frequently?
    a. Mammogram
    b. Pap smear
    c. Bone scan
    d. Colonoscopy

2. Which of the following is an expected laboratory value for a patient taking warfarin (Coumadin)?
    a. aPTT 35 seconds
    b. PT 13 seconds
    c. INR 2.5
    d. Elevated D-dimer

3. Which of the following vital signs would indicate that a patient taking metoprolol (Lopressor) is responding well to treatment?
    a. Blood pressure of 129/78 mmHg and pulse of 61 bpm
    b. Pulse of 98 and respirations of 18 breaths per minute
    c. Blood pressure of 115/76 mmHg and pulse of 48 bpm
    d. Blood pressure of 135/80 mmHg and temperature of 98.5 degrees Fahrenheit

4. Which of the following would indicate albumin is delivering the desired therapeutic effect? (Select ALL that apply.)
    a. Increased respirations
    b. Increased blood pressure
    c. Decreased heart rate
    d. Decreased edema
    e. Decreased skin turgor

5. Which of the following instructions should the pharmacist give to a patient taking liquid ferrous sulfate for iron deficiency anemia? (Select ALL that apply.)
    a. Dilute liquid iron with juice.
    b. Take with vitamin C supplements.
    c. Rinse mouth after swallowing.
    d. Take on an empty stomach.
    e. Limit the intake of muscle, meats, and egg yolks.
    f. Increase fiber intake.

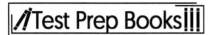

6. While examining a patient's medical record, the pharmacist notices that the patient has seizure disorder listed as a medical condition. Which of the following medications would the pharmacist recognize as a treatment for seizure disorders?
    a. Lorazepam (Ativan)
    b. Oxazepam (Serax)
    c. Flurazepam (Dalmane)
    d. Clonazepam (Klonopin)

7. A patient with Parkinson's disease is prescribed Sinemet (carbidopa/levodopa). Upon review of the patient's medication list, the pharmacist would be concerned if the patient was taking which other drug?
    a. Phenelzine (Nardil)
    b. Metformin (Glucophage)
    c. Tramadol (Ultram)
    d. Psyllium (Vitalax)

8. A provider speaks with the pharmacist regarding the best option for an opioid-acetaminophen medication for a patient with a history of drug addiction. The pharmacist recognizes that which of the following has the greatest risk for abuse and dependency?
    a. Vicodin
    b. Percocet
    c. Hydrocet
    d. Lorcet HD

9. A patient is taking diazepam (Valium) for the management of anxiety disorder. Which of the following are possible side effects of this medication? (Select ALL that apply.)
    a. Lack of appetite
    b. Lightheadedness
    c. Stomach cramping
    d. Drowsiness
    e. Lack of coordination

10. A pharmacist is reviewing a patient's medical history. The pharmacist notes that the patient has a history of multiple sclerosis (MS). Which of the following medications would the pharmacist recognize is indicated for MS?
    a. Tramadol (Ultram)
    b. Cyclobenzaprine (Flexeril)
    c. Diclofenac (Voltaren)
    d. Balsalazide (Colazal)

11. A patient is taking atorvastatin (Lipitor) as a treatment for hypercholesterolemia. Which of the following laboratory parameters would indicate that the medication is achieving the therapeutic goal? (Select ALL that apply.)
    a. Cholesterol level, 190 mg/dL
    b. AST level, 55 U/L
    c. ALT level, 60 U/L
    d. HDL level, 62 mg/dL
    e. LDL level, 90 mg/dL
    f. Triglyceride level, 155 mg/dL

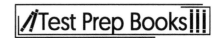

12. A patient is taking levothyroxine (Synthroid) for a diagnosis of hypothyroidism. Which of the following physical manifestations would indicate to the pharmacist that this medication is having the intended effect? (Select ALL that apply.)
    a. Increased weight
    b. Increased appetite
    c. Improved ability to sleep
    d. Increased pulse rate
    e. Increased alertness

13. A patient is prescribed nortriptyline (Pamelor) PO 25 mg TID for depression. Upon reviewing the patient's current medication list, the pharmacist would be concerned with drug interactions if which of the following medications are on the list? (Select ALL that apply.)
    a. Phenelzine (Nardil)
    b. Clonidine (Catapress)
    c. Levetiracetam (Keppra)
    d. Hydrocodone/acetaminophen (Vicodin)
    e. Lamotrigine (Lamictal)

14. A pharmacist is reviewing laboratory parameters for a patient prescribed sirolimus (Rapamune) PO 2 mg/day. Which of the following would alert the pharmacist to question the medication order?
    a. Hemoglobin, 20 g/dL
    b. Sodium level, 145 mEq/L
    c. BUN, 19 mg/dL
    d. ALT level, 135 IU/L

15. A patient has been prescribed nisoldipine (Sular) PO 30 mg/day for the treatment of hypertension. When educating the patient on possible side effects, which of the following should the pharmacist mention? (Select ALL that apply.)
    a. Constipation
    b. Itchiness
    c. Headache
    d. Sinusitis
    e. Anxiety
    f. Palpitations

16. Which of the following clinical manifestations is expected for a patient taking alendronate (Fosamax)?
    a. Absence of Trousseau's sign
    b. Decreased muscle spasms
    c. Decreased muscle weakness
    d. Absence of Chvostek's sign

17. Which of the following lab parameters would indicate that a patient taking epoetin (Procrit) is achieving the goals of therapy? (Select ALL that apply.)
    a. Hematocrit, 34%
    b. Eosinophils, 3%
    c. Neutrophils, 61%
    d. Hemoglobin, 12 g/dL
    e. Red blood cells (RBCs), 5.1 million/mm^3

81

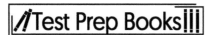

18. Which of the following lab values would indicate a medication is causing nephrotoxicity?
    a. Urine pH, 7.8
    b. Creatinine level, 2.1 mg/dL
    c. BUN, 19 mg/dL
    d. Uric acid, 7.2 mg/dL

19. Which of the following factors influence medication response? (Select ALL that apply.)
    a. Body size
    b. Age
    c. Rh factor
    d. Sex
    e. Route of administration

20. Rank the following sources of evidence from most reliable to least reliable:
    I. Randomized controlled trials
    II. Systematic reviews
    III. Case reports
    IV. Pilot studies
    a. II, I, IV, III
    b. II, IV, I, III
    c. I, IV, II, III
    d. I, II, III, IV

21. A pharmacist is evaluating the therapeutic response in a patient taking Zaroxolyn. Which clinical manifestation indicates the medication is having its intended effect? (Select ALL that apply.)
    a. Systolic blood pressure below 120 mmHg
    b. Absence of edema
    c. Tolerance of oral nutrition
    d. Semi-soft bowel movements
    e. Lack of dyspnea

22. A pharmacist is performing a patient interview to determine cardiovascular risk factors. Which of the following chronic illnesses increases the risk of cardiovascular events?
    a. Osteoporosis
    b. Anorexia
    c. Microalbuminuria
    d. Endometriosis

23. A patient is prescribed ferrous sulfate for the treatment of anemia. The patient asks the pharmacist which foods he should eat to supplement his diet. What food will the pharmacist mention?
    a. Turnips
    b. Spinach
    c. Black beans
    d. Avocados

24. Which of the following laboratory tests should a pharmacist monitor for a patient taking levofloxacin (Levaquin)? (Select ALL that apply.)
    a. Calcium level
    b. Red blood cell count
    c. White blood cell count
    d. Bilirubin level
    e. Albumin level
    f. Hemoglobin level

25. Which of the following lab values is best corrected with indapamide?
    a. Calcium, 5.9 mEq/L
    b. Magnesium, 2.8 mEq/L
    c. Potassium, 4.9 mEq/L
    d. Sodium, 132 mEq/L

26. A pharmacist is reviewing the medication record of a patient taking disopyramide. The pharmacist should inquire further if they notice which of the following medications on the record? (Select ALL that apply.):
    a. Phenytoin
    b. Rifampin
    c. Docusate
    d. Cimetidine
    e. Ketorolac
    f. Bretylium

27. During an initial interview, a patient tells the pharmacist their last blood pressure reading was 138/87. What blood pressure category does this reading fall under?
    a. Normal
    b. Elevated
    c. Stage 1 Hypertension
    d. Stage 2 Hypertension

28. Which of the following medications has the highest potential for abuse?
    a. Tylenol with Codeine
    b. Restoril
    c. Phenergan with Codeine
    d. Duragesic

29. A pharmacist is reviewing the medication record for a patient receiving pantoprazole at 8 mL/hr. The supplied dose is 40 mg/50 mL. How many milligrams is the patient receiving every hour? (Round the final answer to the nearest TENTH.)

30. A pharmacist sees sertaconazole on a patient's medication record. Which condition does this medication treat?
    a. Tinea corporis
    b. Tinea cruris
    c. Interdigital tinea pedis
    d. Tinea capitis

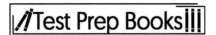

31. What clinical manifestation would be expected for a patient with a calcium level of 3.2 mEq/L?
    a. Hypertension
    b. Diaphoresis
    c. Constipation
    d. Seizures

32. A pharmacist is reviewing a patient's current medication list. Which medication has the greatest risk for noncompliance due to socioeconomic factors?
    a. Bleomycin
    b. Famotidine
    c. Meclizine
    d. Prazosin

33. Which of the following lab values would most accurately indicate that a patient taking methimazole (Tapazole) is responding positively to treatment?
    a. Total T3 level, 100 ng/dL
    b. HGB level, 14.0 g/dL
    c. Total T4 level, 7.0 mcg/dL
    d. TSH level, 1.9 mIU/L

34. Which of the following lab values is directly impacted by patiromer (Veltassa)?
    a. Sodium (Na^+)
    b. Potassium (K^+)
    c. Chloride (Cl^-)
    d. Calcium (Ca^{2+})

35. Why is it important to collect the patient's medical history before filling a prescription?
    a. It is not usually important, unless the patient is elderly.
    b. It can provide an allergy history and prevent dangerous drug reactions.
    c. It can help the pharmacist predict the next medical condition.
    d. It can make it easier to provide refills.

36. On a patient's lab values for the day, one lab parameter has gone up significantly, signaling a possible infectious process at work. Which lab parameter is likely to align with this conclusion?
    a. Blood urea nitrogen
    b. Hematocrit
    c. Neutrophils
    d. Sodium level

37. Which of the following are common barriers to medication adherence in patients? (Select **ALL** that apply.)
    a. Cost
    b. Poor patient-provider communication
    c. Poor patient knowledge of the illness and medication
    d. Dose packaging
    e. Forgetfulness

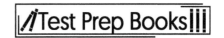

38. Belinda has Type 2 diabetes and has experienced multiple instances of forgetting to take her prescription metformin. When her adult son visits, he usually notices if she misses a dose and reminds her, and she takes her dose as soon as she remembers. However, she has been admitted twice to the emergency department with complications from hyperglycemia. Which intervention would most effectively benefit Belinda?
    a. A health coaching appointment
    b. Remote continuous glucose monitoring
    c. A prescription for rapid-acting insulin
    d. Moving in with her son

39. Jenni is a pharmacist who is reviewing a patient's medical information. This patient has been diagnosed with several conditions affecting the cardiovascular system and needs to start three new medications to manage the diagnoses. Jenni calls the patient's health insurance provider and securely sends them the patient's medical history, diagnosis code, and physician notes. The health insurance provider notices that one diagnosis code is missing and lets Jenni know. Jenni speaks with the patient's physician, obtains the missing diagnosis code, and updates the patient's information with the health insurance company. The health insurance company then approves payment for the medication, and Jenni begins to fill the prescriptions. What key process is Jenni using to support the patient and the physician?
    a. Prior authorization
    b. New patient intake
    c. Revenue cycle
    d. Intervention monitoring

40. Why should pharmacists ask patients to disclose information about non-prescription supplements they are taking? (Select **ALL** that apply.)
    a. Because some supplements can react adversely with prescription medications
    b. To recommend the highest-quality form of a supplement
    c. To understand the primary causes of a patient's health concern
    d. To shift the patient to a food-based source of the supplement instead
    e. To shift the patient to a regulated, FDA-approved therapeutic instead

41. Upon medication pick-up, which of the following is a way to confirm patient identity and maintain high quality of care in a pharmacy setting?
    a. Asking the patient for the generic name of the medication they are picking up
    b. Asking the patient for their prescribing provider
    c. Asking the patient for their date of birth
    d. Asking the patient for their health insurance card

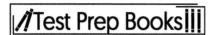

Identifying Drug Characteristics

1. Which of the following medications is the most dangerous for use during pregnancy?
   a. Verapamil (Calan)
   b. Diphenhydramine (Benadryl)
   c. Colchicine (Colcrys)
   d. Nystatin (Mycostatin)

2. Rank the following antidysrhythmic medications by class (I–IV):
   I. Procainamide (Procanbid)
   II. Amiodarone (Cordarone)
   III. Propranolol (Inderal)
   IV. Verapamil (Calan)
   a. I, III, II, IV
   b. III, I, II, IV
   c. I, II, IV, III
   d. III, II, I, IV

3. Which of the following anticonvulsant medication orders has the fastest peak activity?
   a. Phenytoin (Dilantin) 100 mg IV
   b. Fosphenytoin (Cerebyx) 4 mg EQ/kg/day IM
   c. Phenytoin (Dilantin) 300 mg PO
   d. Fosphenytoin (Cerebyx) 5 mg EQ/kg/day IV

4. Which of the following formulations of isosorbides has the shortest duration of action?
   a. Isosorbide dinitrate (ISDN) SL
   b. Isosorbide mononitrate (ISMN) ER
   c. Isosorbide dinitrate (ISDN) PO
   d. Isosorbide mononitrate (ISMN) PO

5. Which of the following local anesthetics has a high potency and long duration?
   a. Lidocaine
   b. Procaine
   c. Bupivacaine
   d. Prilocaine

6. Where are the nicotinic receptors located?
   a. Skeletal muscle
   b. Heart
   c. Glands
   d. Blood vessels

7. Which of the following is a second-generation beta-blocker? (Select ALL that apply.)
   a. Metoprolol
   b. Propranolol
   c. Esmolol
   d. Timolol
   e. Atenolol
   f. Bisoprolol

8. In which part of the digestive system is oral tetracycline (Sumycin) best absorbed?
   a. Esophagus
   b. Large intestine
   c. Small intestine
   d. Stomach

9. Which of the following antihypertensive medications is classified as a diuretic?
   a. Indapamide (Lozol)
   b. Losartan (Cozaar)
   c. Atenolol (Tenormin)
   d. Captopril (Capoten)

10. Rank the following topical steroids based on the strength of their active ingredient (lowest to highest percentage):
   I. Dexamethasone sodium phosphate (Neodecadron)
   II. Fluticasone propionate (Cutivate)
   III. Fluocinolone acetonide (Capex)
   IV. Hydrocortisone valerate (Westcort)
   a. III, I, II, IV
   b. III, II, I, IV
   c. II, III, I, IV
   d. II, I, III, IV

11. Which of the following antitubercular medications is in group III (according to their group (I–IV))?
   a. Ofloxacin
   b. Rifampin
   c. Streptomycin
   d. Ethionamide

12. Which of the following corticosteroids has the shortest systemic duration period?
   a. Betamethasone PO
   b. Cortisone PO
   c. Dexamethasone IM
   d. Methylprednisolone IM

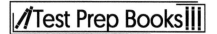
13. Rank the following inhaled corticosteroids by their medication concentration in mcg/puff, from highest to lowest:

        I. Flunisolide (Aerobid) 250

        II. Triamcinolone acetonide (Nasacort) 100

        III. Budesonide (Pulmicort) 200

        IV. Beclomethasone (Qvar) 80

    a. I, IV, II, III

    b. III, IV, II, I

    c. I, III, II, IV

    d. III, I, II, IV

14. What antibody acts as the first line of defense for the immune system?

    a. IgG

    b. IgM

    c. IgA

    d. IgE

15. Oral medications are identified by which of the following? (Select ALL that apply.)

    a. Imprint

    b. Shape

    c. Size

    d. Smell

    e. Color

16. Rank the following antacid products based on their aluminum hydroxide concentration per dose, from the most milligrams to the least milligrams:

        I. Amphojel

        II. Mylanta

        III. Maalox

        IV. Aludrox

    a. IV, I, III, II

    b. I, III, II, IV

    c. II, III, I, IV

    d. III, II, IV, I

17. Which part of the cell is disrupted by micafungin (Mycamine)?

    a. Cytoplasm

    b. Cell wall

    c. Plasma membrane

    d. Ribosome

18. Which of the following hormonal contraceptives is the most concentrated based on estrogen concentration?

    a. Aviane

    b. Ogestrel

    c. Levlen

    d. Brevicon

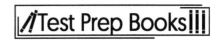

19. Which of the following is a fourth-generation cephalosporins?
    a. Cefotaxime (Claforan)
    b. Cefepime (Maxipime)
    c. Cefoxitin (Mefoxin)
    d. Cefazolin (Ancef)

20. Which of the following subcutaneous insulins is the shortest acting?
    a. Humulin N
    b. Novolin R
    c. Insulin glargine
    d. Insulin aspart

21. Which of the following carries information about the pharmacology of a medication?
        I. Prescription label
        II. PPI
        III. Product monograph
    a. I only
    b. II only
    c. II and III
    d. I, II, and III

22. Which of the following statements is NOT TRUE regarding generic substitution?
    a. Generics are more cost effective.
    b. Medication cannot be substituted if the prescriber writes DAW.
    c. Prescriber approval must be obtained for any generic substitution.
    d. Therapeutically equivalent generics have the same efficacy as their branded counterparts.

23. Which one of the following agencies may initiate a drug recall?
    a. United States Food and Drug Administration (FDA)
    b. Drug Enforcement Administration (DEA)
    c. Occupational Safety and Health Administration (OSHA)
    d. The Joint Commission (TJC)

24. Which of the following agencies oversees the National Medication Errors Reporting Program (MERP)?
    a. Drug Enforcement Administration (DEA)
    b. The Institute of Safe Medication Practices (ISMP)
    c. Occupational Safety and Health Administration (OSHA)
    d. The Joint Commission (TJC)

25. Which of the following medications are cardiovascular agents? (Select **ALL** that apply.)
    a. Chlorothiazide
    b. Methylphenidate
    c. Nitroglycerin
    d. Omeprazole
    e. Abacavir

89

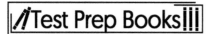

26. Dolly has recently been diagnosed with fibromyalgia, a disease that affects the nervous system and is characterized by musculoskeletal pain, sleep and mood disruption, and fatigue. Which of the following brand-name medications is Dolly's physician most likely to prescribe to her?
    a. Prempro
    b. Ritalin
    c. Humira
    d. Cymbalta

27. In which therapeutic category would the medication doxycycline fall under?
    a. Analgesics
    b. Antivirals
    c. Antibacterials
    d. Antiemetics

28. The medication Eliquis (generic name: apixaban) would be best prescribed to which of the following patients?
    a. Lucia, who was recently diagnosed with Stage II breast cancer
    b. Mickey, who just had a hip replacement
    c. Wren, who is experiencing withdrawals as she recovers from oxycodone addiction
    d. Kenji, who is experiencing symptoms of bone-density loss

29. Which of the following SSRIs would be best recommended for a nursing mother? (Select ALL that apply.)
    a. Nortriptyline
    b. Imipramine
    c. Sertraline
    d. Paroxetine
    e. Nursing mothers should avoid all SSRI medications and resume only when breastfeeding is complete.

30. Mika, a twenty-eight-year-old woman, has been experiencing symptoms of depression lately. These symptoms include prolonged feelings of sadness and hopelessness, extreme fatigue, and loss of interest in activities that used to bring her joy. Her best friend notices the changes in Mika's behavior, and shares a story about how St. John's wort, an herbal supplement, helped when she went through a similar experience. Mika feels that since it is an affordable over-the-counter supplement, it's worth trying. What should Mika know about this supplement before starting a regimen?
    a. It can interact adversely with her hormonal contraceptive.
    b. It has a black box warning.
    c. It is only FDA-approved for women in menopause.
    d. It should only be used in conjunction with FDA-approved antidepressants.

31. Which of the following brand name medications have black box warnings? (Select **ALL** that apply.)
    a. Zoloft
    b. Levaquin
    c. Lipitor
    d. Neurontin
    e. Prescription-strength Tylenol

32. Which of the following drugs works by acting upon ergosterol?
    a. Ramipril
    b. Naproxen
    c. Ketoconazole
    d. Amoxicillin

Developing or Managing Treatment Plans

1. Which of the following laboratory data is important to assess for a patient taking furosemide (Lasix)?
    a. White blood cells
    b. Potassium levels
    c. Hemoglobin
    d. Albumin levels

2. A patient is prescribed codeine (Paveral) 20m PO q6hr PRN for cough. When dispensing this medication, which instructions should the pharmacist give the patient? (Select ALL that apply.)
    a. Change positions slowly
    b. Avoid driving while taking this medication
    c. Monitor daily weight
    d. Take this medication in the morning
    e. Take this medication with food
    f. Increase fluid intake

3. Which of the following are therapeutic uses for fluoxetine (Prozac)? (Select ALL that apply.)
    a. Dysmenorrhea
    b. Major depression
    c. Panic disorders
    d. Bulimia nervosa
    e. Venous thrombosis

4. A pharmacist is teaching a patient to consume adequate amounts of calcium while taking alendronate sodium (Fosamax). The pharmacist will mention which of the following foods?
    a. Swiss chard
    b. Yogurt
    c. Beans
    d. Cream soups

5. Which of the following parameters are used to evaluate the effectiveness of metformin (Glucophage)? (Select ALL that apply.)
    a. HgA1C levels below 7%
    b. Sodium levels below 145 mEq/L
    c. Blood pressure less than 130/80 mmHg
    d. Glucose levels between 90 and 130 mg/dL
    e. Healing of gastric ulcers
    f. Total cholesterol level below 200 mg/dL

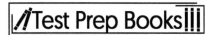

6. Which of the following rapid-acting nitroglycerine (Nitrol) routes should patients take at the first sign of chest pain?
    a. Topical
    b. Sublingual
    c. Transdermal
    d. Oral

7. A pharmacist informs a patient to avoid tyramine-rich foods while taking phenelzine (Nardil). Which of the following symptoms will the patient experience when combining Nardil and tyramine? (Select ALL that apply.)
    a. Nausea
    b. Fever
    c. Headache
    d. Increased heart rate
    e. Increased blood pressure

8. The influenza vaccine would be contraindicated in which of the following patients?
    a. A patient who is allergic to eggs
    b. A patient who has history of anemia
    c. A patient with frequent nausea
    d. A patient who gets frequent colds

9. The movement of medication from the site of administration to the bloodstream is which principle of pharmacokinetics?
    a. Excretion
    b. Distribution
    c. Absorption
    d. Metabolism

10. A primary care provider and a pharmacist are discussing treatment options for a patient with gout. Which of the following medications are options for treatment of this condition? (Select ALL that apply.)
    a. Colchicine
    b. Cyclosporine (Neoral)
    c. Indomethacin (Indocin)
    d. Allopurinol (Zyloprim)
    e. Sulfasalazine (Azulfidine)

11. A pharmacist receives a medication order for a patient with a history of a stroke. The patient is dysphagic and has decreased mobility. Which administration route is contraindicated for this patient?
    a. Parenteral
    b. Transdermal
    c. Sublingual
    d. Oral

12. Which of the following affects pharmacokinetics in older adults? (Select ALL that apply.)
    a. Decreased circulation
    b. Increased protein-binding sites
    c. Decreased body fat
    d. Increased gastric pH
    e. Increased gastric emptying

13. A patient is taking amitriptyline (Elavil) for depression. The pharmacist knows that this medication can cause anticholinergic effects. When educating the patient, which symptoms should the pharmacist mention? (Select ALL that apply.)
    a. Dry mouth
    b. Photophobia
    c. Rigidity
    d. Restlessness
    e. Urinary retention
    f. Involuntary movements

14. Rank the following vitamins by their recommended daily intake for adult males, from most to least milligrams:
        I. Vitamin E
        II. Vitamin B3 (Niacin)
        III. Vitamin B5 (Pantothenic acid)
        IV. Vitamin C
    a. I, II, IV, III
    b. III, I, II, IV
    c. III, II, IV, I
    d. I, III, II, IV

15. A pharmacist notes an order for azithromycin (Zithromax) 1 g PO. The pharmacist recognizes that this prescription will primarily treat which disease?
    a. Syphilis
    b. Human Immunodeficiency Virus (HIV)
    c. Chlamydia
    d. Human papillomavirus (HPV)

16. Moderate-dose dopamine (Intropin) has which of the following pharmacological actions? (Select ALL that apply.)
    a. Vasoconstriction
    b. Renal blood vessel dilation
    c. Increased heart rate
    d. Increased myocardial contractility
    e. Bronchodilation

17. Which of the following minerals has the lowest daily tolerable upper intake level based on their daily tolerable upper intake levels for children over the age of nine?
    a. Calcium
    b. Magnesium
    c. Phosphorus
    d. Fluoride

93

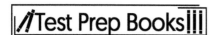

18. Succinylcholine (Anectine) is the preferred medication for which of the following? (Select ALL that apply.)
   a. Lumbar puncture
   b. Seizure control during ECT
   c. Biopsy
   d. Endotracheal intubation
   e. Endoscopic procedure
   f. Chemotherapy

19. A patient is taking oseltamivir (Tamiflu). Which of the following laboratory data should cause the pharmacist concern?
   a. Hemoglobin (g/dL), 15
   b. Hematocrit (%), 48.8
   c. BUN (mg/dL), 93
   d. Serum creatinine (mg/dL), 2.3

20. A patient is taking prochlorperazine (Compazine) for the treatment of psychotic disorder. The pharmacist warns the patient about the most common extrapyramidal reaction, which manifests as compulsive movements. What is the name of that extrapyramidal reaction?
   a. Dystonia
   b. Dyskinesia
   c. Akathisia
   d. Parkinsonism

21. What size needle should be used for a 6-month-old infant receiving the IPV vaccine?
   a. $26G \frac{1}{2}$ in
   b. $25G \frac{5}{8}$ in
   c. 25B 1 in
   d. $23G 1\frac{1}{4}$ in

22. Which of the following are possible adverse effects of torsemide (Demadex)? (Select ALL that apply.)
   a. Hypercalcemia
   b. Edema
   c. Hypotension
   d. Ototoxicity
   e. Hypokalemia

23. Rank the following medications based on their time of onset (fastest to slowest):
   I. Heparin Sub-Q
   II. Haloperidol PO
   III. Glycopyrrolate IV
   IV. Escitalopram PO
   a. I, II, IV, III
   b. III, I, II, IV
   c. III, IV, I, II
   d. I, III, IV, II

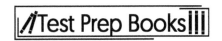

24. A patient requests to speak to a pharmacist for suggestions on over-the-counter medications that will help relieve mild knee pain but not cause stomach irritation. The pharmacist tells the patient the best over-the-counter medication for pain relief without gastric irritation is which of the following?
    a. Aspirin
    b. Acetaminophen (Tylenol)
    c. Ibuprofen (Advil)
    d. Naproxen (Aleve)

25. Rank the following medications from the lowest to the highest drug classification schedule:
        I. Alprazolam (Xanax)
        II. Meperidine (Demerol)
        III. Buprenorphine (Suboxone)
        IV. Robitussin AC
    a. III, I, II, IV
    b. I, III, IV, II
    c. IV, I, III, II
    d. II, III, IV, I

26. A hospitalized patient has an order for rivastigmine (Exelon) to manage his Alzheimer's. The pharmacist knows that which of the following reversal agents needs to be in stock in case of toxicity?
    a. Flumazenil
    b. Naloxone
    c. Protamine sulfate
    d. Atropine

27. A patient taking captopril (Capoten) for hypertension is instructed to avoid potassium-rich foods. The pharmacist should provide the patient a list of potassium-rich foods to avoid that includes which of the following? (Select ALL that apply.)
    a. Apricots
    b. Kiwi
    c. Cream soups
    d. Oysters
    e. Spinach
    f. Potatoes

28. Which of the following medication orders has the fastest onset?
    a. Hydromorphone (Dilaudid) 1 mg SubQ q3 hours for moderate pain
    b. Hydromorphone (Dilaudid) 0.5 mg IV q4 hours for severe pain
    c. Hydromorphone (Dilaudid) 1.5 mg IM q4 hours for severe pain
    d. Hydromorphone (Dilaudid) 4 mg PO q3–4 hours for moderate pain

29. Which of the following medications are used for the treatment of hypertension? (Select ALL that apply.)
    a. Sucralfate (Carafate)
    b. Ramipril (Altace)
    c. Nizatidine (Axid)
    d. Furosemide (Lasix)
    e. Doxazosin (Cardura)

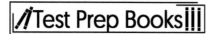

30. Rank the following administration routes for epinephrine (adrenalin) based on their final concentration from most potent to least potent.
        I. Intravenous
        II. Intradermal
        III. Subcutaneous
        IV. Inhalation
    a. III, IV, II, I
    b. IV, II, I, III
    c. III, I, II, IV
    d. IV, III, I, II

31. During a follow-up, a pharmacist is assessing possible complications for a patient taking ceftazidime (Fortaz). The pharmacist should be concerned if the patient reports which of the following side effects?
    a. Dizziness
    b. Yellow discoloration of the eye
    c. Lightheadedness
    d. Altered sense of taste

32. Which of the following side effects are expected for a patient with a serum lithium level of 0.9 mEq/L? (Select ALL that apply.)
    a. Tinnitus
    b. Hand tremors
    c. Ataxia
    d. Metallic taste
    e. Polyuria
    f. Slurred speech

33. A pharmacist is providing education to a patient who has been prescribed sodium bicarbonate. As part of the instructions, the pharmacist tells the patient to avoid foods that will alkalinize the urine, which can lead to renal calculi. Which of the following foods should the pharmacist instruct the patient to avoid?
    a. Milk
    b. Poultry
    c. Rice
    d. Pasta

34. A patient with diabetes is prescribed repaglinide (Prandin) PO 2 mg AC. Upon review of the patient's home medications, which of the following herbal supplements would raise concern for possible hypoglycemia if taken concurrently with repaglinide (Prandin)? (Select ALL that apply.)
    a. Gingko biloba
    b. Ginseng
    c. Garlic
    d. Glucosamine
    e. Basil

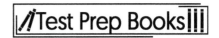

35. Which of the following foods contains the most milligrams per serving of potassium?
    a. 1 cup lentils
    b. 1 cup milk
    c. 1 cup orange juice
    d. 1 cup brewed coffee

36. Which of the following medications decrease the effects of theophylline? (Select ALL that apply.)
    a. Clindamycin (Cleocin)
    b. Lithium
    c. Phenobarbital
    d. Cimetidine (Tagamet)
    e. Propranolol (Inderal)
    f. Phenelzine (Nardil)

37. The action of one drug that facilitates or increases the action of another is known as
    a. synergism.
    b. antagonism.
    c. efficacy.
    d. specificity.

38. Which of the following medications requires a dosage reduction in patients with mild renal failure?
    a. Amiodarone
    b. Haloperidol
    c. Mirtazapine
    d. Acyclovir

39. Which of the following are types of humoral allergic reactions? (Select ALL that apply.)
    a. Delayed hypersensitivity
    b. Anaphylactic
    c. Cytolytic
    d. Arthus
    e. Phototoxic

40. Which of the following anti-seizure medications is a first-choice drug for the treatment of status epilepticus?
    a. Phenytoin
    b. Valproate
    c. Lorazepam
    d. Carbamazepine

41. Which of the following medications has the potential to prolong the Q-T interval (as seen in an electrocardiogram)? (Select ALL that apply.)
    a. Amiodarone
    b. Amitriptyline
    c. Warfarin
    d. Procainamide
    e. Enoxaparin
    f. Quinidine

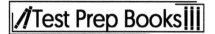

42. Which of the following injectable local anesthetics has the highest safe maximum dose in milligrams?
    a. Procaine
    b. Lidocaine
    c. Dibucaine
    d. Bupivacaine

43. Which of the following anti-depressants is a serotonin and noradrenaline reuptake inhibitor (SNRI)?
    a. Fluvoxamine
    b. Citalopram
    c. Fluoxetine
    d. Venlafaxine

44. A patient is receiving continuous heparin for the treatment of deep vein thrombosis. The pharmacist knows that which of the following medications should be readily available to reverse the effects of heparin?
    a. Vitamin K
    b. Acetylcysteine
    c. Flumazenil
    d. Protamine sulfate

45. In which part of the brain does ondansetron exert its greatest therapeutic effect?
    a. Midbrain
    b. Pons
    c. Medulla oblongata
    d. Cerebellum

46. A provider orders cefazolin 1 g IV × 1 dose prior to a surgical procedure. The patient had a penetrating abdominal injury less than 2 hours ago. How is this operative wound classified?
    a. Dirty
    b. Contaminated
    c. Clean-contaminated
    d. Clean

47. Which of the following therapeutic effects is expected after taking fexofenadine? (Select ALL that apply.)
    a. Relief of heartburn
    b. Decreased itching
    c. Decreased gastric bleeding
    d. Absence of rhinorrhea
    e. Prevention of acid indigestion

48. A pharmacist is reviewing treatment for a patient with a urinary tract infection (UTI). The pharmacist recognizes that which of the following medications treats UTIs?
    a. Tadalafil
    b. Finasteride
    c. Tamsulosin
    d. Nitrofurantoin

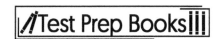

49. A provider and a pharmacist are reviewing antiretroviral treatment guidelines for a patient with the human immunodeficiency virus (HIV). The pharmacist recognizes that which of the following circumstances are indications for initiation of antiretroviral therapy? (Select ALL that apply.)
   a. Pregnancy
   b. Platelet level of 455,000/mm³
   c. CD4 count of 400/mm³
   d. Active tuberculosis infection
   e. Hypertension

50. Esmolol is used to treat which of the following abnormal cardiac rhythms?
   a. Sinus tachycardia
   b. Atrial fibrillation
   c. Premature atrial contractions
   d. Second-degree heart block

51. A patient with hypertension asks a pharmacist for nutritional advice. Knowing that sodium contributes to fluid volume excess, which of the following foods should the patient avoid? (Select ALL that apply.)
   a. Broccoli
   b. Cheese
   c. Ketchup
   d. Banana
   e. Soy sauce
   f. Bacon

52. Rank the following inhaled anti-asthma medications based on their onset from fastest to slowest.
   I. Ipratropium (Atrovent)
   II. Salmeterol (Serevent)
   III. Budesonide (Pulmicort)
   IV. Albuterol (Proventil)
   a. I, IV, II, III
   b. III, IV, II, I
   c. II, IV, I, III
   d. IV, III, II, I

53. A pharmacist is conducting a medication reconciliation for a pediatric patient taking guaifenesin (Robitussin) for a cough. The patient's mother states she administers 2 teaspoons of medication QID. The pharmacist will document that the patient takes how many milliliters of medication in a 24-hour period?

99

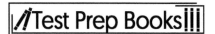

54. Rank the following antitubercular medications based on their recommended maximum daily dose, from the lowest dose to the highest:
    I. Streptomycin IM
    II. Isoniazid PO
    III. Pyrazinamide PO
    IV. Rifampin IV
a. II, IV, III, I
b. III, I, II, IV
c. III, IV, II, I
d. II, IV, I, III

55. Factors that directly influence the rate of medication metabolism include which of the following? (Select ALL that apply.)
a. Blood type
b. Age
c. First-pass effect
d. Placebo effect
e. Half-life
f. Therapeutic index

56. A patient has an order for psyllium (Metamucil) PO 6 grams TID mixed in 120 ml of water with each dose. When providing education to the patient, the pharmacist should instruct the patient to dissolve the medication in how many ounces of water per dose? (Round the final answer to the nearest WHOLE number.)

57. A 45-pound pediatric patient with leukemia is prescribed rasburicase (Elitek) IV 0.2 mg/kg daily $\times$ 5 days for management of elevated uric acid levels. How many total milligrams will this patient receive during the full course of therapy? (Round the final answer to the nearest TENTH).

58. Rank the following medications based on their pH level (lowest to highest):
    I. Pramlintide
    II. Warfarin
    III. Cidofovir
    IV. Micafungin
a. II, III, IV, I
b. IV, III, I, II
c. I, IV, III, II
d. III, IV, II, I

59. A patient was prescribed a medication as an oral suspension 60 milliliters PO BID. When providing instructions, how many tablespoons will the pharmacist instruct the patient to take with each dose? (Round the final answer to the nearest WHOLE number.)

60. A pharmacist and a provider are discussing treatment options for a 175-pound patient with a pulmonary embolism (PE). How many milligrams of fondaparinux should this patient receive daily?
a. 2.5 milligrams
b. 5 milligrams
c. 7.5 milligrams
d. 10 milligrams

100

61. Which of the following medications should be taken first in the morning?
   a. Zolpidem (Ambien)
   b. Simvastatin (Zocor)
   c. Levothyroxine (Synthroid)
   d. Allopurinol (Zyloprim)

62. In which of the following body systems does theophylline (Uniphyl) provide its therapeutic effects?
   a. Digestive system
   b. Nervous system
   c. Endocrine system
   d. Respiratory system

63. Where should the first dose of the DTaP vaccine be administered?
   a. Vastus lateralis site
   b. Deltoid site
   c. Ventrogluteal site
   d. Dorsogluteal site

64. Rank the following antidysrhythmics based on their therapeutic serum drug level range in mcg/ml, from lowest to highest:
   I. Phenytoin
   II. Propranolol
   III. Mexiletine
   IV. Procainamide
   a. I, IV, III, II
   b. III, II, IV, I
   c. II, III, IV, I
   d. IV, I, III, II

65. A pharmacist notes an order for Penicillin G 2.4million units IM × 1. Which of the following lab results will this prescription treat?
   a. Herpes 1, 2.22 high
   b. Chlamydia, positive
   c. Hepatitis B, positive
   d. Syphilis, reactive

66. Where should a patient be instructed to administer their enoxaparin (Lovenox) injection?
   a. Abdominal wall
   b. Lower back
   c. Back of the arm
   d. Upper thigh

67. Which of the following heart rhythms does diltiazem (Cardizem) treat?
   a. Atrial fibrillation (AFib)
   b. Sinus bradycardia
   c. Supraventricular tachycardia (SVT)
   d. Normal sinus rhythm

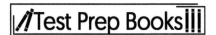

68. What type of dosage form is dissolved under the tongue?
    a. Buccal
    b. Inhalation
    c. Subcutaneous
    d. Sublingual

69. A patient has brought in a prescription for Diazepam. Which of the following conditions is the most likely reason that the patient needs this prescription?
    a. Hypertension
    b. ADHD
    c. Epilepsy
    d. Depression

70. Which of the following is TRUE regarding dietary supplements?
    a. The Dietary Supplement Health and Education Act of 1994 states dietary supplements must be labeled as such.
    b. Dietary supplements undergo the same rigorous FDA evaluation processes as legend drugs.
    c. Dietary supplements are deemed safe and effective by the FDA.
    d. Any product claims for a dietary supplement made by its manufacturer must be substantiated.

71. Which dietary supplement is recommended for a woman of childbearing age to help prevent birth defects?
    a. Vitamin D
    b. Calcium
    c. Folic acid
    d. Echinacea

72. Which of the following is TRUE regarding narrow therapeutic index medications?
    a. Patients taking these medications require minimal monitoring.
    b. Achieving an optimal therapeutic dose can be difficult.
    c. These types of medications must always be administered intravenously.
    d. They are generally considered safer than medications with a higher therapeutic index value.

73. For which of the following types of medication must INR values be closely monitored?
    a. Blood thinners
    b. Statins
    c. Antibiotics
    d. Anticonvulsants

74. Which of the following are signs that a patient is having an allergic reaction after administering a drug?
    a. Aching and stiffness
    b. Coughing and fever
    c. Fever and chills
    d. Itching and rash

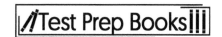

75. Which term refers to a route of medication administration other than through the gastrointestinal tract?
    a. Parenteral
    b. Enteral
    c. Motor
    d. Buccal

76. Paxlovid is a relatively new medication that is now being used under FDA emergency-use authorization to prevent high-risk patients from developing severe complications from COVID-19. Which of the following patients is a good candidate for Paxlovid if they are diagnosed with COVID-19?
    a. Tony, an eleven-year-old patient with Type 1 diabetes
    b. Melanie, a fifty-year-old patient with non-alcoholic fatty liver disease
    c. Susan, a twenty-three-year-old pregnant woman
    d. Eli, a sixty-year-old man with Stage I colon cancer

77. Which of the following is an evidence-based, non-drug therapy for Parkinson's disease? (Select **ALL** that apply.)
    a. Tai chi
    b. Speech therapy
    c. Coenzyme Q10 supplementation
    d. Massage
    e. Yoga

78. Radhika recently moved to a new state due to a job transfer. She takes several medications on a regular basis to help with menopause symptoms, bone density, and a chronic metabolic condition. After getting recommendations from her new neighbors, she visits a local community pharmacy where she hopes to transfer her prescriptions. The pharmacist on duty gets the name and contact information of Radhika's former prescribing physician, her new prescribing physician, and her former pharmacy. After receiving Radhika's medication list, she notices that her new physician has prescribed her a topical estrogen compound that is similar to one prescribed by her former physician, but the old prescription still has several active refills available. Radhika follows up with the new physician for more information, and then speaks with Radhika about which medication is the better fit for her condition. She then cancels all available refills for the medication that Radhika is no longer using. Which task has the pharmacist just completed?
    a. cGMP certification
    b. New patient intake
    c. Medication reconciliation
    d. Sterile compound waste management

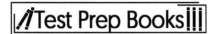
79. Antonio is a pharmacist in the middle of his workday. An elderly patient is standing in line behind several other patients, coughing violently and wheezing. Antonio asks the pharmacy intern he is supervising to help the next patient, and Antonio pulls the coughing patient aside. The patient says she has asthma and needs a refill on her inhaler medication, which she has consumed faster than usual. She is wheezing harshly between words as she tries to communicate her needs. Antonio can tell that the patient is having significant respiratory problems but does not appear to be having an asthma attack. He asks if his pharmacy intern can administer a rapid influenza test on the patient, and she agrees. The test is positive, and Antonio refers her to the local emergency department, with which his pharmacy has a strong working relationship. The patient's husband is able to drive her to the emergency department, and she is taken in promptly for treatment. She is later diagnosed with pneumonia. Based on his knowledge and capacity, what was Antonio able to do?
   a. Medication reconciliation
   b. Triage
   c. A dosing adjustment
   d. Refer-to-pharmacy

Performing Calculations

1. A patient is prescribed acetaminophen (Tylenol) 650 mg PO q4-6 hours for fever above 39°C. When providing home instructions, the pharmacist tells the patient the medication should be taken when their temperature is higher than how many degrees Fahrenheit? (Round the final answer to the nearest TENTH).

2. A patient is prescribed pramlintide (Symlin) 90 mcg Sub-Q TID. The availability is 0.06 mg/ml. How many milliliters must be dispensed for this patient in a 24-hour period? (Round the answer to the nearest WHOLE number.)

3. A 185-pound patient is prescribed prazosin (Minipress) 0.3 mg/kg PO daily. The pharmacist should dispense how many milligrams per dose?
   a. 56 mg
   b. 25 mg
   c. 28 mg
   d. 280 mg

4. A pharmacist receives an order for furosemide 1.5 mg/kg/day PO suspension in two divided doses for a patient who weighs 55 lbs. The medication is supplied as furosemide 40 mg/5 ml. How many milliliters should be dispensed per dose? (Round the final answer to the nearest TENTH.)

5. A patient has an order for hydromorphone (Dilaudid) 200 mcg IV q 4 hrs as needed for severe pain. The vial is supplied as 2 mg/ml. How many milliliters will the patient receive with each dose? (Round the final answer to the nearest TENTH.)

6. A 27-pound patient has an order for Ampicillin PO suspension 25 mg/kg/day. The available medication is supplied as Ampicillin 100 mg/ml. How many milliliters will the patient receive in one day? (Round the answer to the nearest WHOLE number.)

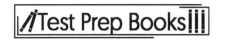

prescribed Colace 200 mg PO BID. The available medication is 500 mg/tsp. How many milliliters should be dispensed for this patient daily?

a. 4 milliliters
b. 2 milliliters
c. 5 milliliters

(Motrin) reports having a temperature of 101.2 °F. What temperature in °C should the pharmacist document in the patient's medical record? (Round the final answer

Augmentin 250 mg PO TID. The label reads 125 mg/5 ml. How many a 24-hour period? (Round the final answer to the nearest WHOLE number.)

has an order for Solu-Medrol 40 mg IV q4hrs. The medication is supplied as 100 mg/2 ml. How many milliliters should be dispensed per dose?

a. 0.4 ml
b. 8 ml
c. 1.25 ml
d. 0.8 ml

11. A prescription order calls for 600 mg of acetaminophen to be administered QID for 5 days. Oral acetaminophen suspension provides 30 mg/mL. How many milliliters should be dispensed for this patient? (Answer must be numeric; round the final answer to the nearest WHOLE number.)

12. A patient has an order for haloperidol (Haldol) 2 mg IM every 4 hours as needed for agitation. Haloperidol is available in 5 mg/mL. What volume of medication will be dispensed with each dose? (Answer must be numeric; round the final answer to the nearest TENTH.)

13. A provider prescribes Dilaudid (hydromorphone) 0.5 mg IV q2 hours for severe pain. The vial is labeled Dilaudid (hydromorphone) 200 mcg/mL. How many milliliters should be dispensed per dose? (Answer must be numeric; round the final answer to the nearest TENTH.)

14. A primary provider prescribes enoxaparin (Lovenox) 1 mg/kg BID SQ for a patient with a DVT. The patient weighs 175 pounds. How many milligrams per dose should be dispensed for the patient?
a. 175 mg
b. 80 mg
c. 88 mg
d. 385 mg

15. A patient has an order for dexamethasone (Decadron) 2.5 mg IV q8 hours. The available concentration is 4 mg/mL. How many milliliters need to be dispensed for each dose? (Answer must be numeric; round the final answer to the nearest TENTH.)

16. Azithromycin (Zithromax) PO 12 mg/kg daily for 5 days is ordered for a patient with pharyngitis. The patient weighs 77 pounds. How many milligrams will the patient receive per dose? (Answer must be numeric; round the final answer to the nearest WHOLE number.)

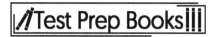
17. A provider prescribes phenytoin (Dilantin) PO 200 mg/day for a pediatric patient with seizure disorder. The oral suspension is supplied as 125 mg/5 mL. How many milliliters will need to be dispensed for this patient for a week's supply of medication? (Answer must be numeric; round the final answer to the nearest WHOLE number.)

18. Calculate the basal metabolic rate (BMR) of a 47-year-old male who weighs 180 pounds and is 5 feet 11 inches tall. (Round the final answer to the nearest WHOLE number.)

19. A 110-pound patient receiving chemotherapy has an order for ondansetron (Zofran) 0.15 mg/kg 30 minutes prior to treatment and repeated 4 hours later. How many total milligrams of Zofran will the patient receive?
    a. 16.5 mg
    b. 33 mg
    c. 15 mg
    d. 7.5 mg

20. A patient diagnosed with sinus bradycardia has a prescription for atropine 0.5 mg IV PRN x1. The vial shows a concentration of 200 mcg/mL. How many milliliters should be dispensed for each dose? (Answer must be numeric; round the final answer to the nearest TENTH.)

21. A prescriber orders hyoscyamine (Gastrosed) IV 0.25 mg TID for a patient with abdominal cramping. The medication is available as 0.5 mg/mL. How many milliliters will the patient receive in 1 day? (Answer must be numeric; round the final answer to the nearest TENTH.)

22. A 117-pound patient is prescribed iron sulfate 3 mg/kg/day divided into 4 doses. How many milligrams will the patient be taking per dose? (Answer must be numeric; round the final answer to the nearest WHOLE number.)

23. A 54-pound patient has been prescribed ciprofloxacin (Cipro) PO 15 mg/kg BID for 14 days for a urinary tract infection. How many milligrams of medication will the patient receive per day? (Answer must be numeric; round the final answer to the nearest WHOLE number.)

24. Calculate the basal metabolic rate (BMR) of a 50-year-old female who weighs 140 pounds and is 5 feet 6 inches tall. (Round the final answer to the nearest WHOLE number.)

25. Calculate the daily caloric need of a patient with a basal metabolic rate (BMR) of 1750 and a moderate activity level. (Round the final answer to the nearest WHOLE number.)

26. A provider orders a continuous infusion to administer 100 milligrams of medication every hour. The medication is supplied in a bag of 50 mg/100 mL. At what rate should the medication be set to administer the ordered dose?
    a. 200 mL/hr
    b. 50 mL/hr
    c. 100 mL/hr
    d. 20 mL/hr

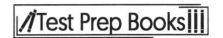
27. A patient has an order for a continuous infusion of enteral feeding. The can of enteral formula supplies 300 calories for every 250 milliliters of nutrition. The patient requires a daily intake of 1800 calories. At what rate should the infusion pump be set to deliver the daily caloric need? (Round the final answer to the nearest WHOLE number.)

28. A 190-pound patient is on a continuous heparin infusion after achieving therapeutic range. The provider orders 16 units/kg/hr. How many units of heparin will the patient receive in a 24-hour period? (Round the final answer to the nearest WHOLE number.)

29. A pharmacist is labeling a medication to include the infusion rate. The order reads to administer 200 mg IV × 1 dose. The medication is supplied in a bag of 150 mg/50 mL. What infusion rate should the pharmacist note on the label? (Round the final answer to the nearest TENTH.)

30. What is the site for peripheral parenteral nutrition (PPN) administration?
    a. Median vein
    b. Femoral vein
    c. Central vein
    d. Subclavian vein

31. A provider writes an order for meropenem 125 mg/hr IV. The medication is available as 1 gm/250 mL. At what rate should the infusion pump be set to administer the ordered dose? (Round the final answer to the nearest WHOLE number.)

32. A pharmacist notices alemtuzumab being administered at 15 mL/hr. The supplied dose is 30 mg/100 mL. How many milligrams are being administered every hour? (Round the final answer to the nearest TENTH.)

Compounding, Dispensing, or Administering Drugs or Managing Delivery Systems

1. A pediatrician has prescribed a patient cephalexin (Keflex) 600 mg PO daily divided in 3 doses. The oral suspension is supplied as 100 mg/5 mL. When providing instructions to the patient's parents, the pharmacist would instruct the parents to administer how many teaspoons of medication per dose? (Answer must be numeric; round the final answer to the nearest WHOLE number.)

2. A pharmacist is conducting a follow-up on a patient taking cimetidine (Tagamet). Which of the following statements would indicate that the patient understands the use of this medication?
    a. "I take this medication only when I have heartburn."
    b. "I take the medication on an empty stomach."
    c. "I have increased my fiber intake while taking this medication."
    d. "I take aspirin for pain as needed."

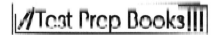

3. A patient is recently prescribed an ipratropium (Atrovent) inhaler for chronic emphysema. Which of the following teaching points regarding inhalers should the pharmacist discuss with the patient?
   a. Hold your breath for 10 seconds after breathing in the medication.
   b. Do not shake the medication.
   c. Press on the inhaler and breathe the medication in quickly.
   d. Wait 1 minute before taking a second inhalation of the medication.

4. A patient is prescribed oxymetazoline (Afrin). How should it be administered?
   a. Orally
   b. Intranasally
   c. Intravenously
   d. Intramuscularly

5. A patient is prescribed metronidazole (Flagyl) PO 500 mg BID for 7 days. The tablets available are 250 mg each. How many tablets should be dispensed to fulfill this prescription? (Answer must be numeric; round the final answer to the nearest WHOLE number.)

6. Which of the following systemic antifungal medications has the greatest protein-binding percentage?
   a. Voriconazole (Vfend)
   b. Flucytosine (Ancobon)
   c. Terbinafine (Lamisil)
   d. Fluconazole (Diflucan)

7. Which of the following vitamins are water-soluble? (Select ALL that apply.)
   a. Vitamin K
   b. Vitamin A
   c. Folic acid
   d. Vitamin B_{12}
   e. Vitamin B_5
   f. Niacin

8. A pharmacist is assessing a patient's knowledge regarding the administration of NPH insulin. Which of the following patient responses would indicate that the patient is administering this medication accurately?
   a. "I administer my insulin cold right out of the refrigerator."
   b. "I administer my insulin in different parts of the body every day."
   c. "I store my insulin at 30 degrees Fahrenheit."
   d. "I agitate the vial before drawing up the medication."

9. A patient is prescribed 11 units of NPH insulin qAC. The patient tells the pharmacist he eats 3 meals per day. The availability is 100 units/mL in 10-mL vials. How many vials should be dispensed for a 30-day supply? (Answer must be numeric.)

10. A prescriber orders captopril (Capoten) PO 50 mg to be given STAT and 25 mg subsequently BID. Tablets are available in 12.5 mg. How many tablets will the patient receive the day of the order? (Answer must be numeric; round the final answer to the nearest WHOLE number.)

11. Which of the following medications has the shortest plasma half-life?
    a. Aspirin
    b. Penicillin-G
    c. Digoxin
    d. Doxycycline

12. What method is used to administer formoterol (Foradil)?
    a. Topical application
    b. Oral liquid
    c. Metered dose inhaler
    d. Syringe and needle

13. A provider has ordered 40 milliliters of a 3% topical ointment. The available stock doses are 40 milliliters of 2% and 40 milliliters of 3.5% ointments. How much volume of the 2% stock ointment should be used to fulfill the prescription? (Round the final answer to the nearest WHOLE number.)

14. A pharmacist is reviewing an order for nitroprusside 0.3 mcg/kg/min to be administered to a 150-pound patient for a maximum of 10 minutes. How many milligrams must the pharmacist dispense to fulfill the order? (Round the final answer to the nearest TENTH.)

15. A 130-pound patient has just been diagnosed with diabetes type 1. The provider prescribes NPH insulin 0.5 units/kg/day. The medication is supplied as 100 units/mL. How many milliliters must the pharmacist dispense to cover a 30-day supply of NPH insulin? (Round the final answer to the nearest WHOLE number.)

16. Rank the following fluoroquinolones based on their half-life (shortest to longest):
    I. Ciprofloxacin
    II. Levofloxacin
    III. Gemifloxacin
    IV. Moxifloxacin
    a. IV, II, III, I
    b. II, I, III, IV
    c. I, III, II, IV
    d. III, I, II, IV

17. A patient with dysphagia is prescribed 125 milligrams of a medication PO daily. The medication is in tablet form of 250 mg/tablet. The pharmacist needs to compound the medication into an oral suspension. The available formulation is 25 mg/mL in a 40 milliliter suspension. How many tablets will the pharmacist need in order to compound the 40 milliliter suspension? (Round the final answer to the nearest WHOLE number.)

18. A patient requests for a supplied medication to be converted into an oral solution for easier administration. The patient's medication order is to take 200 milligrams of medication PO daily. The tablets are supplied as 100 mg/tablet. The available formulation is 20 mg/mL in a 30 milliliter suspension. How many milliliters of the oral suspension should the pharmacist instruct the patient to take? (Round the final answer to the nearest WHOLE number.)

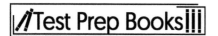

19. A provider has ordered enteral feeding for a patient who suffered a stroke. The pharmacist knows that which of the following enteral tubes is best used for the absorption of calcium and glucose?
    a. Nasogastric (NG) tube
    b. Jejunostomy tube
    c. Percutaneous endoscopic gastrostomy (PEG) tube
    d. Nasoduodenal (ND) tube

20. What personal protective equipment (PPE) will a pharmacist require in order to compound sterile medication products? (Select ALL that apply.)
    a. Boxed gloves
    b. Autoclave
    c. Hair cover
    d. Goggles
    e. Face mask

21. A pharmacist must compound medication tablets into an oral suspension for a patient with difficulty swallowing. The patient's medication order reads to administer 100 milligrams BID. The tablets are supplied as 100 mg/tablet. The available formulation is 30 mg/mL in a 20 milliliter suspension. How many tablets must the pharmacist use to compound 20 milliliters of solution? (Round the final answer to the nearest WHOLE number.)

22. Which of the following are routes of administration for ergotamine? (Select ALL that apply.)
    a. Intranasal
    b. Ophthalmic
    c. Intravenous
    d. Intraosseous
    e. Subcutaneous
    f. Oral

23. A patient has an order for atropine sulfate 200 mcg IM × 1 dose. The medication is supplied as 0.1 mg/mL. How many milliliters will need to be dispensed to fulfill the order? (Round the final answer to the nearest WHOLE number.)

24. An 11-pound pediatric patient received an order for oral suspension amoxicillin 50 mg/kg/day for 7 days. The oral suspension concentration is 50 mg/mL. How many milliliters should be dispensed for this patient? (Answer must be numeric; round the final answer to the nearest WHOLE number.)

25. A patient who weighs 27 pounds is prescribed phenobarbital (Luminal) 5 mg/kg/day divided in 2 doses for the management of seizure disorder. The medication is available in 50-mg/mL vials. How many milliliters will this patient receive on a daily basis? (Answer must be numeric; round the final answer to the nearest TENTH.)

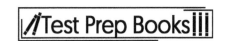
Developing or Managing Practice or Medication-Use Systems to Ensure Safety and Quality

1. A patient diagnosed with type II diabetes has been started on insulin therapy. The pharmacist confirms the patient's understanding of insulin lispro if which of the following statements is made?
    a. "I need to eat within 15 minutes of administering insulin lispro."
    b. "I need to inject insulin lispro at bedtime."
    c. "Insulin lispro should be injected into the muscle."
    d. "I should inject insulin lispro into the skin at a 15 degree angle."

2. A pharmacist receives an order for magnesium hydroxide (Milk of Magnesia) PO 30 ml daily. When dispensing the medication, the pharmacist will tell the patient to take how many tablespoons daily? (Round the final answer to the nearest WHOLE number.)

3. Rank the following childhood vaccines based on their recommended administration date from earliest to latest.
    I. *Haemophilus influenzae* type B
    II. Hepatitis B
    III. Measles-mumps-rubella (MMR)
    IV. Influenza
    a. II, I, IV, III
    b. III, IV, I, II
    c. II, III, I, IV
    d. III, I, II, IV

4. Which term is used to describe quality of care over time?
    a. Standard of care
    b. Quality improvement
    c. Continuity of care
    d. Risk management

5. Which of the following is the preferred method of transmission of prescriptions to a pharmacy?
    a. Writing
    b. Telephoning
    c. Faxing
    d. Electronic prescribing

6. Which is NOT an effective strategy for preventing errors when receiving a verbal prescription?
    a. Collecting treatment indication
    b. Reading back prescription
    c. Spelling the drug's name
    d. Using abbreviations

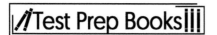

7. There is an interruption in the patient's care when their case is shifted from one health care environment to another in a way that causes ambiguity over who is responsible for care. What is this called?
   a. Continuity of care
   b. Fluidity of care
   c. Fragmentation of care
   d. Division of care

8. Which of the following ratios best defines value-driven health care?
   a. Quality/cost
   b. Cost/quality
   c. Safety/revenue
   d. Provider/reimbursement

9. Which organization is best known for driving quality standards in pharmacies, including standards related to medication safety and appropriate use?
   a. The Centers for Disease Control and Prevention
   b. The Institute for Healthcare Improvement
   c. The United States Drug Enforcement Agency
   d. The Pharmacy Quality Alliance

10. Continuity of care is associated with an increase in which of the following outcomes? (Select **ALL** that apply.)
   a. Health equity
   b. Health data security
   c. Clinical readmissions
   d. Cost savings
   e. Medication adherence

11. Which of the following is an example of a pharmacy providing a public health prevention service? (Select **ALL** that apply.)
   a. Pharmacists provide immunizations during a two-hour clinic at a worksite.
   b. Pharmacists deliver a federally recognized diabetes education program.
   c. Pharmacists provide individualized coaching appointments to help patients develop health goals.
   d. Pharmacies sell over-the-counter medications.
   e. Pharmacies accept FSA and HSA funds for retail health purchases.

12. Which of the following people most likely has a role in the field of pharmacy informatics?
   a. Lois, a trained pharmacist whose main job responsibility is to recruit and support interns
   b. Tai, a trained pharmacy technician who publishes one health education newsletter per week
   c. Emmie, a trained pharmacist who monitors drug inventory, counts, dispensation, and audits
   d. Isaac, a trained business professional who manages office tasks

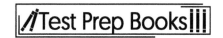

13. Which of the following agreements allows a pharmacist to make certain medical decisions, such as medication substitutions and chronic care management education, in partnership with a licensed physician?
    a. 1099 contract
    b. Collaborative practice agreement
    c. Memorandum of understanding
    d. Non-compete agreement

14. Barney and Justine are the owners of an independent pharmacy. Twice a year, they set up a training conference for their entire staff that focuses on antibiotic education and advances in therapeutics that more effectively fight bacterial infections. The training takes place during a weekend in a relaxing setting that promotes team building and focused work. What is this training an example of?
    a. Value-driven healthcare
    b. Pharmaceutical sales
    c. Stewardship
    d. Scope of practice

15. Which specialty of pharmacy focuses on tailored medications and is especially helpful for vulnerable populations?
    a. Compounding
    b. Ambulatory
    c. Retail
    d. Pharmacology

16. Which of the following is an example of pharmacy-based screening initiative?
    a. A patient's blood pressure is taken prior to medication pick-up.
    b. A patient is able to receive a rapid test for COVID-19 in their car.
    c. A patient answers intake questions prior to their medication being called in.
    d. A patient is given a satisfaction survey in the pharmacy waiting room.

Answer Explanations #1

Obtaining, Interpreting, or Assessing Data, Medical, or Patient Information

1. B: The human papillomavirus (HPV) is a sexually transmitted disease that can cause cervical cancer in women. High-risk strains change the morphology of cervical cells into cancerous cells that can be removed if present. Routine Papanicolaou smear tests (Pap smears) are recommended for HPV-positive patients to track changes. Choice A is not correct. Mammograms are screening tests to detect breast cancer. Choice C is not an appropriate diagnostic test for HPV. Bone scans help diagnose bone disorders such as osteoarthritis. Choice D is a screening test used to detect rectal polyps and assist in diagnosing colon cancer.

2. C: Warfarin therapy dosing is regulated according to the international normalized ratio (INR). Effective warfarin therapy is characterized by INR levels greater than 2.0. Choice A is not used to evaluate warfarin therapy; aPTT is used in heparin administration. Choice B is not correct. The normal prothrombin time is 10 to 14 seconds. The intended value when taking warfarin is approximately 18 seconds. Choice D is not a preferred lab value; an elevated D-dimer indicates blood clotting, the opposite of warfarin's intended therapy.

3. A: Metoprolol is a beta-blocker antihypertensive medication that lowers blood pressure and blocks the effects of the adrenaline hormone epinephrine. A patient taking metoprolol should expect to see a blood pressure closer to the normal range of 120/80 mmHg. Beta-blockers also slow down the heart, so a decreased heart rate is expected. Choice B is not correct; metoprolol does not have a direct effect on respirations and would not be used to assess efficacy of therapy. Choice C is incorrect; although the blood pressure is normal, a heart rate less than 60 beats per minute is considered abnormal. Choice D is not correct because 135/80 mmHg is considered stage 1 hypertension, and temperature is not a direct indicator of effective metoprolol therapy.

4. B and D: Albumin is a type of protein administered intravenously to correct fluid volume deficit and hypoalbuminemia. Albumin helps to expand circulating blood volume by exerting oncotic pressure. Increase in circulating volume would result in increased blood pressure. Fluid transferred from the tissues into the circulatory system would decrease edema. Choice A is not correct. Albumin does not directly affect the respiratory system. Increased respirations would be an indication of fluid volume excess, an unintended response. Choice C does not align with an increase in circulatory volume. Choice E is incorrect; decreased skin turgor is an indication of dehydration.

5. A, C, D, and F: Iron may cause teeth staining if taken in liquid form. Diluting the iron in water or juice, drinking it with a straw, and rinsing the mouth after swallowing can minimize this risk. Stomach acid increases the absorption of iron. Patients should be instructed to take iron on an empty stomach to maximize absorption. Iron increases the risk of constipation; increasing water and fiber intake are encouraged to prevent constipation. Choice B is not correct; vitamin C increases the risk of side effects and should be avoided when taking iron. Choice E is incorrect because foods high in iron should be encouraged to correct the deficiency. These foods include yeast, muscle meats, liver, and egg yolks.

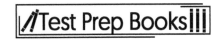

6. D: Clonazepam (Klonopin) has a primary indication of seizure prevention. Klonopin is an anti-convulsant benzodiazepine that produces sedative effects in the central nervous system and decreases abnormal electrical activity by presynaptic inhibition. Choices *A, B,* and *C* are also benzodiazepines that have different therapeutic effects. Choice *A* has a primary therapeutic effect of managing anxiety and preoperative sedation. Choice *B* is used to manage anxiety and symptomatic alcohol withdrawal. Choice *C* is used for the short-term management of insomnia.

7. A: Phenelzine (Nardil) is a monoamine oxidase (MAO) inhibitor. MAO inhibitors cause tyramine to be absorbed systemically. Tyramine is a precursor to norepinephrine, which causes increased rate and contractility of the heart. Concurrent use of a dopamine agonist with an MAO inhibitor can result in hypertensive reactions. Choice *B* is a biguanide used to treat diabetes; it does not have a significant drug interaction with dopamine agonists. Choice *C* is a centrally acting analgesic used to treat moderate to moderately severe pain; there is no significant drug interaction with dopamine agonists. Choice *D* is a bulk-forming laxative used to treat simple or chronic constipation; there are no significant interactions between psyllium and Sinemet.

8. B: Opioid medications are ranked according to a drug schedule. The lower the schedule number, the higher the risk of abuse and dependency. Percocet is a Schedule II medication that includes 5 mg of oxycodone in addition to 325 mg of Tylenol. Choices *A, C,* and *D* are all Schedule III drugs. Vicodin Hydrocet, and Lorcet HD include 5 mg of hydrocodone and 500 mg of Tylenol. Hydrocet is dispensed in capsule form, whereas Vicodin and Lorcet HD are dispensed as tablets.

9. B, D, and E: Lightheadedness, drowsiness, and lack of coordination are all possible side effects of central nervous system depression. Diazepam (Valium) is a benzodiazepine that enhances the action of gamma-amino butyric acid (GABA) in the central nervous system. GABA reduces the excitability of nerve cells throughout the body and is commonly used to stabilize mood disorders. Choices *A* and *C* are gastrointestinal effects that do not occur with Valium.

10. B: Cyclobenzaprine (Flexeril) is a skeletal muscle relaxant that reduces muscle spasticity. Multiple sclerosis is a disease process that destroys the myelin sheath. Myelin covers and insulates nerves found in the brain and spinal cord. Destruction of the sheath results in muscle weakness and spasms. Choice *A* is an analgesic commonly prescribed for moderate to moderately severe pain; this would not be indicated for the relief of muscle spasms. Choice *C* is an NSAID used in the treatment of rheumatoid arthritis.; inflammation is not characteristic of MS. Choice *D* is a gastrointestinal anti-inflammatory drug used in the treatment of mild to moderate ulcerative colitis; this is not an indication for MS.

11. A, D, and E: Atorvastatin is a hydroxymethylglutaryl-coenzyme A (HMG-CoA) reductase inhibitor used in the primary treatment of dyslipidemia. Statins inhibit HMG-CoA that is required for synthesis of cholesterol in the liver. A decrease in the production of cholesterol lowers all forms of low-density lipoprotein (LDL). LDL can potentially lead to fatty plaques within the arteries, or *atherosclerosis*. The intended goal of a medication like atorvastatin is to decrease total cholesterol (less than 200 mg/dL), decrease LDL (less than 100 mg/dL), and increase high-density lipoprotein (HDL) (greater than 60 mg/dL). HDL is considered a good form of cholesterol that is broken down and excreted in the liver. Choices *A* and *B* are liver function tests that are necessary to monitor throughout drug therapy. Elevated AST and ALT enzyme levels are indicative of liver injury or toxicity. AST levels should be less than 46 U/L and ALT levels less than 30 U/L. Choice *F* is a type of lipid found in the blood that is stored and released as energy between meals. High levels of triglycerides increase the risk of heart disease. Normal levels should be less than 150 mg/dL.

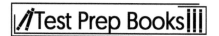

12. B, D, and E: Synthetic levothyroxine replaces the deficiency in thyroid hormone and is the drug of choice for hypothyroidism. Hypothyroidism causes decreased cardiovascular function, metabolism, energy level, mood, and muscle function. Levothyroxine helps improve these symptoms. Increased appetite resolves the metabolic symptoms. Increased pulse rate helps restore cardiovascular function, and increased alertness helps patients improve their mood. Choices *A* and *C* are intended effects for antithyroid medications.

13. A, B, and D: Nortriptyline (Pamelor) is a tricyclic antidepressant that potentiates the effect of serotonin and norepinephrine. Serotonin is a neurotransmitter that helps transmit feelings of pleasure, reward, and euphoria. A high-alert drug interaction is concurrent use of monoamine oxidase (MAO) inhibitors. MAO inhibitors block the breakdown of norepinephrine, which leads to increased contractility of the heart. Phenelzine (Nardil) is an MAO inhibitor that can cause hypertension, seizures, and death if used in combination with another antidepressant. Nortriptyline prevents the therapeutic response of antihypertensives. Concurrent use with clonidine (Catapres), an antihypertensive, may cause a hypertensive crisis. Nortriptyline can cause drowsiness, lethargy, and fatigue. Drug interaction with opioids can cause central nervous system depression. Hydrocodone/acetaminophen (Vicodin) is an opioid analgesic. Choices *C* and *E* are anticonvulsants that do not have a significant drug interaction with tricyclic antidepressants.

14. D: Sirolimus (Rapamune) is an immunosuppressant drug used to prevent organ rejection in transplants. Sirolimus is contraindicated in hepatic impairment because it is heavily metabolized by the liver and can lead to toxicity. Alanine aminotransferase (ALT) enzyme levels help determine the extent of liver damage. Normal levels of ALT are 10 to 30 IU/mL. Choice *A* is not correct. Hemoglobin is a protein that carries oxygen within red blood cells. The normal upper level is 18 g/L. The slight abnormality would not affect a patient taking Rapamune. Choice *B* is incorrect because sodium levels should range between 135 and 145 mEq/L. This is a normal finding. Choice *C* is used to assess renal function. BUN levels should range between 10 and 20 mg/dL; 19 mg/dL is a normal finding.

15. C, D, and F: Calcium channel blockers are used in the management of hypertension and other cardiovascular disorders, such as tachydysrhythmias and angina pectoris. The main mechanism of action is dilation of peripheral arteries and decreased vascular resistance by relaxing vascular smooth muscle. Central nervous system side effects include headache and dizziness. Nose and throat side effects include pharyngitis and sinusitis. Cardiovascular adverse effects include heart palpations, peripheral edema, and hypotension. Choices *A*, *B*, and *E* are not side effects expected when taking nisoldipine (Sular).

16. C: Alendronate (Fosamax) is a bisphosphonate medication used in the treatment of hypercalcemia. Increased levels of calcium in the blood result in the inability of nerves to respond to stimuli and a decreased ability of the muscles to relax and contract. This leads to muscle weakness. Therapeutic effects of Fosamax include a decrease in muscle weakness. Choices *A*, *B*, and *D* are all expected therapeutic effects for calcium preparations used in the treatment of hypocalcemia. Low calcium causes tetany, a muscle spasm that is present when tapping on the side of the face (Chvostek's sign) and compressing the upper arm and watching for carpal spasm (Trousseau's sign).

17. A, D, and E: Epoetin (Procrit) is a hematopoietic agent used in the treatment of anemia. It stimulates the bone marrow to produce red blood cells (RBCs). The expected goal of therapy is to have an increase in RBC and its components. The normal RBC count is 4.2 to 6.2 million/mm^3. Hematocrit measures the volume of RBCs to the total circulating blood volume in the body. Patients taking epoetin will have their dose adjusted depending on the hematocrit percentage. The suggested value is between 30% and 36% to allow for maturation of RBCs. Hemoglobin is the concentration of oxygen saturation in RBCs. The

116

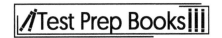

normal value range is 12 to 18 g/dL. Choices *B* and *C* are components of white blood cells (WBCs) used in the immune response. Neutrophils are granulocytes that help resolve infections and repair damage to tissues by foreign bacteria. Eosinophils fight infection and play a part in the inflammatory process. Epoetin's main mechanism of action is stimulating the formation of RBCs.

18. B: *Nephrotoxicity* is the term used to describe damage to the kidneys. The extent of kidney damage can be assessed by renal laboratory studies. Creatinine levels are determined by the clearance of muscle and protein by-products. The normal level is 0.5 to 1.3 mg/dL. Levels of 2.1 mg/dL can signal renal dysfunction. Choice *A* is not correct. Urine pH is the acidity of the urine. Normal urine acidity should have a value of 4.5 to 8. The given value of pH is normal. Choice *C* is incorrect. A BUN test measures the amount of urea nitrogen in the body. A level of 6 to 20 mg/dL is considered normal. Choice *D* is not correct. Uric acid is an insoluble compound as a result of nitrogen waste. The normal values are 2.7 to 8.5 mg/dL.

19. A, B, D & E. There are various factors that influence the way the body will respond to medication. Although every medication has the same intended effect, each patient has varying factors that can affect the way the drug will function. Body size can influence the medication concentration at the site of action. Body weight and surface area are important factors to consider when selecting a dose for a medication. Medication dosages should also be adjusted based on age. Children and infants do not have fully developed organs and metabolize medications slower. Sex is another factor that influences drug response. Females require dosages on the lower end of the spectrum due to their overall smaller body size and hormonal composition. The route of administration greatly affects how a medication will take effect. Parenterally administered medications produce a rapid drug response while oral administration will take longer to deliver the therapeutic effect. Choice *C* is not correct. The Rh factor is a protein found on the surface of red blood cells that determines the compatibility between blood products. This does not influence medication response.

20. A: Evidenced-based medicine is the practice of developing new medications through scientific investigation and extensive research. Before a medication can be deemed safe, multiple studies and trials must occur. The extent of evidence is categorized from Grade I to Grade IV. Grade I is the most reliable type of evidence and forms the basis for clinical decisions. Systematic reviews are categorized as Grade I evidence. Multiple randomized controlled trials are categorized as Grade II evidence but can be refuted by other studies that use similar parameters. Pilot studies are Grade III evidence and lack rigorous testing and require further investigation. Case reports are the least reliable evidence. Case reports are categorized as Grade IV and are based on subjective clinical experience that requires further research and testing.

21. A, B, & E: Zaroxolyn is a thiazide diuretic that helps decrease the excess fluid in the body tissues by preventing too much absorption of sodium. Zaroxolyn is used to treat fluid overload in patients with high blood pressure, kidney disorders, and congestive heart failure. The intended response is normal blood pressure (systolic at or below 120 mmHg), lack of fluid retention (no edema), and absence of fluid overload in the lungs (no shortness of breath). Choices *C* and *D* are not correct. Zaroxolyn does not have a direct effect on the gastrointestinal system.

22. C: Microalbuminuria is characterized by increased levels of albumin in the urine. Increased permeability of the kidneys can lead to an increased excretion of albumin from the body. Microalbuminuria is indicative of kidney disease. Kidney damage is a precursor to cardiovascular disease. Choice *A* is not correct. Osteoporosis occurs when bones become brittle and porous. This condition does not have a direct correlation to cardiovascular disease. Choice *B* is not correct. Anorexia

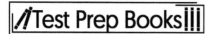

is the term used to define an eating disorder that leads to abnormally low body weight. A risk factor for cardiovascular events is obesity, the opposite of anorexia. Choice *D* is not correct. Endometriosis is a condition in which uterine tissue grows outside of the uterine cavity. This condition is not directly related to cardiovascular events.

23. C: Black beans are a rich source of iron. 1 cup of black beans contains approximately 10 milligrams of iron. The recommended daily intake of iron for a male is 20 milligrams. Choices *A*, *B*, and *D* are foods rich in vitamin K. Vitamin K is essential for blood clotting. 1 medium turnip contains approximately 0.4 milligrams of iron. 1 cup of spinach and 1 cup of avocado both have approximately 0.8 milligrams of iron.

24. C, D, & E: Levofloxacin (Levaquin) is a fluoroquinolone used in the treatment of bacterial infections. White blood cell count is a crucial laboratory value to assess. White blood cells are part of the immune system and fight infection alongside levofloxacin. All fluoroquinolones can cause increased levels of bilirubin and albumin. Bilirubin is a pigmented by-product of red blood cell breakdown. Albumin is a protein necessary for fluid balance. Choices *A*, *B*, and *F* are laboratory values that can be affected particularly by moxifloxacin. Moxifloxacin is a second-generation fluoroquinolone used in the treatment of skin and respiratory infections. This medication can increase calcium levels and decrease red blood cell and hemoglobin levels. Calcium is important for bone structure, while red blood cells and hemoglobin are important for oxygen transport throughout the body.

25. B: Indapamide is a thiazide diuretic used in the treatment of fluid overload. It primarily increases the excretion of sodium by preventing its reabsorption. Indapamide also promotes the excretion of chloride, potassium bicarbonate, and magnesium. The lab value of magnesium is out of range. The normal magnesium level is 1.5–2.5 mEq/L. Hypermagnesemia can lead to vomiting, neurological impairment, and hypotension. Calcium is not excreted by thiazide diuretics. Although the calcium level is high, a diuretic will not correct the imbalance. The normal calcium level is 4.5–5.5 mEq/L. The potassium leve does not need to be corrected. The normal potassium level is 3.5–5.0 mEq/L. The sodium level is out of range. The normal sodium level is 135–145 mEq/L. Administering indapamide will cause further hyponatremia and can lead to coma and death.

26. A, B, D, & F: Drug interactions can lead to additive or decreased therapeutic effects. Disopyramide is a Class I antidysrhythmic used in the prevention of ventricular tachycardia. Disopyramide decreases myocardial excitability and suppresses ventricular arrhythmias. Phenytoin is an anti-epileptic medication used in the treatment of seizures. Rifampin is an antitubercular medication used in the treatment of tuberculosis. Both medications decrease the effects of disopyramide by accelerating the metabolism of antiarrhythmics in the liver. A quick metabolism decreases the duration and serum concentration of the drug. Cimetidine is a histamine antagonist used in the treatment of peptic ulcers. It increases the effects of disopyramide by inhibiting hepatic metabolism. Decreased metabolism increases the serum concentration of the drug. Bretylium is a class III antiarrhythmic also used in the treatment of ventricular arrhythmias. When combined with disopyramide, it can have additive cardiac depressant effects. Choices *C* and *E* are incorrect. Docusate is a stool softener used in the treatment of constipation. Ketorolac is a non-steroidal anti-inflammatory drug (NSAID) used as an analgesic. Neither of these medications have a direct interaction with disopyramide.

27. C: The 2018 American Heart Association blood pressure guidelines categorize the presence of hypertension based on systolic and diastolic readings. Having a systolic blood pressure between 130–139 mmHg or a diastolic blood pressure between 80–89 mmHg is classified as stage 1 hypertension. Choice *A* is not correct. Normal blood pressure is having a systolic reading of less than 120 mmHg and a

118

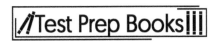

diastolic reading of less than 80 mmHg. Choice *B* is incorrect. Elevated blood pressure is classified as having a systolic blood pressure of 120–129 mmHg and a diastolic reading of less than 80 mmHg. Choice *D* is incorrect. Stage 2 hypertension is characterized by a systolic reading of 140 mmHg or higher or a diastolic reading of 90 mmHg or higher.

28. D: Medications approved for treatment are placed in controlled substance schedules based on their potential for abuse and likelihood of causing dependence if used for a prolonged period of time. Controlled substances can lead to psychological and physical dependence. Schedule I substances are not approved for medical treatment and are considered street drugs, such as heroin, peyote, and cannabis. Schedule II medications have a high potential for abuse and include narcotics such as Duragesic (fentanyl), morphine, and oxycodone. Schedule III medications have a lower risk of physical dependence compared to schedule II. Medications containing codeine must have no more than 90 milligrams of codeine per dosage units. Schedule III medications include Tylenol with Codeine and buprenorphine. Schedule IV medications have a lower abuse potential than schedule III drugs. Examples include benzodiazepines and sedatives such as temazepam (Restoril), alprazolam (Xanax), and lorazepam (Ativan). Schedule V medications contain limited amounts of narcotic and have a low risk of abuse. For medications containing codeine, there must be no more than 200 milligrams of codeine per 100 grams of medication. Schedule V drugs include Phenergan with Codeine and Robitussin AC.

29. 6.4 milligrams: The first step is to find how many hours it will take to infuse the supplied dose. The rate of infusion is 8 milliliters every hour. The supplied dose is 50 milliliters. It will take 6.25 hours to infuse the supplied dose of 40 milligrams: $50 \div 8 = 6.25$. To find how many milligrams are being infused every hour, the supplied dose should be divided by the number of hours it will take to infuse the total volume: $40 \div 6.25 = 6.4$. The patient is receiving 6.4 milligrams every hour. Rounded to the nearest tenth, 6.4 remains as 6.4 milligrams.

30. C: Interdigital tinea pedis, commonly known as athlete's foot, is a fungal infection that affects the skin membranes in between the toes. Sertaconazole is a topical medication that treats fungal infections on the feet. Choice *A* is incorrect. Tinea corporis, commonly known as ringworm, affects the skin on the face, torso, and limbs. Tinea corporis is treated with medications such as ketoconazole and tolnaftate. Choice *B* is incorrect. Tinea cruris, commonly known as jock itch, is a fungal infection that affects the groin area. Humidity and lack of ventilation can cause and exacerbate tinea cruris. Tinea cruris is treated with medications such as econazole and miconazole. Choice *D* is incorrect. Tinea capitis is a fungal infection that affects the scalp. It can lead to inflammation of hair follicles and hair loss. Tinea capitis is treated with systemic medications such as terbinafine and fluconazole.

31. D: A calcium level of 3.2 mEq/L is considered hypocalcemia. Normal calcium levels are between 4.5–5.5 mEq/L. Patients with low levels of calcium will exhibit signs of tetany—involuntary contraction of muscles that increases the action potential of cells. Seizures are uncontrolled muscle movements due to electrical disturbances in the brain. Choice *A* is not correct. Decreased levels of calcium lead to hypotension—decreased blood pressure. Choice *B* is not correct. Excessive sweating is not a known clinical manifestation of low calcium levels. Diaphoresis is controlled by the endocrine glands. Choice *C* is incorrect. Decreased calcium leads to abdominal cramping. Constipation can be caused by high levels of calcium—hypercalcemia.

32. A: Bleomycin in an antineoplastic medication used in the treatment of cancers, including lymphomas, squamous cell carcinomas, and teratocarcinomas. Medications that treat complex conditions are usually tier 5 medications, which are significantly more expensive, and even the tier 5 generic drugs are expensive. Choices *B*, *C*, and *D* treat common conditions and have generic alternatives

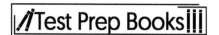

that are more cost-effective. Famotidine is an antiulcer agent used in the treatment of gastroesophageal reflux disease (GERD). Meclizine is an antiemetic medication used to treat motion sickness. Prazosin is an antihypertensive medication used in the treatment of high blood pressure.

33. D: Methimazole (Tapazole) is an antithyroid medication used in the treatment of hyperthyroidism. Hyperthyroidism is defined as an excessive secretion of thyroid hormone. As a result of the excess, the pituitary gland will decrease its production of the thyroid-stimulating hormone (TSH). Thus, levels of TSH will be decreased in patients with hyperthyroidism. Antithyroid medications aim to increase the levels of TSH. The normal level is 0.5 to 4.2 mcg/dL. Choices *A* and *D* are hormones that function to regulate the body's heart rate, metabolism, and temperature. The values provided are within normal limits. In patients with hyperthyroidism, T3 and T4 levels will not be affected and do not require correction. Choice *B* does not evaluate the efficacy of Tapazole; hemoglobin (HGB) is a protein responsible for the transfer of oxygen via red blood cells throughout the body.

34. B: Patiromer (Veltassa) is a potassium binder medication that treats hyperkalemia. Potassium is an electrolyte necessary for adequate contraction of smooth and skeletal muscles throughout the body. Potassium also maintains a steady electrical rhythm of the heart. Potassium plasma levels above 5.0 mEq/L can cause muscle weakness, fatigue, decreased heart rate, and abnormal heart rhythms. The digestive tract is lined with smooth muscle and enables potassium absorption. Veltassa prevents the absorption of potassium into the bloodstream by binding itself to potassium ions in the digestive tract and excreting them through the feces. This mechanism decreases potassium levels in the body.

35. B: Collecting the patient's history can help identify allergic reactions or drug-drug interactions. Although in some cases having the patient's history can help track which medications may need to be refilled, it's not the primary intent.

36. C: Neutrophils are the major component of the white blood cells. When their count is elevated, that means the white blood cells are hard at work fighting an infectious process. Further investigation could support this conclusion. Blood urea nitrogen is a waste product of the body. An elevated level would suggest failing kidneys but not an infection. Hematocrit is a component of red blood cells and is not part of the body's immune system. A high sodium level is an electrolyte abnormality that may have to do with the renal system or overall patient fluid status but not an infectious process.

37. A, B, C, E: High costs are a barrier to medication adherence because patients are unlikely to buy medications that they cannot afford. Poor patient-provider communication is a barrier to medication adherence because patients may not realize or acknowledge the importance of a medication without provider support and collaboration; additionally, the patient may face a lifestyle barrier that remains unaddressed if the provider does not notice it. If a patient does not have adequate knowledge or understanding of their illness and how the medication is helping their health, they are less likely to take the medication as prescribed. Forgetting to take a medication is common and normal, as this is a new habit that the patient needs to develop. Based on these four reasons, Choices *A, B, C,* and *E* can be selected as barriers to medication adherence. Dose packaging, on the other hand, has been shown to help medication adherence. Dose packaging provides individual units of medication for patients to ease the burden of remembering to take medications and the act of dosing medications out individually. This packaging process is especially helpful in medication adherence for patients who are on multiple medications. Therefore, Choice *D* can be eliminated.

38. B: Remote continuous glucose monitoring systems detect a patient's blood glucose levels continuously throughout the day. They are equipped to alert both the patient and the provider if

120

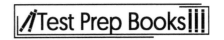

glucose levels are moving out of a healthy range, and this can notify the patient to quickly administer the necessary intervention (e.g., remembering to take a medication before too much time elapses). A health coaching appointment may help Belinda with lifestyle habits to help manage her disease, but this solution takes time and typically involves more than one coaching session. Therefore, Choice A can be eliminated.

In Type 2 diabetics, rapid-acting insulin is typically prescribed as an injection to be taken prior to a large, carbohydrate-rich meal to ensure that the patient can digest high levels of glucose rapidly. Patients must remember to administer the medication in order to receive the benefits. This behavior is one that Belinda is struggling with; additionally, the question does not indicate that she is struggling with specific meals only. As this additional prescription may not be an appropriate solution for her, Choice C can be eliminated. Moving is a major and often stressful lifestyle change that may not offer a solution quickly, so Choice D can be eliminated.

39. A: Prior authorization is the process of communicating a patient's medical information, diagnoses, and treatment plan to their health insurance company to receive reimbursement approval for a medical procedure or medication(s) prior to administering the procedure or medication(s). This lets the patient know that certain or all costs are covered and provides more accurate information about what their out-of-pocket costs may be. Prior authorization involves all the tasks that Jenni completed, such as sharing diagnostic codes and communicating directly with the health insurance company. New patient intake for this patient was likely completed by administrative staff when the patient first arrived at the medical facility and includes information such as demographics, family information, and so on. Jenni did not complete these tasks, so Choice B can be eliminated. While all healthcare facilities manage revenue cycles, which track how patients access health services all the way to the distribution of payment, this is normally completed by healthcare administrators and non-clinical staff rather than a pharmacist, physician, or the patient. Choice C can be eliminated. The patient has not yet received any medication nor begun the intervention, so Choice D does not yet apply and can be eliminated.

40. A, B, C: Vitamin, mineral, and herbal supplements can interact with prescription medications, so it is important for a pharmacist to be aware of any supplements that a patient is consuming. Pharmacists have expert knowledge on drug manufacturing processes. Supplements are not regulated by the FDA, but many supplement companies voluntarily undergo third-party lab testing with transparent results and apply for other credentialing to provide evidence for the quality of their products. Pharmacists can help guide patients to the most reputable and reliable supplement manufacturers. The supplements a patient is taking can provide information about their health goals, beliefs, and concerns.

By knowing these pieces of information, a pharmacist can speak with a patient about whether or not the supplements they are taking will help achieve their desired outcomes. The pharmacist can also provide better solutions where applicable. Choices A, B, and C are reasons that pharmacists should know what supplements a patient is taking. Pharmacists should not automatically assume that a food source or FDA approved medication will support the patient's health goals or desired health outcomes, so these should not be the primary reason for learning more about what supplements the patient is taking. Therefore, Choices D and E can be eliminated.

41. C: When combined with patient name, their date of birth is a reliable patient identifier to ensure a patient or affiliated caregiver picks up the correct medication. This ensures a high-quality process—that the correct medication is dispensed for a patient, and that the medication is given to the right person. In general, at least two patient identifiers should be used before the interaction is complete. Other valid identifiers include a valid identification card, home address, or telephone number. A patient should not

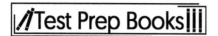

be expected to know the generic name of their medication, so Choice *A* can be eliminated. Many patients at a pharmacy can be referred by the same provider, so this is not a good patient identifier. Choice *B* can be eliminated. A health insurance card typically only provides a patient's name and no other identifier. Utilizing a name as a sole identifier can result in dispensation errors and is not considered a practice that promotes quality healthcare. Choice *D* can be eliminated.

Identifying Drug Characteristics

1. C: Medications are assigned a pregnancy category. Nystatin is an antifungal used to treat vaginal candidiasis. It is a pregnancy category A drug. Diphenhydramine is an antihistamine used in the treatment of allergies. It is a pregnancy category B drug. Verapamil is a calcium channel blocker used in the treatment of hypertension and dysrhythmias. It is a pregnancy category C drug. Colchicine is an anti-gout medication used to treat acute attacks of gouty arthritis. It is a pregnancy category D drug.

2. A: Anti-dysrhythmic medications are classified according to their mechanism of action and how they affect the conducting system of the heart. Procainamide (Procanbid) is a class I sodium channel blocker drug. Propranolol (Inderal) is a class II beta-blocker medication. Amiodarone (Cordarone) is a class III potassium channel blocker medication, and verapamil (Calan) is a class IV calcium channel blocker drug.

3. A: Phenytoin and fosphenytoin are anticonvulsant medications used in the treatment of seizures. Their peak activity varies and is dependent on the route of administration. The fastest peak activity is achieved by intravenous administration of phenytoin (Dilantin). The peak activity is rapid. Intravenous fosphenytoin (Cerebyx) has a peak activity of 15 to 60 minutes. Intramuscular fosphenytoin (Cerebyx) reaches its peak activity in 30 minutes. The slowest peak activity is achieved with oral phenytoin (Dilantin) at 1.5 to 3 hours.

4. C: Isosorbides are nitrates used in the management of angina (chest pain). Isosorbide dinitrate is used to prevent attacks of angina. Isosorbide mononitrate widens the blood vessels and makes blood flow easier. Their formulations determine the duration of medication in the system. Isosorbide mononitrate (ISMN) ER is an extended-release formulation with a duration of 12 hours. Isosorbide mononitrate (ISMN) PO is an oral formulation with a duration of 7 hours. Isosorbide dinitrate (ISDN) PO is an oral formulation with a duration of 4 hours. Isosorbide dinitrate (ISDN) SL is a sublingual medication with a duration of 1 to 2 hours.

5. C: Local anesthetics provide loss of sensory perception by blocking nerve impulses to different areas of the body. The effect they produce is reversible, and they are often used after minor surgeries or invasive procedures. Local anesthesia only affects areas of the body in which it is applied or injected. The extent to which they block nerve impulses is known as potency. The duration refers to how long it takes for sensory perception to return. Bupivacaine is an anesthetic commonly used during dental work and childbirth. It has a high potency and long duration. Choice *A* is incorrect. Lidocaine is a common skin-numbing agent for procedures such as biopsies and catheter insertions. Choice *B* is not correct. Procaine is a low-potency, short duration anesthetic used to numb teeth and reduce pain caused when penicillin is injected into the muscle. Choice *D* is incorrect. Prilocaine is commonly used for peripheral nerve blocks and spinal and epidural anesthesia.

6. A: Nicotinic receptors are channel proteins that trigger neuromuscular transmissions when acetylcholine attaches to them. Acetylcholine is a neurotransmitter that causes contraction of smooth muscles, increases bodily secretions, and dilates blood vessels. Nicotinic receptors are considered

122

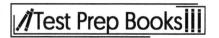

ionotropic. Ionotropic receptors allow positively charged ions, such as sodium, to flow through them without secondary messengers. Nicotinic receptors are found in skeletal muscle. The heart, glands, and blood vessels contain muscarinic receptors. Muscarinic receptors require a second messenger to transport ions when activated by acetylcholine.

7. A, C, E, & F: Second-generation beta-blockers are cardioselective medications. Cardioselective medications bind to Beta 1 (B1) receptors and inhibit their action. B1 receptors are found in the heart and increase the rate and contractility of the heart when stimulated. Second-generation beta-blockers include metoprolol, esmolol, atenolol, and bisoprolol. Choices *B* and *D* are incorrect. Propranolol and timolol are first-generation beta-blockers that are nonselective. In addition to inhibiting B1 receptors, nonselective beta-blockers like propranolol and timolol target Beta 2 (B2) receptors found in the bronchioles of the lungs and fibers of skeletal muscles. B2 receptors cause relaxation of the muscles in the airway and dilation in the periphery.

8. D: Tetracycline (Sumycin) is an anti-infective medication used in the treatment of various infections, including skin conditions such as acne. Between 60–80% of the medication is absorbed after oral administration. Tetracycline is an acidic medication that is readily absorbed in the stomach. Gastric acid has a pH level of approximately 1.5–3.5. Acidic medications are absorbed in the stomach. If taken with enough fluid, medications bypass the esophagus into the stomach. The small intestine absorbs most nutrients and medications with a neutral or basic pH level. The large intestine is primarily responsible for absorbing excess water.

9. A: Indapamide (Lozol) is a thiazide diuretic used in the treatment of high blood pressure. Thiazide diuretics prevent the over-absorption of sodium in the body and decrease fluid retention in the tissues. Decreased volume leads to decreased vessel resistance resulting in decreased blood pressure. Choice *B* is incorrect. Losartan (Cozaar) is an angiotensin blocker. Angiotensin is a protein that causes constriction of the blood vessels and leads to increased resistance and pressure. Choice *C* is not correct. Atenolol is a beta blocker also used in the treatment of high blood pressure. Beta blockers prevent the release of hormones such as adrenaline and noradrenaline. These hormones cause an increase in the heart rate and narrow the blood vessels, which increases blood pressure. Choice *D* is incorrect. Captopril (Capoten) is an angiotensin converting enzyme (ACE) inhibitor. ACE inhibitors prevent the conversion of angiotensin I to angiotensin II. Angiotensin II is a potent vasoconstricting hormone that raises blood pressure.

10. B: The strength of topical steroids is determined by the volume of the active ingredient in a mass of solvent. For example, grams of solute (medication) in grams of solvent (creams or ointments). Fluocinolone acetonide (Capex) is formulated in a shampoo used in the treatment of scalp dermatitis. Its corticosteroid strength is 0.01%. Fluticasone propionate (Cutivate) is a topical cream used in the treatment of skin dermatitis. Its corticosteroid strength is 0.05%. Dexamethasone sodium phosphate (Neodecadron) is an ophthalmic solution for the treatment of conjunctivitis. Its corticosteroid strength is 0.1%. Hydrocortisone valerate (Westcort) is a topical cream used in the treatment of itching and skin inflammation. Its corticosteroid strength is 0.2%.

11. A: Ofloxacin is a group III medication. Ofloxacin is a fluoroquinolone primarily used to treat skin and urinary tract infections. Group III medications are used to treat drug resistant tuberculosis. Rifampin is an antibiotic in group I used as a first-line treatment for tuberculosis. Rifampin is administered with other group I antitubercular medications such as isoniazid and pyrazinamide for a period of several months. Streptomycin is a group II injectable antitubercular medication. Group II medications are potent and bactericidal but must be injected for therapeutic effects. Ethionamide is a group IV antitubercular

123

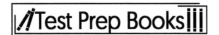

medication. Group IV medications are less effective for treatment of drug resistant tuberculosis and are used as second-line medications.

12. B: Corticosteroids are immunosuppressive medications used to treat inflammatory conditions that result from the body's immune response. The systemic duration period refers to the time a medication's effect lasts within the body. Cortisone is a short-acting corticosteroid used in the management of adrenal insufficiency. When taken orally, it has a duration of 1.25–1.5 days. Dexamethasone is a long-acting corticosteroid used in the management of cerebral edema. When administered parenterally, it has a duration of 2.75 days. Betamethasone is a long-acting corticosteroid used in the treatment of various systemic and local chronic diseases such as allergies and autoimmune conditions. When taken orally, it has a duration of 3.25 days. Methylprednisolone is an intermediate-acting corticosteroid used to treat chronic inflammatory diseases and in management of acute spinal cord injuries. When administered intramuscularly, it has a long duration of 1–4 weeks.

13. C: Inhaled corticosteroids are used in the treatment of mild to severe asthma. Medications are pre-filled into an inhaler, which releases a standard dose with each puff. Patients should be educated on the use of an inhaler and the proper number of puffs to administer based on their dosage range. Flunisolide (Aerobid) provides the most micrograms of medication with each puff (250). Budesonide (Pulmicort) delivers 200 mcg of medication with each puff. Triamcinolone acetonide (Nasacort) provides 100 mcg of medication with each puff. Beclomethasone (Qvar) delivers the smallest dose per puff (80 mcg).

14. B: Antibodies are proteins that bind with and eliminate antigens to help fight off infection. Antigens are found on invasive organisms, such as viruses, bacteria, and fungi. IgM is the largest antibody found in the blood and is the first line of defense for the immune system when an infection is detected. IgG is a small antibody that can cross the placenta. They are a secondary form of antibody protection. IgA antibodies are found on various body surfaces, such as blood, saliva, and tears. They primarily provide viral protection. IgE are antibodies found in the mucous membranes, skin, and lungs. They protect against environmental allergens, such as spores, pet dander, and pollen.

15. A, B, C, & E: Physical attributes of a medication identify the type of drug it is. Each medication that is approved for use by the Food and Drug Administration (FDA) must include identifying characteristics to include the shape, size, color, and imprint. Shapes can include rectangles, hexagons, ovals, and circles. Sizes range from a few millimeters to a couple of centimeters in size. The bigger the tablet, the harder it will be to swallow via the oral route. There are many different pigmentations and colors that identify a medication. Imprints can be in the form of numbers, letters, or logos. Each medication on the market must have distinctive features and cannot copy the exact physical attributes of another medication. This allows for proper tracking in case of toxicity, unlabeled uses, or accidental ingestion. Choice *D* is not correct. The majority of tablets should not have a smell; it is not a physical attribute that identifies a unique medication.

16. A: Antacids react with gastric acid to neutralize the acidic pH of hydrochloric acid. They provide an alkaline environment to help treat heartburn and gastritis. Aluminum-based antacids have a slow onset and a low neutralizing capability. Combination products contain different doses of aluminum hydroxide. Aludrox contains the highest concentration of aluminum hydroxide per dose (307 mg). Amphojel contains 300 mg of aluminum hydroxide per dose. Maalox contains 225 mg of aluminum hydroxide per dose. Mylanta has the least amount of aluminum hydroxide per dose (200 mg).

17. B: Micafungin (Mycamine) is an antifungal medication used in the treatment of candidiasis infections. Mycamine acts by inhibiting the synthesis of glucan, which is a type of glucose polymer that is

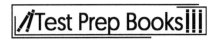

required for the formation of a fungal cell wall. The cell wall protects and supports the components inside the cell that are necessary for replication. Without a cell wall, the cell collapses and is unable to divide and form new cells. The fungus is eliminated by destroying the walls of fungal cells already present in the body. The other parts of the cell are not directly affected by Mycamine.

18. B: The majority of hormonal contraceptives contain a synthetic form of estrogen (ethynyl estradiol) and progestin (norethindrone). All the listed contraceptives are monophasic. They contain a fixed amount of synthetic estrogen and progestin. Ogestrel is the most concentrated and contains 50 mcg of ethinyl estradiol. Brevicon contains 35 mcg of ethinyl estradiol. Levlen contains 30 mcg of ethinyl estradiol. Aviane contains the least amount of estrogen, with 20 mcg of ethinyl estradiol.

19. B: First-generation cephalosporins are effective against streptococci infections except methicillin-resistant *Staphylococcus aureus* (MRSA). Cefazolin is the drug of choice for prophylaxis in surgical procedures. Second-generation cephalosporins are active against some gram-negative organisms and more effective against anaerobic organisms than first-generation drugs. Third-generation cephalosporins extend the spectrum of activity against gram-negative organisms. They are able to treat resistant strains not treated by first- or second-generation cephalosporins. Fourth-generation cephalosporins have a greater stability against breakdown by beta-lactamase enzymes and greater potency than first-, second-, or third-generation cephalosporins.

20. D: Insulins are characterized by their alteration in amino acid sequence that allows them to act quickly or over a longer period of time. Insulin analogs mimic human insulin and lower the glucose level in the blood. Insulin aspart has a rapid onset of 15 minutes and a duration of 3 to 5 hours. Novolin R has a short onset of 30 to 60 minutes and a duration of 5 to 7 hours. Humulin N has an intermediate onset of 1 to 2 hours and a duration of 18 to 24 hours. Insulin glargine is a long-acting insulin with an onset of 1 hour and lasts 24 hours within the body.

21. C: The PPI (patient package insert) carries detailed information about the medication including the pharmacology. The product monograph or product insert (PI) or prescribing information (PI) carries various details of the medication including pharmacology, toxicology, and clinical studies.

22. C: Choice *C* is the correct choice because prescriber approval is only required when substituting a narrow therapeutic index medication, as NTIs have a variable window between efficacy and toxicity. Generic medications help to keep drug costs down; they can be significantly less expensive than the brand name versions, so Choice *A* is true of generic substitution. Prescribers can avoid generic substitution by writing "Dispense as Written" on a prescription when they feel the brand medication is the best therapeutic option for the patient; therefore, Choice *B* is also true of generic substitution. To be considered the therapeutic equivalent formulation of a brand name drug, the generic formulation must meet the same efficacy and safety parameters as the brand medication; thus, Choice *D* is true of generic substitution as well.

23. A: The FDA has the authority to initiate a drug recall, whether class I, II, or III. Reasons for drug recalls vary and may include health hazards, mislabeling, contamination, and manufacturing defects. In recent years, there has been a surge in drug recalls initiated by the FDA. The agencies in Choices *B, C,* and *D* do not have the authority to initiate a drug recall.

24. B: The Institute of Safe Medication Practices (ISMP) oversees the MERP. The service provides for confidential and voluntary reporting of medication errors. The MERP performs analyses of the errors

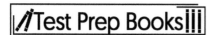

reported and circulates recommendations for their prevention to drug manufacturers and regulatory organizations. The ISMP also manages the National Vaccine Errors Reporting Program (VERP).

25. A, C: Chlorothiazide is a diuretic that can be used to manage fluid that contributes to high blood pressure. Nitroglycerin is a vasodilator that is used to treat chest pain and other symptoms of coronary artery disease. Therefore, Choices *A* and *C* are correct. Methylphenidate is a nervous system agent used to treat symptoms associated with attention deficit disorder, so Choice *B* can be eliminated. Omeprazole is a proton pump inhibitor used to treat symptoms such as acid reflux. As it is a gastrointestinal agent, Choice *D* can be eliminated. Abacavir is an antiviral that acts on the immune system, primarily to suppress human immunodeficiency virus. Therefore, Choice *E* can be eliminated.

26. D: Cymbalta is an FDA-approved anti-depressant specifically approved for use in treating fibromyalgia. It is used to alleviate symptoms of pain and mood dysfunction. Prempro is a brand-name drug used to treat symptoms associated with menopause, such as hot flashes, so it is unlikely that Dolly's doctor would prescribe this medication to treat fibromyalgia. Choice *A* can be eliminated. Ritalin is a brand-name drug used to treat symptoms associated with attention deficit disorder, such as impulsivity and loss of focus. It would not be the first line of treatment for fibromyalgia, so Choice *B* can be eliminated. Humira is a brand name drug used to help relieve symptoms of rheumatoid arthritis. While this medication is used to treat pain, it is unlikely that Dolly's doctor would prescribe this medication over one that is specifically approved to treat symptoms of fibromyalgia. Therefore, Choice *C* can be eliminated.

27. C: Doxycycline is a generic antibiotic that is primarily used to treat various bacterial infections. The therapeutic category of analgesics comprises medications used to treat pain, and includes medications such as morphine, oxycodone, and acetaminophen. Choice *A* can be eliminated. Antivirals include medications such as baloxavir and peramivir and are used to suppress viral infections. Choice *C* can be eliminated. Anti-emetics are a therapeutic category primarily used to prevent nausea and vomiting. Medications include ondansetron and dexamethasone. Choice *D* can be eliminated.

28. B: Eliquis is a prescription thrombolytic, a drug category that helps break down blood clots to decrease stroke risk. It is commonly prescribed and administered just after joint-replacement surgeries, as clotting is common after these procedures. Patients may need to take thrombolytics for up to three months after joint-replacement procedures. A breast cancer patient would most likely be prescribed chemotherapy and anti-nausea medications, which Eliquis is not. Therefore, Choice *A* can be eliminated. Patients who are in opioid withdrawal typically are prescribed opioid partial agonist-antagonists, or opioid antagonists. Eliquis does not fall into these drug classes, so Choice *C* can be eliminated. Patients experiencing bone density loss may be prescribed medications that slow down the rate at which bone density is lost, or extra-strong vitamin and mineral supplements (e.g., calcium and vitamin D). Eliquis does not produce these results, so Choice *D* can be eliminated.

29. C, D: Both sertraline and paroxetine are SSRIs that have empirical evidence supporting safety when used by breastfeeding mothers to treat depression. They are two of four medications recommended specifically to treat depression in breastfeeding mothers. Therefore, both of these answer choices are correct. Nortriptyline and imipramine are the other two medications recommended for use in breastfeeding mothers due to their safety profile; however, these medications are not SSRIs. They are tricyclic antidepressants. Therefore, Choices *A* and *B* can be eliminated. Since there are SSRIs that nursing mothers can use safely, Choice *E* can be eliminated.

126

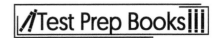

30. A: St. John's wort is a plant that has been shown in some trials (although not consistently) to be an effective supplement to treat depression. However, results have been inconsistent, and the supplement is not FDA-approved for use in the United States. It can interact adversely with several prescription medications, including birth control. It has been shown to reduce effectiveness in birth control and result in breakthrough bleeding as well as unplanned pregnancies. Therefore, Mika would not want to use this medication while taking a hormonal contraceptive. This supplement does not have a black box warning, which is for FDA-approved pharmaceuticals that can cause extremely adverse side effects. Choice *B* can be eliminated. St. John's wort is not FDA-approved for any demographic, so Choice *C* can be eliminated. St. John's wort should never be used alongside prescription antidepressants, as this can be extremely dangerous and even life threatening. Therefore, Choice *D* can be eliminated.

31. A, B, C, D, E: A black box warning is the most critical warning the FDA can include on approved drugs. A black box warning indicates that serious adverse reactions can occur across various contexts. Over four hundred prescription drugs have black box warnings. These drugs are safe to use in most instances, but have the potential to cause life threatening injuries if misused. Zoloft (an antidepressant) has a black box warning because it can increase suicidal ideation in some patients. Levaquin (an antibiotic) has a black box warning because it increases the risk of tendon issues, including ruptures, in some patients. Lipitor (a statin) has a black box warning because it can affect cognition in some patients. Neurontin (an anti-convulsant) has a black box warning because it can increase the risk of respiratory distress in some patients. Prescription-strength Tylenol (acetaminophen) has a black box warning because it can cause liver injuries in some patients; however, over-the-counter acetaminophen does not carry this warning. Therefore, all of these options are correct.

32. C: Ergosterol is found in the cell membranes of fungi and helps maintain the membrane structure. It is a steroid found only in living fungi. Anti-fungal medications such as ketoconazole work by inhibiting ergosterol and ultimately inhibiting or ending a fungal infection. Ramipril is an ACE inhibitor that acts upon enzymes associated with vasoconstriction, and is not associated with ergosterol, so Choice *A* can be eliminated. Naproxen is an anti-inflammatory that acts upon enzymes associated with creating inflammation, so Choice *B* can be eliminated. Amoxicillin is an antibiotic that works on enzymes within bacterial cell walls to prevent bacterial infections, so Choice *D* can be eliminated.

Developing or Managing Treatment Plans

1. B: Furosemide (Lasix) is a loop diuretic used in the treatment of fluid overload. Lasix causes diuresis. During fluid excretion, electrolyte imbalances may occur. Lasix is not a potassium-sparing diuretic; therefore, potassium levels should be monitored to avoid hypokalemia. Choices *A*, *C*, and *D* are not affected by Lasix. White blood cells are part of the immune response and can be affected by medications such as antibiotics and antifungals. Hemoglobin aids in transporting oxygen throughout the body. Abnormal hemoglobin levels may be treated with medications such as iron. Albumin is a protein that is produced in the liver and aids in fluid balance. Loop diuretics such as Lasix exert their action in the kidneys.

2. A, B, E, and F: Codeine (Paveral) is an opioid agonist used primarily in the treatment of pain. When administered in smaller doses, it provides antitussive effects to suppress the cough reflex. Opioids cause decreased peristalsis and can lead to constipation. Patients should be encouraged to take the medication with meals and increase their fluid intake to prevent constipation. Codeine binds to receptors in the central nervous system and can produce sedative effects. Patients should be advised to

127

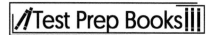

change positions slowly to avoid dizziness, and for safety reasons they should be discouraged from driving. Choices *C* and *D* are not affected by codeine. Weight change is not expected, and codeine may be taken around the clock as ordered.

3. B, C, and D: Fluoxetine (Prozac) is a selective serotonin reuptake inhibitor (SSRI) used in the treatment of depressive disorders, obsessive-compulsive disorders, panic disorders, and bulimia nervosa. Fluoxetine inhibits the reuptake of serotonin in the central nervous system and decreases the behaviors associated with the mentioned conditions. Choice *A* is the term used to describe pain during menstruation. Dysmenorrhea is treated with analgesic medications. Choice *E* is a blood clot that usually forms in the peripheral extremities. Venous thrombosis is treated with anticoagulant medications.

4. D: Alendronate sodium (Fosamax) is a bisphosphonate used in the treatment of osteoporosis. Fosamax inhibits bone reabsorption and prevents the breakdown of bone tissue. Patients are encouraged to consume calcium-rich foods to support calcium stores within the bone. Choices *A*, *B*, and *C* are all vitamin K–rich foods. Vitamin K helps to support blood clotting.

5. A, C, D, and F: Metformin (Glucophage) is a biguanide anti-diabetic medication used primarily in the treatment of diabetes type 2. Glucophage is also used to decrease insulin resistance and metabolic syndrome in patients with polycystic ovarian syndrome (PCOS). For diabetic management, expected values are hemoglobin A1C levels below 7% and glucose levels less than 130 mg/dL. HgA1C measures the average serum glucose levels over a period of a couple of months. For the management of PCOS, the goal is to decrease the metabolic syndrome (high blood pressure, obesity, high cholesterol, and insulin resistance). Choice *B* is an electrolyte that is not directly affected by Glucophage. Choice *E* is not an intended response to an anti-diabetic medication. Gastric ulcers are treated with medications that decrease gastric acid, such as pantoprazole (Protonix).

6. B: Nitroglycerine (Nitrol) is an antianginal nitrate medication used in the treatment of acute and long-term chest pain. Acute anginal attacks are treated with rapid-acting formulations such as sublingual and translingual routes. With the sublingual route, patients place the medication underneath their tongue until it dissolves. Choices *A* and *C* refer to applying medicine directly to the skin. These are slow routes that are used for long-term prophylaxis. Choice *D* is used for long-term prophylaxis of chest pain. Oral ingestion provides a slow onset and a long duration.

7. A, C, D, and E: Phenelzine (Nardil) is a monoamine oxidase inhibitor (MAOI) used in the treatment of eating disorders, depression, and obsessive-compulsive disorder (OCD). Nardil blocks MAO in the brain and increases the availability of serotonin and norepinephrine. Norepinephrine is a neurotransmitter that has vasoconstrictive effects, and tyramine also causes vasoconstriction. When tyramine is mixed with medications such as Nardil, vasoconstriction increases and can cause a hypertensive crisis. Symptoms of a hypertensive crisis include headache, nausea, and an elevated heart rate and blood pressure. Patients should be encouraged to avoid tyramine-rich foods such as aged cheese, bananas, red wine, and salami. Choice *B* can develop if Nardil is combined with an analgesic known as meperidine (Demerol).

8. A: The influenza vaccine is grown in eggs and may contain some of the proteins found in egg products. Patients with egg allergies may develop a reaction after administration of the flu vaccine, so a skin test should be performed prior to administration. Choice *B* is not correct. Vaccines help the body create immunity against viruses. Decreased red blood cells associated with anemia do not play a direct role in immunity. Choice *C* is not correct. Nausea is a gastrointestinal symptom unassociated with the immune

128

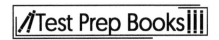

system. Choice *D* is not correct. Patients who experience frequent colds should be encouraged to receive the influenza vaccine to protect them against various strains respiratory viruses.

9. C: The movement of medication from its site of administration—such as the GI tract, skin, or muscle—into the bloodstream is known as absorption. Factors influencing absorption include the amount of medication, the route of administration, and the rate of medication absorption. Choice *A* refers to the elimination of a medication from the body. The majority of medications are excreted via the kidneys. Choice *B* refers to the transportation of a medication to its site of action via bodily fluids. Distribution is affected by factors such as circulation, plasma protein binding, and lipid solubility. Choice *D* is the process by which the liver inactivates medications and decreases the risk of toxicity in the body. Factors that influence metabolism include age, therapeutic index, and nutritional status.

10. A, C, and D: Antigout medications work by preventing infiltration of leukocytes and decreasing inflammation, inhibiting uric acid production, or inhibiting uric acid reabsorption in the renal tubules. Colchicine and indomethacin (Indocin) decrease inflammation and prevent leukocyte infiltration. Allopurinol (Zyloprim) prevents the production of uric acid. Choices *B* and *E* are medications used in the treatment of rheumatoid arthritis. Cyclosporine (Neoral) is an immunosuppressive used to decrease the inflammatory response in patients with arthritis. Sulfasalazine (Azulfidine) slows the degeneration of the joints and prevents the progression of rheumatoid arthritis.

11. D: The term *dysphagia* means the inability to swallow. Medications that are administered orally require the patient to have an intact gag reflex. Patients who are unable to swallow have a risk of aspiration if oral medications are administered. Choice *A* is administered via injections or directly into the vascular space. These medications are not contraindicated for a patient with decreased mobility or dysphagia. Choice *B* is applied directly to the skin. Transdermal patches release medication over time. There is no risk to a patient who is unable to swallow or has decreased mobility. Choice *C* is not correct. Sublingual medications should be placed underneath the tongue until they dissolve. Patients taking sublingual drugs do not swallow them.

12. A and D: Aging affects multiple responses in the body. Cardiovascular blood flow decreases through the major organs including the liver and kidneys. Active substances in medications take longer to reach their target tissues when blood flow is inadequate. Gastric acid becomes more alkaline during aging. The increase in pH buffers medications in the stomach and can delay their intended response. Choice *B* is not correct. Aging decreases the protein-binding sites, which delays the therapeutic effect. Choice *C* is not correct. Aging results in decreased lean body mass, decreased water content, and increased body fat. Medications take longer to metabolize with increased tissue and decreased muscle. Choice *E* is incorrect. Aging causes a decrease in gastric emptying. Medications not properly metabolized can lead to an accumulation and cause adverse effects.

13. A, B, and E: Medications such as amitriptyline (Elavil) can produce anticholinergic effects. Elavil blocks the muscarinic receptors found in the smooth muscle of various organs. Muscarinic receptors are responsible for recognizing the neurotransmitter acetylcholine. Acetylcholine is responsible for the contraction of smooth muscle, dilation of vessels, and increase in bodily secretions. Inhibition of acetylcholine results in dry mouth, sensitivity to sunlight, and retention of urine. Choices *C*, *D*, and *F* are extrapyramidal symptoms (EPSs) associated with medications used to treat mental disorders such as haloperidol and thioridazine. EPSs are abnormal body movements including rigidity, uncontrollable restlessness, involuntary fine motor movements, and spasticity.

129

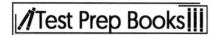
14. B: All vitamins have a recommended daily intake. Ingesting more than the recommended range increases the possibility of toxicity and organ dysfunction. Vitamin B5 is also known as pantothenic acid and is essential for the metabolism of fat, proteins, and carbohydrates. The recommended daily intake for adult males is 5 mg. Vitamin E is an antioxidant that helps maintain the integrity of cell membranes. The recommended daily intake is 15 mg. Vitamin B3, also known as niacin, is essential for fat synthesis. The recommended daily intake is 16 mg. Vitamin C is essential for skin integrity, wound healing, and immunity. The recommended daily intake is 90 mg.

15. C: Chlamydia is a sexually transmitted disease that can affect the reproductive system and fertility if not treated. The recommended treatment is a single dose of azithromycin (Zithromax). Choice *A* is not correct. The choice of treatment for syphilis, another sexually transmitted infection, is penicillin. Choices *B* and *D* are viruses. Zithromax is an antibacterial medication. HIV is treated with antiretroviral medications such as zidovudine (Retrovir) and abacavir (Ziagen). There is no medical treatment for HPV. Medical management for HPV includes treating cancerous cells as they appear and promoting safe sex practices.

16. B, C, and D: Dopamine (Intropin) is an adrenergic agonist medication used in the treatment of shock and heart failure. In moderate doses (2 to 10 mcg/kg/min), it helps to dilate the vessels within the arteries of the kidney to regulate the blood pressure within the body. Intropin also increases the heart rate and myocardial contractility to improve cardiac output and assist with organ perfusion throughout the body. Choice *A* is not correct. Vasoconstriction results from activation of alpha-1 receptors. These receptors are activated with high doses of Intropin (>10 mcg/kg/min). Choice *E* is not a pharmacological action produced by dopamine. Bronchodilation occurs with the activation of alpha-2 receptors.

17. D: Minerals support growth in children and maintain normal body functioning. Overdoses of minerals can be toxic and cause life-threatening adverse effects such as kidney and liver failure. Upper intake limits are established to prevent organ dysfunction. Fluoride is a mineral that helps strengthen teeth. The daily upper intake level for children over the age of 9 years is 10 mg. Magnesium is a mineral that helps promote bone structure. Its daily upper intake level is 350 mg. Calcium is a necessary mineral that supports bone health and maintains normal functioning of the central nervous system. Its daily upper intake level is 2.5 g (2,500 mg). Phosphorus is a mineral that provides muscle contractions and repairs tissue cells. Its daily upper intake level is 4g (4,000 mg).

18. B, D, and E: Succinylcholine (Anectine) is a neuromuscular blocking agent used in conjunction with anesthesia to produce relaxation of the muscles during procedures such as surgery and invasive tests. Anectine helps relax muscle contractions that occur during seizure activity in patients receiving electroconvulsive therapy. Anectine is also used during endotracheal intubation to facilitate muscular relaxation of the airway. Endoscopic procedures use invasive tools and require sedation. Anectine is used to relax muscles for easier passage of the scope. Choices *A*, *C*, and *F* do not require neuromuscular blocking agents. Lumbar punctures and biopsies are performed using topical anesthetics such as lidocaine. Chemotherapy is administered intravenously and does not require anesthesia or muscular blocking medications.

19. D: Oseltamivir (Tamiflu) is an antiviral medication used in the treatment of influenza infections. Over 99% of the medication is excreted via the urine. Intact renal function is required to avoid toxic effects to the kidneys. Patients with renal impairment require dosage adjustments. Serum creatinine levels directly evaluate renal function. Normal serum creatinine levels are 0.6 to 1.3 mg/dl. Elevated levels indicate renal dysfunction.

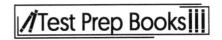

20. C: Phenothiazine medications such as prochlorperazine (Compazine) can result in extrapyramidal symptoms. Extrapyramidal symptoms are abnormal movements in the body. Compulsive, involuntary restlessness is known as akathisia, and it is the most common extrapyramidal effect experienced with Compazine. Choices *A* and *B* are symptoms that are less commonly experienced with phenothiazines. Dystonia is uncoordinated, bizarre movements of the eyes, face, and neck. Dyskinesia is involuntary rhythmic body movements. Choice *D* is characterized by loss of movement, muscular rigidity, and a shuffling gait.

21. C: Vaccines administered in infants should be given in the anterolateral aspect of the thigh muscle. A 1-inch needle is sufficiently long to penetrate the skin and reach into the muscle. Needles of $\frac{1}{2}$ in and $\frac{5}{8}$ in are too short in length to reach the muscle. The needle that is $1\frac{1}{4}$ in is too long and can cause damage to underlying structures.

22. C, D, and E: Torsemide (Demadex) is a loop diuretic used in the treatment of fluid overload conditions such as pulmonary edema, hypertension, and kidney disease. Loop diuretics cause diuresis. Excessive fluid loss can lead to a decrease in blood pressure and loss of electrolytes such as potassium. Medications such as torsemide may also cause damage to the cell junctions in the blood vessels found within the cochlea. Damage to these blood vessels can result in hearing loss. Choice *A* is incorrect. Loop diuretics help to treat high calcium due to kidney stone formation. Choice *B* is incorrect. Edema is an accumulation of fluid within the tissues. Demadex is given to correct this imbalance.

23. B: Glycopyrrolate is an anticholinergic antispasmodic medication used to inhibit salivation and decrease respiratory secretions. It has a quick onset of 1 to 10 minutes when administered intravenously. Heparin is an anticoagulant medication used in the treatment of blood clotting disorders. It has an onset of 20 to 60 minutes when administered subcutaneously. Haloperidol is an antipsychotic medication used in the treatment of psychotic disorders such as schizophrenia. It has an onset of 2 hours when administered orally. Escitalopram is a selective serotonin reuptake inhibitor (SSRI) used in the treatment of depression. Antidepressants have a long onset of 1 to 4 weeks when administered orally.

24. B: Acetaminophen is a pain reliever and fever reducer that is commonly prescribed as an analgesic. It is used as a substitute for nonsteroidal anti-inflammatories (NSAIDs) because it does not interfere with blood clotting or cause gastrointestinal effects. Choices *A, C,* and *D* are all NSAIDs. NSAIDs inactivate both COX-1 and COX-2 enzymes. COX-1 decreases gastric acid secretion and protects the mucosa. COX-2 causes vasodilation and inflammation. Inhibition of COX-1 leads to stomach irritation.

25. C: Substances are classified by schedules that determine their potential risk for abuse and dependency. The lower the schedule number, the higher the risk of dependency. Schedule I substances are not indicated for medical use and include "street" drugs such as heroin, LSD, and peyote. Schedule II medications have a high potential for abuse and can lead to physical and psychological dependence. These medications include hydromorphone (Dilaudid), oxycodone (Percocet), and meperidine (Demerol). Schedule III narcotics have less potential for abuse than Schedule II substances and have a moderate to low physical dependence. These medications include ketamine, combination products with less than 15 mg of hydrocodone, and buprenorphine (Suboxone). In comparison, Schedule IV medications have a low potential for abuse. These include clonazepam (Klonopin), midazolam (Versed), and alprazolam (Xanax). Schedule V medications contain limited quantities of narcotic medications and have a low potential for abuse. These medications include Phenergan with codeine, ezogabine, and Robitussin AC.

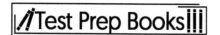
26. D: Atropine is the reversal agent for cholinesterase inhibitors. Medications such as rivastigmine (Exelon) decrease the inactivation of acetylcholine by acetylcholinesterase. Acetylcholine is a neurotransmitter that maintains brain and muscle function. Excessive levels of rivastigmine can cause adverse effects, such as bradycardia, urinary urgency, and increased gastric secretions. Decreased muscle function can occur with toxic levels. Atropine counteracts the effects by blocking muscarinic receptors. Choice *A* is the reversal agent for benzodiazepines; flumazenil helps block the binding of benzodiazepines to the GABA receptor sites. Choice *B* is the reversal for opioid narcotics; Narcan competes for the same receptor site as narcotics and therefore decrease the adverse effects of opioids, such as respiratory depression and sedation. Choice *C* is the reversal agent for heparin; protamine sulfate binds with heparin to inactive the effects of blood thinning.

27. A, B, E, and F: Angiotensin-converting-enzyme (ACE) inhibitors excrete sodium and water while retaining potassium through the effects of the kidney. Elevated potassium levels can cause cardiac dysrhythmias, nausea, and weakness. Fruits such as apricots and kiwi are rich in potassium. Vegetable greens such as spinach and white potatoes also contain high amounts of potassium. Choices *C* and *D* are considered calcium-rich foods and do not interfere with ACE inhibitors.

28. B: Intravenous medications have the fastest onset when administered via this route. Directly introducing medications into the bloodstream will have quick effects. Dilaudid administered via the IV route will have an onset of between 10 and 15 minutes. Choices *A* (subcutaneous) and *C* (intramuscular) will have onsets within 15 minutes of administration. Choice *D* (orally) will have the longest onset at 30 minutes.

29. B, D, and E: Hypertension can be treated with several different types of medications. Choice *B* is an angiotensin-converting enzyme (ACE) inhibitor that blocks the enzyme that converts angiotensin I to angiotensin II. Angiotensin II is a strong vasoconstrictor. Choice *D* is a loop diuretic that prevents sodium and chloride from being reabsorbed in the kidney and produces strong diuresis. Choice *E* is an antiadrenergic agent that blocks the activity of the sympathetic nervous system (SNS). The SNS increases the heart rate, force of contraction in the myocardium, and cardiac output. Choices *A* and *C* are medications affecting the digestive system. Nizatidine (Axid) is a histamine2 receptor antagonist (H2RA) that inhibits the secretion of gastric acid and decreases the acidity, amount, and pepsin content of gastric juices. Axid is used in the treatment of peptic ulcer disease. Sucralfate (Carafate) is used in the treatment of active duodenal ulcers. It promotes healing by binding to gastric ulcers and forming a protective barrier between gastric acid and the stomach mucosa.

30. D: Epinephrine (adrenalin) is an adrenergic medication that is commonly used in cardiac arrest, anaphylactic shock, and conditions with acute bronchospasms. At high doses, epinephrine is used as a vasoconstrictor to shunt blood toward the central vital organs. The concentration varies depending on the route that is used for administration. The most potent concentration is via the inhaled route. Inhaled epinephrine is used during laryngeal edema and acute bronchospasms. Its final concentration is 1%. Subcutaneous epinephrine may be used for acute asthma attacks to produce bronchodilation. Its final concentration is 0.5%. Intravenous epinephrine is used during cardiac arrest to stimulate the heart and cause peripheral vasoconstriction. Its final concentration is 0.01%. Intradermal epinephrine is used in combination with local anesthetics and is the least potent form. Its final concentration is 0.001%.

31. B: Ceftazidime (Fortaz) is a third-generation cephalosporin used in the treatment of bacterial infections, such as meningitis, pneumonia, and urinary tract infections. Once absorbed, cephalosporins have maximum concentrations in the liver. Yellow discoloration of the eye is also known as *jaundice*. Jaundice is an accumulation of bilirubin and can be a sign of medication toxicity. Choices *A* and *C* are

132

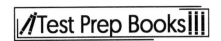

central nervous system symptoms and are not associated with the use of Fortaz. Choice *D* is not correct. An altered sense of taste is not a defined side effect for this medication.

32. B, D, and E: Lithium carbonate (Eskalith) is a medication used in the treatment of bipolar disorder. It is a metallic salt that occurs naturally and has a narrow range between therapeutic and toxic levels. Toxicity occurs when serum levels surpass 2.5 mEq/L. Common side effects that occur when serum lithium levels are between 0.6 and 1.2 mEq/L include hand tremors, a metallic taste in the mouth, polyuria, fatigue, edema, and polydipsia. Choices *A, C,* and *F* occur when serum lithium levels are between 1.5 and 2.5 mEq/L.

33. A: Sodium bicarbonate acts as an alkalotic medication to buffer acidic metabolic conditions. It is a common therapy for neutralizing gastric acid. Excessive use of sodium bicarbonate may cause formation of stones in the kidneys and hypercalcemia. Milk is considered an alkalinizing food and should be avoided when taking this medication. Choices *B, C,* and *D* are all acidic foods that can have an opposite intended effect.

34. B, C, and E: Repaglinide (Prandin) is an antidiabetic medication that stimulates the release of insulin from the pancreas and helps reduce blood glucose levels. Ginseng is a plant root that has been shown to lower blood glucose levels. If taken concurrently with Prandin, additive hypoglycemic events may occur. Garlic is an herb that may increase the production of serum insulin. It has a similar mechanism of action to Prandin and can cause additive hypoglycemic effects. Basil is an herb that may lower blood sugar when taken as a supplement in large amounts. When taken with Prandin, blood sugar levels may decrease more than expected. Choices *A* and *D* may cause hyperglycemia, the opposite of the intended effect. Gingko biloba increases hepatic metabolism of insulin, and glucosamine can cause impaired insulin secretion.

35. A: The National Institutes of Health provides a list of food sources containing potassium. If a patient requires potassium restriction or supplementation, a pharmacist would need to be aware of these values; 1 cup of lentils contains 731 mg of potassium per serving, 1 cup of orange juice contains 496 mg of potassium per serving, 1 cup of milk contains 366 mg of potassium, and 1 cup of brewed coffee contains the least amount of potassium at 116 mg per serving.

36. B, C, and E: Theophylline is a xanthine used for bronchodilation and as a secondary drug for asthma, emphysema, and bronchitis if primary medications are not effective. Lithium is a mood stabilizer used in the treatment of bipolar disorder. If taken concurrently with Foradil, lithium increases the excretion of theophylline and decreases the effectiveness. Phenobarbital is a barbiturate used in the treatment of seizures. When taken concurrently, it increases the metabolism of theophylline and decreases its effectiveness. Propranolol (Inderal) is a beta-blocker used in the treatment of hypertension. Using it with theophylline can cause bronchoconstriction, the opposite intended effect. Choices *A* and *D* can decrease theophylline clearance and increase plasma levels. Clindamycin (Cleocin) is an anti-infective used in the treatment of various infections. Choice *D* is a histamine antagonist used in the prevention of gastric ulcers. Choice *F* is a monoamine oxidase (MAO) inhibitor that is used in the treatment of depression. When taken concurrently with theophylline, it increases the metabolism of catecholamines, which can increase blood pressure.

37. A: Synergism is when the action of one drug facilitates or increases the action of another. Choice *B* is not correct. Antagonism is when one medication decreases the mechanism of action of another. Choice *C* is not correct. Efficacy is defined as the intended therapeutic effect of a medication. Choice *D* is

133

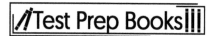

incorrect. Specificity refers to the range of actions produced by a medication. Some medications produce only one action, while others exert effects on multiple organs in the body.

38. D: Acyclovir is an anti-viral medication used in the treatment of herpes infections. Over 90% of the medication is excreted unchanged via the kidneys. Administration of acyclovir in patients with renal dysfunction may cause organ failure. Dosage adjustments are required. Choice *A* is not correct. Amiodarone is an antiarrhythmic used in the treatment of life-threatening ventricular arrhythmias. Amiodarone is to be used cautiously in patients with congestive heart failure, liver disease, and thyroid disorders. Choice *B* is incorrect. Haloperidol is an antipsychotic medication used in the treatment of psychosis and schizophrenia. Special precautions are indicated in patients with cardiac disease, liver dysfunction, and bone marrow suppression. Choice *C* is not correct. Mirtazapine is an antidepressant medication used in conjunction with psychotherapy to treat depression. Mirtazapine is to be used cautiously in pregnant patients or patients with a history of seizures.

39. B, C, & D: Allergic reactions to medications occur via two types of immune responses: humoral or cellular. In a humoral response, antibodies and immunoglobulins in the body destroy antigens through chemical processes. During an anaphylactic reaction, reaginic antibodies known as IgE are produced and attach themselves to the surface of mast cells. This reaction causes the release of histamine, leukotrienes, and prostaglandins which cause itching, bronchospasms, swelling, and vascular dilation. During a cytolytic reaction, IgG and IgM antibodies bind to the target cells and cause disruption of the cells. This results in liver, kidney, and muscle damage. During an Arthus reaction, a widespread inflammatory response occurs as a result of IgG antibodies. Clinical manifestations include a rash, fever, and inflammation of heart and renal tissues. Choice *A* is not correct. Delayed hypersensitivity is a cell-mediated immune response. In delayed hypersensitivity, cells destroy antigens by surrounding them with T-lymphocytes—white blood cells that target and eliminate infected cells. Choice *E* is not a type of humoral response. Phototoxicity refers to localized tissue damage caused by UV radiation.

40. C: Lorazepam is a sedative used in the treatment of anxiety, insomnia, and seizures. Its mechanism of action potentiates the neurotransmitter gamma-aminobutyric acid (GABA), which decreases neuron excitability. Lorazepam is one of the first-choice medications for the treatment of status epilepticus. Status epilepticus is sustained seizure activity lasting over 30 minutes, or more than two seizures with loss of consciousness. Lorazepam is 75–90% effective in treating status epilepticus. Choice *A* is not correct. Phenytoin should only be used as an alternative when seizures do not stop after the administration of lorazepam. Phenytoin can cause vascular complications such as hypotension and cardiac arrhythmias. Choice *B* is incorrect. Valproate is the drug of choice for treating myoclonic seizures. Myoclonic seizures are brief, jerk-like movements of the muscles that last a few seconds. Choice *D* is not correct. Carbamazepine is the drug of choice for treating complex partial seizures. These types of seizures are characterized by the inability to control movements and absence of speech.

41. A, B, D, & F: The QT interval seen in an electrocardiogram depicts the time it takes between ventricular contraction and relaxation. A prolonged QT interval means the heart takes longer to electrically recharge between heart beats. A prolonged QT interval can lead to a condition known as torsades de pointes—an emergent form of ventricular tachycardia that can cause sudden cardiac arrest. Procainamide and quinidine are class I antiarrhythmics that prolong the refractory period of the heart and suppress the atrioventricular node. Amiodarone is a class III antiarrhythmic that prolongs the repolarization rate of the heart. Amitriptyline is a tricyclic antidepressant medication that also has the potential to prolong the QT interval. Tricyclic antidepressants increase the levels of serotonin and norepinephrine in the bloodstream. Choices *C* and *E* are anticoagulant medications used in the

134

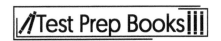

treatment of blood clotting disorders. These medications do not have the characteristics to alter ventricular contraction and relaxation.

42. A: Local anesthetics are injected into the tissues to numb the site for procedures such as bone marrow biopsies, dental work, and minor surgical procedures. Although tissue toxicity risk is low, local anesthetics may still produce adverse effects if administered in large doses. Absorption and metabolism are affected by body mass and may cause central nervous system adverse effects if injected as a nerve block. Adverse effects include visual disturbances, muscle twitching, and involuntary movements. Dibucaine is the most potent local anesthetic and can cause toxicity if administered in large doses. It is used for spinal anesthesia, and the recommended maximum dose is 50 milligrams. Bupivacaine is a long-acting anesthetic used as a nerve block, epidural, and spinal anesthetic. Its recommended maximum dose is 100 milligrams. Lidocaine is a commonly used topical and injectable anesthetic used for surface procedures, nerve blocks, and epidurals. Its maximum dose is 300 milligrams. Procaine is the oldest synthetic anesthetic introduced. It is uncommonly used in conjunction with penicillin for intramuscular injection. Its maximum dose is 400 milligrams.

43. D: Venlafaxine is both a serotonin and noradrenaline reuptake inhibitor. Serotonin is a neurotransmitter responsible for regulating mood and cognition and is the reward center of the brain. Noradrenaline is a hormone and neurotransmitter responsible for mental vigilance and concentration. Decreased amounts of both neurotransmitters contribute to depression. Venlafaxine prevents the reuptake of these substances back into the presynaptic cells and allows for higher concentrations in the bloodstream. Choices *A*, *B*, and *C* are selective serotonin reuptake inhibitors (SSRIs). These medications only prevent the reabsorption of serotonin.

44. D: Heparin is a blood thinner that is administered parenterally (intravenously and subcutaneously). It is used in the treatment of venous thrombosis and clotting disorders. Toxicity can result in internal bleeding. Protamine sulfate is a low molecular weight protein that neutralizes heparin when administered intravenously. 1 milligram of protamine sulfate is required to neutralize 100 units of heparin. Choice *A* is not correct. Vitamin K is the reversal agent for the oral anticoagulant warfarin (Coumadin). Choice *B* is not correct. Acetylcysteine is the antagonist for acetaminophen (Tylenol). Choice *C* is incorrect. Flumazenil is the reversal agent for benzodiazepine medications, such as alprazolam, lorazepam, and diazepam.

45. C: Ondansetron is an anti-emetic medication used as a treatment for vomiting. Vomiting results from stimulation of the chemoreceptor trigger zone located in the medulla oblongata. Substances such as medications can easily stimulate the medulla oblongata as it is not protected by a blood-brain barrier. The midbrain is responsible for motor movement and sensory processing. The pons controls respirations, the swallow reflex, equilibrium, and several sensory functions. The cerebellum is responsible for coordination of body movements, balance, and speech.

46. B: A penetrating wound is considered a contaminated wound. Any potential contamination from the gastrointestinal tract into the abdominal cavity requires surgery to cleanse the area. The injury happened less than 2 hours ago. This differentiates a contaminated wound from a dirty wound. Choice *A* is not correct. A dirty wound is classified as a purulent wound or penetrating injury greater than 4 hours old. Choice *C* is incorrect. Clean-contaminated wounds have no opening of the viscera and no contact with infected structures. Choice *D* is not correct. Clean wounds are classified as nontraumatic procedures with unexposed viscera and no infection present.

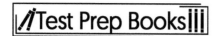

47. B & D: Fexofenadine is an antihistamine used in the treatment of seasonal allergies. Its brand name is Allegra, and it is a common over-the-counter medication. Histamine is a component of the immune response and causes an inflammatory process when an allergen is present. Symptoms of seasonal allergies due to pollen or mold include sneezing, watery eyes, and excess nasal drainage (rhinorrhea). Fexofenadine blocks the effects of histamine and relieves its clinical manifestations. The medication is also used to treat idiopathic urticaria. This condition results in hives with a cause unknown. Fexofenadine relieves the itching associated with hives. Choices *A, C,* and *E* are therapeutic effects of H2 histamine antagonists such as cimetidine, famotidine, and ranitidine. H2 histamine receptors are found in the gastric lining and secrete gastric acid. Excess acid can lead to ulcerations, indigestion, and heartburn.

48. D: Nitrofurantoin is an antibiotic medication used primarily in the treatment of urinary tract infections. Nitrofurantoin interferes with bacterial enzymes that cause invasion of organisms in the urinary tract. Choices *A, B,* and *C* are medications used to treat prostatic enlargement. Choice *A* is a vasodilator used primarily in the treatment of erectile dysfunction. Due to its vasodilation properties, it is also used to treat the symptoms of an enlarged prostate such as incomplete bladder emptying, hesitation, and dribbling. Choice *B* is an androgen inhibitor that treats benign prostatic hyperplasia. It inhibits the enzyme responsible for converting the hormone testosterone into a metabolite in the prostate. It reduces the size of the prostate that can interfere with urinary flow. Finasteride is also used to treat male pattern baldness. Choice *C* is a peripherally acting antiadrenergic. Tamsulosin decreases the contractions of the smooth muscle in the prostate and results in decreased symptoms of BPH.

49. A, C, & D: Antiretroviral therapy (ART) is a combination of medications that inhibit the replication of HIV. Medications such as zidovudine, abacavir, and lamivudine work together to prevent the virus from multiplying and destroying the body's immune system. The World Health Organization established recommended guidelines for initiating ART. Pregnancy carries a risk of passing the virus to the unborn fetus. Therapy initiation is recommended. There is strong evidence that supports starting ART in patients with a CD4 count between 350–500/mm^3. CD4 refers to the T helper cell count. T helper cells help the immune system fight off infection. The normal CD4 count is between 500–1,600/mm^3. Tuberculosis is an opportunistic infection that commonly occurs in patients who have a weakened immune system. Patients with a concurrent HIV infection require treatment to improve their lifespan. Choices *B* and *E* are not circumstances that require initiation of ART. Platelets help the blood to clot. Although the platelet level is slightly higher than normal, there is no correlation with an HIV infection. The normal platelet count is 150,000–450,000/mm^3. Hypertension is a common co-morbidity with no direct correlation to the weakened immune system in patients with HIV.

50. A: Esmolol is a class II antiarrhythmic beta blocker used in the treatment of sinus tachycardia and supraventricular arrhythmias. Esmolol blocks the action of myocardial adrenergic receptors. These receptors increase the rate of the heart and conduction of the atrioventricular node. Sinus tachycardia is an increased rate of the heart greater than 100 beats per minute. Choice *B* is not correct. Atrial fibrillation is uncoordinated and weak contractions of the atria in the heart. Atrial fibrillation can lead to blood clot formation and is treated with blood thinners. Choice *C* is not correct. Premature atrial contractions (PACs) occur when an early or extra atrial beat is triggered before receiving a signal from the sinus node. PACs are common and generally not treated unless the rhythm progresses into atrial fibrillation. Choice *D* is incorrect. A second-degree heart block occurs when atrial impulses through the AV node become delayed or blocked. Second-degree heart blocks can progress into heart failure and sudden cardiac arrest. This type of heart block is treated with the anticholinergic medication atropine.

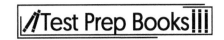

51. B, C, E, & F: Sodium rich foods can increase fluid volume within the body. Sodium attracts water, increasing the amount that is distributed throughout the tissues. Increased volume leads to swelling and high blood pressure. The recommended daily intake of sodium should be no more than 1500 milligrams. Cheese contains large amounts of sodium. One slice of American cheese contains approximately 460 milligrams of sodium. Condiments such as ketchup and mustard contain large amounts of salt, sugar, and seasonings. Ketchup contains approximately 150 milligrams of sodium for every tablespoon. Soy sauce is another condiment with a high sodium content. Soy sauce contains approximately 300 milligrams of sodium in each tablespoon. Bacon is a salt-cured pork product that also contains a significant amount of salt. Every slice contains approximately 175 milligrams of sodium. Choices *A* and *D* do not contain large amounts of sodium. Broccoli contains approximately 20 milligrams of sodium for every 2 spears. Bananas are a potassium-rich food with a very small sodium content. One medium banana contains 1 milligram of sodium.

52. B: Bronchodilators relieve the constriction that occurs in the airways in patients who have asthma. There are various types of antiasthma medications with a difference in onset, peak, and duration. Budenoside (Pulmicort) is a corticosteroid that reduces inflammation in the airways when used topically with inhalation. Its onset time is immediate with rapid peak action. Albuterol (Proventil) and Salmeterol (Serevent) are adrenergic medications that produce bronchodilation. Proventil has an onset of 5 minutes after inhalation with a peak of 1.5 to 2 hours. Serevent has an onset of 13 to 20 minutes with peak activity after 3 to 4 hours. Ipratropium (Atrovent) is an anticholinergic medication that blocks the action of acetylcholine, a neurotransmitter that produces bronchoconstriction and mucus secretion. It has an onset of 15 minutes and a peak time of 1 to 2 hours.

53. 40 milliliters: The amount being administered needs to be converted to milliliters: 1 teaspoon = 5 ml. With every dose, the patient is receiving 10 milliliters of medication. The patient receives four doses of medication in one day; QID means four times a day. The milliliters per dose need to be multiplied by four to find the total volume in 24-hour period ($10 \text{ ml} \times 4 = 40 \text{ ml}$).

54. D: Antitubercular medications are used to treat tuberculosis. Antitubercular medications can be hepatotoxic if taken in large doses. Isoniazid is a primary drug that inhibits the formation of cell walls. Its recommended dose is 300 mg a day. Rifampin is a primary drug that inhibits the synthesis of ribonucleic acid (RNA). Its recommended maximum daily dose is 600 mg. Streptomycin is a primary drug that is used when tuberculosis is resistant to isoniazid or rifampin. Its maximum daily dose is 1 gram. Pyrazinamide is a bactericidal medication used in combination with isoniazid and rifampin. Its recommended daily dose is 2 grams.

55. B, C, E, and F: Medications are primarily metabolized in the liver. Metabolism helps to inactivate medications to aid the kidneys in excreting them via the urine. Metabolism also decreases the risk of toxicity by inactivating medications. Age affects the metabolism of medications. Infants have limited ability to metabolize medication. Since liver function tends to decrease with age, careful consideration must be taken when administering medications to older patients. Medications that are inactivated during their first pass through the liver are known as first-pass medications. Sublingual and intravenous routes are preferred for first-pass medications. The half-life of a medication is the time it takes for an active substance to decrease in concentration by 50% within the circulation. Liver and kidney function may affect a medication's half-life. The therapeutic index refers to the medication's ability to reach serum peak levels. Medications that have a high therapeutic index have a wide safety margin and do not require frequent laboratory monitoring. Choice *A* is important when administering blood products; it

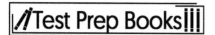

does not directly affect the metabolism of medications. Choice *D* is a term used when medication effects are experienced as a result of psychological factors as opposed to chemical and physical factors.

56. 4 ounces: The order says to dissolve each dose in 120 ml of water. The volume needs to be converted to ounces (1 oz = 30 ml) To find the total volume, the ordered volume needs to be divided by 30 (120 ml/30 ml = 4 oz). The ordered dose and frequency are not relevant to the question.

57. 20.5 mg: The patient's weight needs to be converted to kilograms: 1 kg = 2.2 lbs. The patient weighs 20.45 kg (45 lb × 2.2 lbs = 20.45 kg). The order calls for 0.2 mg per kilogram of weight. The patient's weight needs to be multiplied by 0.2 mg to find the daily dose. The patient will receive 4.09 mg of medication per day:

$$0.2 \text{ mg} \times 20.45 \text{ kg} = 4.09 \text{ mg}$$

The patient will receive 5 total doses (once per day). The daily dose needs to be multiplied by five to find the total dose (4.09 mg × 5 = 20.45 mg). The question asks to round the final answer to the nearest tenth, and 20.45 mg rounds to 20.5 mg.

58. C: The pH level of medications determines its acidity. A neutral pH is 7.0. Numbers below 7.0 are considered acidic and are absorbed more readily within the stomach and initial part of the small intestine when administered orally. Medications with a pH level above 7.0 are considered alkaline and are absorbed further down the small intestine when administered orally. Pramlintide is an antidiabetic medication used in the treatment of hyperglycemia when adequate blood glucose levels cannot be achieved with insulin therapy. It has an acidic pH level of 4.0. Micafungin is an antifungal medication used primarily in the treatment of esophageal candidiasis. When reconstituted for parental administration, its pH is between 5.0–7.0. Cidofovir is an antiviral medication used in the treatment of cytomegalovirus. It has a slightly alkaline pH of 7.4. Warfarin is an anticoagulant medication used in the preventative treatment of blood clots. It has an alkaline pH level of approximately 8.1–8.3.

59. 4 tablespoons: To find the household equivalent, the dose needs to be converted to tablespoons. 30 mL = 2 tbsp. The ordered dose is 60 milliliters. The ordered dose is divided by the metric dose and multiplied by 2 to find the number of tablespoons needed: 2 × (60 ÷ 30) = 4. The patient will need to take 4 tablespoons with each dose. Rounded to the nearest whole number, 4 remains as 4 tablespoons. The ordered frequency is not relevant to the question.

60. C: Fondaparinux is a low molecular weight heparin used in the treatment of deep vein thrombosis and pulmonary embolism. The dosage is based on the patient's weight in kilograms. The patient weighs 175 pounds. The weight is converted to kilograms: 1 kg = 2.2 lbs. The patient weighs 79.5 kilograms: 175 ÷ 2.2 = 79.5. Patients with a weight between 50–100 kilograms are prescribed 7.5 milligrams of fondaparinux daily. Choice *A* is incorrect. 2.5 milligrams is a dose recommended for prophylaxis after surgery. The patient in the scenario actively has a disease process. Choice *B* is incorrect. 5 milligrams should be prescribed for patients under 50 kilograms. Choice *D* is incorrect. 10 milligrams should be prescribed for patients over the weight of 100 kilograms.

61. C: Levothyroxine (Synthroid) is a thyroid hormone medication used in the treatment of hypothyroidism. It is recommended to be taken on an empty stomach before breakfast. Fasting increases the absorption of the medication and administering it early in the morning allows for peak activity during day. Allopurinol (Zyloprim) is an antihyperuricemic medication used in the treatment of gouty arthritis. One of the side effects of Zyloprim is upset stomach. Taking this medication with or shortly after a meal will decrease the risk of gastrointestinal side effects. Simvastatin (Zocor) is a lipid-

138

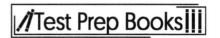

lowering medication used in the treatment of high cholesterol. Most cholesterol is produced in the evening hours of the day. Zocor is recommended to be taken during the evening to enhance its cholesterol level–reducing mechanism. Zolpidem (Ambien) is a sedative used in the treatment of insomnia. It promotes sleep and is recommended to be taken right before bedtime.

62. D: Theophylline (Uniphyl) is a xanthine bronchodilator used in the long-term treatment of asthma and COPD. Uniphyl works by increasing diaphragmatic contractility and reversing airway obstruction caused by narrowing of the bronchial tubes. It exerts its therapeutic effects in the lungs and respiratory system.

63. A: The injection should be given in the vastus lateralis. The first dose of the diphtheria, tetanus, and pertussis (DTaP) vaccine should be administered in infants at the age of 2 months. At this age, the largest muscle mass is found in the vastus lateralis site in front of the thigh. The arm is the deltoid site. This site is recommended until children are above the age of 1 year. The outer aspect of the buttock is the ventrogluteal site. This area does not contain a sufficient amount of muscle mass in infants. The posterior buttock is the dorsogluteal site. This site is not recommended due to its proximity to the sciatic nerve. Injection into the sciatic nerve can cause nerve irritation and possible damage.

64. C: Recommended serum drug levels vary between medications. Serum levels must remain stable to produce therapeutic effects and minimize the risk of toxicity and adverse effects. Propranolol is a Class II beta blocker used in the treatment of tachydysrhythmias. Its recommended serum range is 0.05 to 0.1 mcg/ml. Mexiletine is a Class IB antidysrhythmic used in the treatment of ventricular fibrillation and ventricular tachycardia. Its recommended serum drug level range is 0.5 to 2.0 mcg/ml. Procainamide is a Class IA antidysrhythmic used in the treatment of atrial fibrillation and atrial flutter. Its recommended serum range is 4 to 8 mcg/ml. Phenytoin is a Class IB drug used in the treatment of dysrhythmias caused by digoxin intoxication. It is also an anticonvulsant medication. Its recommended serum range is 10 to 20 mcg/ml.

65. D: Syphilis is a sexually transmitted disease that causes chancre sores. If untreated, it can progress to secondary and latent stages. Late-stage syphilis can cause neurological impairment. The choice of treatment for syphilis is a penicillin G intramuscular injection. In a laboratory record, it will appear as reactive. The normal finding is non-reactive. Chlamydia is treated with antibiotics. Hepatitis B and Herpes 1 are treated with antivirals to stop replication. Antivirals are not a cure.

66. A: Lovenox is a low-molecular-weight heparin anticoagulant used in the prevention of deep vein thrombosis (DVT). It is a subcutaneous medication administered via injection. As per manufacturer recommendations and to enhance the absorption of Lovenox, the medication should be administered in the left or right side of the abdominal wall only.

67. C: Diltiazem (Cardizem) is a calcium channel blocker used in the treatment of supraventricular tachycardia (SVT). SVT consists of an abnormally high heart rate and shows a regular rate with a hidden P wave and a normal QRS interval on the EKG strip. Atrial fibrillation (AFib) is a tremor-like movement of the atria of the heart and is characterized by an irregular rate, no P wave, and a normal QRS interval. Sinus bradycardia is characterized by a slower than normal P wave and QRS interval. Normal sinus rhythm is the expected rhythm of the heart and does not require treatment.

68. D: Sublingual means under the tongue. Inhalation is through the nose or the mouth. Subcutaneous is an injection that goes under the skin. Buccal refers to the cheek inside the mouth, but not under the tongue.

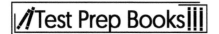
69. C: Epilepsy is caused by overactive neuronal signaling in the brain, so a central nervous system depressant can calm such activity. Hypertension, ADHD, and depression do not improve with this type of medication and potentially, it can be harmful.

70. A: The FDA regulates dietary supplements under the Dietary Supplement Health and Education Act of 1994 guidelines, which means Choice *A* is correct because it states "Dietary Supplements" must be present on the product labeling. Manufacturers and distributers are required to verify that their products are safe and effective, and that their products meet FDA and DSHEA regulations. The FDA does not require manufacturers of dietary supplements to adopt the same practices as drug manufacturers. In addition, manufacturers cannot make claims that dietary supplements be used for the treatment or cure of a condition or ailment; therefore, Choices *B, C,* and *D* are incorrect.

71. C: Choice *C*, folic acid, is a B vitamin that all people need for healthy blood cells, but it is especially important for women of child bearing age because it can help to prevent birth defects that may develop early in a pregnancy, often before a pregnancy is detected. Choices *A* and *B*, Vitamin D and calcium are both supplements that support healthy bone development. Choice *D* is not correct because echinacea is an herbal dietary supplement used as a natural cold remedy.

72. B: Choice *B* is the correct choice because narrow therapeutic index medications require close, frequent monitoring and have several risk factors associated with their administration. Choices *A* and *D* are therefore incorrect. Choice *C* is incorrect because narrow therapeutic index medications are available in various dosage forms including intravenously, oral tablets or capsules, injectables, suspensions, etc.

73. A: Choice *A* is correct because monitoring INR values is the standard method for determining if blood thinners have reached a therapeutic level. Choice *B* is incorrect because statins are not monitored via INR values but instead require annual bloodwork to screen cholesterol values. Antibiotics do not typically require monitoring, so Choice *C* is incorrect. Anticonvulsants require monitoring of bloodwork, but INR values do not apply here, so Choice *D* is incorrect.

74. D: Itching and the development of a rash are signs that the patient is having an allergic reaction to a medication. These two symptoms are signs that the body's inflammatory response has been kicked into overdrive because of a drug allergy. The other symptoms listed are not commonly associated with an allergic reaction.

75. A: *Parenteral* is the term that refers to any route outside of the gastrointestinal tract, also referred to as the *alimentary canal*. *Motor* is not a viable answer choice. *Enteral* also refers to the GI tract or intestines. *Buccal* refers to the cheeks, or inner oral cavity.

76. D: Paxlovid is best used in patients who have risk factors for severe disease, such as a weakened immune system, chronic diseases, and/or are elderly. As an older man with Stage I colon cancer, Eli likely has a weak immune system and would be at high risk of developing severe complications from COVID-19. He does not have any contraindications for the medications, as the other patients listed do. Tony is too young, as the medication is indicated for use in patients who are twelve or older. Choice *A* can be eliminated. Patients with any kind of liver dysfunction or disease should not take Paxlovid due to one of its active pharmaceutical ingredients, which specifically works by suppressing liver enzymes. Patients who already have weakened livers are likely to have significant adverse effects from Paxlovid. Therefore, Choice *B* can be eliminated. This medication should also not be used in pregnant women, so Susan would not be a good candidate. Choice *D* can be eliminated.

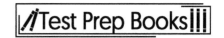

77. A, B, D, E: Parkinson's disease is a disorder of the nervous system that negatively affects movement and speech. Tai chi, formal speech therapy, massage, and yoga have all been studied in patients with Parkinson's disease and have shown to support improvement of symptoms or slow the progression of symptoms. Coenzyme Q10 supplementation is hypothesized to support a person's energy and movement; however, clinical trials have not shown significant findings that would support including this as an evidence-based, non-drug therapy for patients with Parkinson's disease.

78. C: Medication reconciliation is the practice of systematically reviewing a patient's medication list in order to reduce and eliminate medication errors. Medication errors can be costly and harmful to patient health. Medication reconciliation is best performed at transition of care, such as if a patient moves facilities (e.g., switching pharmacies). cGMP, or Current Good Manufacturing Processes, refer to quality standards that pertain to how drugs are developed, manufactured, stored, transported, and dispensed. Facilities and distributors that meet these stringent standards can become cGMP certified. This does not pertain to the pharmacist's interaction with Radhika, so Choice *A* can be eliminated. New patient intake in a pharmacy primarily involves collecting patient demographic information, allergies, and other identifying information. It is typically used to enter a patient into a medical facility's patient record system, and does not typically include in-depth information gathering and review of the patient's current medication list. Therefore, Choice *B* can is not the best option and can be eliminated. There is no indication that the pharmacist is disposing of medication for Radhika, so Choice *D* can be eliminated.

79. B: Antonio noticed that a patient in the facility appeared visibly ill and in need of immediate attention. He was able to triage, or prioritize, her care based on need and expedite her care to the emergency room, where she could get the diagnosis and care she needed. If the patient did not seek additional care or if she waited to see her primary care provider, her condition could have significantly progressed. Antonio did not review the patient's full medication list for duplicate, expired, or contraindicated medications, so Choice *A* can be eliminated. He did not change the dosing of any of her medications, so Choice *C* can be eliminated. Refer-to-pharmacy is a new electronic method of referring patients in emergency and hospital settings remotely to a connected pharmacy so that medication dispensation, reconciliation, and counseling can be performed in a more efficient manner. However, Antonio is referring the patient to the hospital and not vice versa, so Choice *D* can be eliminated.

Performing Calculations

1. 102.2°F: To convert Celsius degrees to Fahrenheit, the temperate should initially be multiplied by the standard number of 1.8:

$$39°C \times 1.8 = 70.2$$

The result should then be added to the standard number of 32:

$$70.2 + 32 = 102.2°F$$

2. 5 milliliters: The ordered dose is in micrograms. The available dose is in milligrams. The ordered dose needs to be converted to milligrams: 1 mg = 1,000 mcg. The ordered dose is 0.09 mg:

$$\frac{90 \text{ mcg}}{1,000} = 0.09 \text{ mg}$$

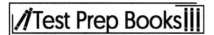

For every milliliter, there are 0.06 mg of medication. The ordered dose needs to be divided by the available dose to find out the volume.

$$\frac{0.09 \text{ mg}}{0.06 \text{ mg}} = 1.5 \text{ ml}$$

The order is to administer this medication three times a day. TID means three times a day. The total volume in one day is 4.5 ml (1.5 ml × 3 = 4.5 ml). The question asks to round to the nearest whole number, and 4.5 ml rounds to 5 ml.

3. B: The ordered dose is 0.3 mg/kg. The patient's weight needs to be converted to kilograms: 1 kg = 2.2 lb. The patient weighs 84 kilograms (185 lbs/2.2 = 84.0 kg). The weight needs to be multiplied by 0.3 mg to find the total milligrams per dose:

$$0.3 \text{ mg} \times 84 \text{ kg} = 25.2 \text{ mg}$$

The answer, 25.2 mg, rounds to 25 mg.

4. 2.3 milliliters: The patient's weight needs to be converted to kilograms to find the daily dose: 1 kg = 2.2 lbs. The patient weighs 25 kg:

$$\frac{55 \text{ lbs}}{2.2} = 25 \text{ kg}$$

Based on the order, the daily dose is 37.5 mg (1.5 mg × 25 kg = 37.5 mg). The order reads to divide the daily dose into two doses. The patient will receive 18.75 mg per dose:

$$\frac{37.5 \text{ mg}}{2} = 18.75 \text{ mg}$$

For every 5 ml of medication, the supplied dose is 40 mg. According to dimensional analysis, the number of milligrams per dose needs to be multiplied by 5 ml and divided by 40 mg. The patient will receive 2.34 ml per dose:

$$\frac{18.75 \text{ mg} \times 5 \text{ ml}}{40 \text{ mg}} = 2.34 \text{ ml}$$

The question asks to round to the nearest tenth, and 2.34 ml rounds to 2.3 ml.

5. 0.1 milliliters: The ordered dose needs to be converted into milligrams: 1 mg = 1,000 mcg. Then the ordered dose needs to be divided by 1,000. The patient will receive 0.2 mg of medication per dose.

$$\frac{200 \text{ mcg}}{1,000 \text{ mcg}} = 0.2 \text{ mg}$$

For each milliliter, the available dose is 2 mg. Therefore, the ordered dose needs to be divided by the supplied dose to find the volume (0.2 mg/2 mg = 0.1 ml).

6. 3 milliliters: The patient's weight needs to be converted to kilograms to figure out the daily dose (1 kg = 2.2 lbs). The patient weighs 12.2 kg. To figure out the total dose per day, the patient's weight needs to be multiplied by twenty-five. The patient will receive 305 mg of medication in one day.

142

$$12.2 \text{ kg} \times 25 \text{ mg} = 305 \text{ mg}$$

For every milliliter, the dose of medication is 100 mg. The ordered dose needs to be divided by the available dose to find the total milliliters per day (305 mg/100 mg = 3.05 ml). The question asks to round to the nearest whole number, and 3.05 ml rounds to 3 ml.

7. A: The available medication needs to be converted to milliliters (1 tsp = 5 ml). For every 5 milliliters, the dose contains 500 mg. The ordered dose is 200 mg. According to dimensional analysis, the ordered dose needs to be multiplied by the supplied volume and divided by the supplied dose. For every dose, the patient will receive 2 milliliters:

$$\frac{200 \text{ mg} \times 5 \text{ ml}}{500 \text{ mg}} = 2 \text{ ml}$$

The medication is ordered BID, which means twice a day. The patient will receive 4 milliliters a day:

$$2 \text{ ml} \times 2 = 4 \text{ ml}$$

8. 38.4 °C: To find the patient's temperature in degrees Celsius, the standard factor of thirty-two should be subtracted from the temperature in degrees Fahrenheit (101.2 − 32 = 69.2). The result should be divided by the standard factor of 1.8 to find the temperature in degrees Celsius:

$$\frac{69.2}{1.8} = 38.44$$

The question asks to provide the result to the nearest tenth, and 38.44 rounds to 38.4.

9. 30 milliliters: The medication is to be given three times a day; TID means every 8 hours. The patient will receive a total of 750 mg in a 24-hour period:

$$250 \text{ mg} \times 3 = 750 \text{ mg}$$

The supplied dose is 125 mg for every 5 milliliters. To find how many milligrams are available per milliliter, the dose needs to be divided by the volume. There are 25 mg for every 1 ml:

$$\frac{125 \text{ mg}}{5 \text{ ml}} = 25 \text{ mg}$$

The daily dose needs to be divided by 25 mg to find the total volume:

$$\frac{750 \text{ mg}}{25 \text{ mg}} = 30 \text{ ml}$$

10. D: The supplied dose is 100 mg for every 2 milliliters. To find the total dose per milliliter, the supplied dose needs to be divided by the supplied volume. Each milliliter contains 50 mg of medication:

$$\frac{100 \text{ mg}}{2} = 50 \text{ mg}$$

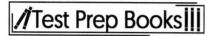

The ordered dose is 40 mg. To find the total volume per dose, the ordered dose needs to be divided by the supplied dose:

$$\frac{40 \text{ mg}}{50 \text{ mg}} = 0.8 \text{ ml}$$

The question asks you to round to the nearest tenth, and 0.8 ml remains as 0.8 ml. The frequency is not relevant to the question.

11. 400 mL: The total milliliters required to fill this medication order is 400 mL; 20 mL is required with every dose. The patient will take 4 doses a day (20 mL × 4 = 80 mL) for 5 days (80 mL × 5 = 400 mL).

12. 0.4 mL: The volume of medication that is required for every injection will be 0.4 mL. The concentration of medication is 5 mg/mL. For every 1 mL of volume, the patient would receive 5 mg of the medication. The ordered dose is 2 mg; 2 mg would have to be divided into 5 mg to obtain the correct volume of medication (2 ÷ 5 = 0.4).

13. 2.5 mL: The vial is dispensed in micrograms; 1,000 mcg = 1 g. The order is for 0.5 mg, which equals 500 mcg. The concentration of medication is 200 mcg/mL. With each milliliter, the patient would receive 200 mcg of medication; 200 mcg should be divided into 500 mcg to obtain the correct volume (200 ÷ 500 = 2.5).

14. B: The patient's weight needs to be converted to kilograms; 2.2 kg = 1 lb. The patient weighs 79.5 kg (175 ÷ 2.2 = 79.5). The question specifies to round to the nearest whole number; 79.5 rounds up to 80. The order is for 1 mg/kg per dose to be administered every 12 hours. With each dose, the patient should receive 80 mg (1 × 80 = 80).

15. 0.6 mL: The patient will need to receive 0.6 mL of medication with each dose. With each milliliter, the patient would receive 4 mg of medication. The ordered dose is 2.5 mg. To find out how many milliliters are required, 2.5 mg would need to be divided into 4 mg (2.5 ÷ 4 = 0.6 mL).

16. 420 mg: The patient will receive a total of 420 mg per dose. The patient's weight needs to be converted to kilograms; 2.2 kg = 1 lb. The patient weighs 35 kg (77 lb ÷ 2.2 = 35 kg). The dose calls for 12 mg for every kilogram of weight. The patient's weight in kilograms needs to be multiplied by 12 to obtain the total dose:

$$12 \text{ mg} \times 35 = 420 \text{ mg}$$

17. 56 mL: The pharmacist will need to dispense 56 mL of medication to cover the dose over a period of 1 week. To determine how many milliliters the patient will require in 1 day, the concentration can be further broken down into 1-mL doses. For every 1 mL of medication, the patient would receive 25 mg of medication:

$$125 \text{ mg} \div 5 \text{ mL} = 25 \text{ mg/mL}$$

The patient requires 200 mg of medication per day. To determine the volume, 200 mg will be divided by 25 (200 mg ÷ 25 mg = 8 mL). The patient requires 8 mL of medication per day. For a week's supply, the daily milliliters need to be multiplied by 7 days:

$$8 \text{ mL} \times 7 \text{ days} = 56 \text{ mL}$$

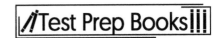

18. 1770: The patient is a male. To find the amount of calories burned in a 24 hour period, the standard formula $66 + ((6.23 \times \text{weight in pounds}) + (12.7 \times \text{height in inches}) - (6.8 \times \text{age in years}))$ is used. The weight is multiplied by the standard factor of 6.23: $6.23 \times 180 \text{ lbs} = 1121.4$. The height in inches is multiplied by the standard factor of 12.7:

$$12.7 \times 71 \text{ in} = 902.41$$

The age is multiplied by the standard factor of 6.8:

$$6.8 \times 47 \text{ yrs} = 319.6$$

The results from the height and weight are added together: $1121.4 + 902.41 = 2023.81$. The result from the age formula is subtracted from the added result: $2023.81 - 319.6 = 1704.21$. This result is added to the standard factor of 66: $66 + 1704.21 = 1770.21$. Rounded to the nearest whole number, 1770.21 is 1770. The final formula is:

$$66 + ((6.23 \times 180) + (12.7 \times 71)0 - (6.8 \times 47))$$

19. C: The patient will receive 2 doses of the medication throughout the chemotherapy session (30 minutes before and 4 hours after). To figure out how many milligrams will be administered per dose, the patient's weight needs to be converted to kilograms (1 lb = 2.2 kg). The patient weighs 50 kg (110 lb ÷ 2.2 kg = 50 kg). The patient will receive 7.5 mg of medication per dose (0.15 mg × 50 kg = 7.5 mg). To find out how many total milligrams the patient will receive in the session, the dose should be multiplied by 2:

$$7.5 \text{ mg} \times 2 \text{ doses} = 15 \text{ mg}$$

20. 2.5 mL: To find the total volume of medication to be administered per dose, micrograms needs to be converted to milligrams; 1000 mcg = 1 mg. For every milliliter in the vial, the dosage is 0.2 mg:

$$200 \text{ mcg} \div 1,000 \text{ mcg} = 0.2 \text{ mg}$$

To find the total volume required to fulfill the order, the dosage per millimeter should be divided into the ordered dose:

$$0.5 \text{ mg} \div 0.2 \text{ mg} = 2.5 \text{ mL}$$

21. 1.5 mL: For every milliliter, the patient will receive 0.5 mg of medication. The order is for 0.25 mg per dose. To determine how many milliliters per dose are required, the available medication needs to be divided into the ordered dose. The patient will receive 0.5 mL per dose (0.25 mg ÷ 0.5 mg = 0.5 mL). To determine how many milliliters the patient will receive in 1 day, the volume per dose needs to be multiplied by 3. TID means 3 times a day. The patient will receive 1.5 mL in 1 day:

$$0.5 \text{ mL} \times 3 = 1.5 \text{ mL}$$

22. 40 mg: To find out how many milligrams the patient will take in 1 day, the patient's weight needs to be converted to kilograms; 2.2 kg = 1 lb. The patient weighs 53.1 kg (117 lb ÷ 2.2 kg = 53.1 kg). The patient's weight needs to be multiplied by the ordered dose to determine how many milligrams they will take in 1 day. The patient will take 159.3 mg of medication in 1 day:

$$53.1 \text{ kg} \times 3 \text{ mg} = 159.3 \text{ mg}$$

145

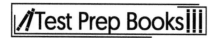

To determine how many milligrams the patient will take in 1 dose, the total dosage should be divided by the 4 ordered doses (159.3 mg ÷ 4 = 39.8 mg); 39.8 mg rounds to 40. The patient will take 40 mg per dose.

23. 735 mg: To find out how many milligrams of medication the patient will receive per dose, the weight needs to be converted to kilograms; 1 lb = 2.2 kg. The patient weighs 24.5 kg (54 lb ÷ 2.2 kg = 24.5 kg). The ordered dose is 15 g per kilogram. The patient will take 367.5 mg of medication per dose (15 mg × 24.5 kg = 367.5 mg). To find out how many milligrams the patient will receive per day, the dose needs to be multiplied by 2. BID means twice a day. The patient will receive 735 mg a day:

$$367.5 \text{ mg} \times 2 = 735 \text{ mg}$$

The length of treatment is not relevant to the question.

24. 1339: The patient is a female. To find the amount of calories burned in a 24 hour period, the standard formula 655 + ((4.35 × weight in pounds) + (4.7 × height in inches) − (4.7 × age in years)) is used. The weight is multiplied by the standard factor of 4.35: 4.35 × 140 lbs = 609. The height in inches is multiplied by the standard factor of 4.7: 4.7 × 66 in = 310.2. The age is multiplied by the standard factor of 4.7: 4.7 × 50 yrs = 235. The results from the height and weight are added together: 609 + 310.2 = 919.2. The result from the age formula is subtracted from the added result: 919.2 − 235 = 684.2. This result is added to the standard factor of 655: 655 + 684.2 = 1339.2. 1339.2 rounded to the nearest whole number is 1339. The final formula is:

$$655 + ((4.35 \times 140) + (4.7 \times 66) - (4.7 \times 50))$$

25. 2713 calories: Standard factors are assigned to different activity levels. For a moderately active lifestyle, the standard factor is 1.55. The BMR is multiplied by 1.55 to find the daily caloric need: 1.55 × 1750 = 2712.5 calories. 2712.5 rounded to the nearest whole number is 2713.

26. A: Infusion pumps are equipped to deliver medication in milliliters per hour. The first step is to find how many milligrams are available in each milliliter of solution. The supplied dose is 50 mg/100 mL. There are 0.5 milligrams of medication in each milliliter of solution: 50 ÷ 100 = 0.5. The ordered dose is 100 milligrams per hour. The ordered dose needs to be divided by the supplied dose to find the rate of administration: 100 ÷ 0.5 = 200. Rounded to the nearest whole number, 200 remains 200 mL/hr.

27. 63 mL/hr: Infusion pumps are set to deliver volume in milliliters per hour. To determine the number of cans needed in 24 hours, the patient's daily caloric need is divided by the supplied calories per container: 1800 ÷ 300 = 6. The patient will require 6 cans daily. Every can provides 250 milliliters of volume. To determine the total volume required in a 24 hour period, the number of cans per day is multiplied by the volume per can: 250 × 6 = 1500. The patient will require 1500 milliliters in 24 hours. To determine the infusion rate, the total volume is divided by 24 hours: 1500 ÷ 24 = 62.5. The rate is 62.5 mL/hr. 62.5 rounded to the nearest whole number is 63.

28. 33,162 units: To find how many units the patient will receive every hour, the weight is first converted to kilograms. 1 kg = 2.2 lbs. The patient weighs 86.36 kilograms: 190 ÷ 2.2 = 86.36. To find the total units per hour, the weight is multiplied by the ordered dose: 16 × 86.36 = 1381.76. The patient will receive 1381.76 units per hour. To find how many units the patient will receive in a day, the total dose per hour is multiplied by 24:

$$24 \times 1381.76 = 33,162.24$$

146

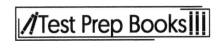

The patient will receive 33,162.24 units per day. 33,162.24 rounded to the nearest whole number is 33,162 units.

29. 66.7 mL/hr: Infusion rates are set to deliver medications in milliliters per hour. The supplied dose is 150 mg/50 mL. To find how many milligrams are available in each milliliter of solution, the available dose is divided by the available volume: $150 \div 50 = 3$. There are 3 milligrams of medication in each milliliter of solution. The ordered dose is 200 milligrams. The ordered dose is divided by the supplied dose to find the rate of administration: $200 \div 3 = 66.66$. 66.66 rounded to the nearest tenth is 66.7.

30. A: Peripheral parenteral nutrition (PPN) is a short-term administration of nutrition through a short catheter placed in a peripheral vein. The catheter length is no longer than 2 inches. This type of nutrition is used for patients who require small concentrations of fat, proteins, and carbohydrates. The area in the neck is used as a central line access. The internal jugular is considered a central venous access site and is used for total parenteral nutrition (TPN). Central veins have a wider diameter and can accommodate a higher concentration of nutrients. The area in the clavicle is also used for TPN. The subclavian vein is wide enough to absorb lipids. The area in the groin is the femoral vein. Femoral vein access is used during cardiac arrest to administer vasopressors. It is also used for patients receiving dialysis treatment.

31. 31 mL/hr: The first step is to ensure all units match. The ordered dose is in milligrams. The supplied dose is in grams. The supplied dose needs to be converted to milligrams. 1 gm = 1000 mg. The supplied dose is 1000 mg/250 mL. To find how many milligrams are in each milliliter of solution, the supplied dose is divided by the supplied volume: $1000 \div 250 = 4$. There are 4 milligrams of medication in each milliliter of solution. The ordered dose is 125 milligrams every hour. To find how many milliliters should be infused every hour, the ordered dose is divided by the milligrams in each milliliter: $125 \div 4 = 31.25$. The rate should be set at 31.25 mL/hr. Rounded to the nearest whole number, 31.25 is 31 mL/hr.

32. 4.5 milligrams: The pharmacist first needs to find how many hours it will take to infuse 30 milligrams. The rate of infusion is 15 milliliters every hour. The supplied dose is 100 milliliters. It will take 6.66 hours to infuse the supplied dose of 30 mg: $100 \div 15 = 6.66$. To find how many milligrams are being infused every hour, the supplied dose is divided by the number of hours it will take to infuse the total volume: $30 \div 6.66 = 4.50$. The patient is receiving 4.50 milligrams every hour. Rounded to the nearest tenth, 4.50 is 4.5 milligrams.

Compounding, Dispensing, or Administering Drugs or Managing Delivery Systems

1. 2 teaspoons: The patient will receive 200 mg of medication with every dose ($600 \text{ mg} \div 3 = 200 \text{ mg}$). For every 5 mL, the medication contains 100 mcg. In order to receive the accurate dose, the patient would need to take 10 mL of the medication ($100 \text{ mg} \div 5 \text{ mL} = 200 \text{ mg} \div 10 \text{ mL}$); 1 teaspoon is equivalent to 5 mL. The parents would need to administer 2 teaspoons to deliver the accurate dose:

$$5 \text{ mL} \times 2 \text{ teaspoons} = 10 \text{ mL}$$

2. C: Cimetidine (Tagamet) is a histamine H2 antagonist that treats and prevents gastric and duodenal ulcers. It reduces gastric secretion in the stomach and helps heal ulcerations. Constipation is one of the side effects of Tagamet. Increasing fiber in the diet to bulk up stool and prevent constipation is encouraged. Choice *A* is not correct. Medication should be taken as directed for the entire course of therapy; taking the medication only when symptoms are present will not prevent ulcerations. Choice *B* is

147

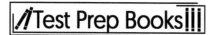

incorrect because Tagamet should be administered with meals to prevent heartburn from food or beverages. Choice *D* is not correct because nonsteroidal anti-inflammatory medications such as aspirin can cause gastric bleeding and worsen the existing ulcerations.

3. A: Ipratroprium is an anticholinergic drug that blocks the action of acetylcholine. Acetylcholine causes bronchoconstriction. Ipratroprium dilates the bronchial airways and improves pulmonary function. In order for the medication to reach the most distal airways, patients should hold their breath for at least 10 seconds to exert maximum effect. Choice *B* is incorrect because inhalers should be shaken well immediately before use to disperse the medication evenly. Choice *C* is not correct; patients should be instructed to inhale slowly over a period of 3 to 5 seconds to absorb the medication appropriately. Choice *D* is incorrect; patients should be instructed to wait 3 to 5 minutes before taking another inhalation of the medication to allow for proper inhalation of each dose.

4. B: Oxymetazolin (Afrin) is a medication used for the treatment of nasal decongestion. It shrinks blood vessels to decrease stuffy nose in patients who have allergies or a common cold. The medication is administered intranasally.

5. 28 tablets: The number of tablets required to fulfill the total dose is 28. Each tablet is 250 mg. To find out how many tablets are required per dose, the dose should be divided by the availability (500 mg ÷ 250 mg = 2 tablets). To determine how many tablets the patient will take in 1 day, the tablets per dose need to be multiplied by the frequency. BID = twice a day = 12 hours. The total required tablets per day is 4 (2 tablets × 2 = 4 tablets). To determine the total tablets, the daily amount should be multiplied by 7 days:

$$4 \text{ tablets} \times 7 \text{ days} = 28 \text{ tablets}$$

6. C: Antifungal medications work to eliminate fungal cells that invade the normal cellular structure. Antifungal medications work by binding to plasma proteins and disrupting the membrane of fungal cells. The percentage of protein-binding determines how effectively a medication is able to disturb the structure of the fungal cells. Flucytosine (Ancobon) is primarily used in yeast infections and minimally binds to proteins. Fluconazole (Diflucan) is a broad-spectrum antifungal used to treat localized infections. It has a protein binding percentage of 11% to 12%. Voriconazole (Vfend) is used for candidiasis in the esophagus and has a protein binding percentage of 58%. Terbinafine (Lamisil) is a medication used primarily in the treatment of ringworm and has a protein binding percentage of 99%.

7. C, D, E, and F: Water-soluble vitamins are excreted from the body if an excess amount is ingested. They are not stored in the body for later use. Folic acid is essential for growth and metabolism of all body cells. Vitamin B_{12} is essential for the formation of red blood cells and metabolism of proteins, fats, and carbohydrates. Vitamin B_5 allows energy to be released from carbohydrates and synthesizes cholesterol. Niacin helps maintain the integrity of the nervous system, digestive tract, and integumentary system. Choices *A* and *B* are fat-soluble vitamins. Fat-soluble vitamins are absorbed from the intestine in the presence of bile salts. Excess doses can accumulate and cause toxicity. Vitamin K is essential for blood clotting and helps activate clotting factors. Vitamin A is required for normal vision and development of bone growth.

8. D: NPH insulin is a modified insulin. Insoluble proteins are added to prolong its drug action. Agitating or rolling the vial between the hands will prevent settling of the particles. Choice *A* is not correct. Insulin should be administered at room temperature to avoid the risk of delayed absorption or lipodystrophy. Lipodystrophy causes atrophy of the subcutaneous tissue and delays absorption. Choice *B* is not correct.

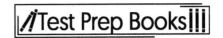

Sites should be rotated within the same anatomical landmarks. Random rotations throughout the body increase the risk of hypoglycemic effects. Choice *C* is not correct because insulin should not be stored below freezing temperatures (32 degrees Fahrenheit). Temperature extremes can decrease the potency of the medication.

9. 1 vial: To determine how many units of insulin the patient will require per day, the ordered dose should be multiplied by 3. The ordered frequency is "before meals." AC means before meals. The patient eats 3 meals per day. The patient will require 33 units of NPH insulin per day (11 units × 3 = 33 units). To find out the total dose required for dispensing, the daily dose needs to be multiplied by 30 (33 units × 30 days = 990 units). The patient requires 990 units in 30 days. Each milliliter contains 100 units of insulin. The vial has a total volume of 10 mL. There is a total of 1,000 units per vial:

$$10 \text{ mL} \times 100 \text{ units} = 1,000 \text{ units/vial}$$

The patient will have enough medication to fulfill his ordered dose with 1 vial of insulin.

10. 8 tablets. The patient will receive 3 doses of medication the day of the order. STAT = immediately. BID = twice a day. The available tablets have a concentration of 12.5 mg. For the STAT order, the patient will receive 4 tablets (50 mg ÷ 12.5 mg = 4 tablets). For each remaining dose, the patient will receive 2 tablets (25 mg ÷ 12.5 mg = 2). The patient will receive 2 doses (2 tablets × 2 = 4 tablets). The total number of tablets the day of the order is 8 (4 + 4 = 8).

11. B: The plasma half-life is defined as the time it takes for a medication's plasma concentration to reduce by half. Medications with a short half-life have a faster effect but remain in the bloodstream a shorter period of time. Alternatively, medications with a longer half-life take more time to work but remain in the bloodstream for longer periods of time. Penicillin-G is an antibiotic used to treat bacterial infections. It has a short half-life of 30 minutes. Aspirin is a non-steroidal anti-inflammatory drug used in the treatment of fever, pain, and swelling. It has a half-life of 4 hours. Doxycycline is an antibiotic used in the treatment of bacterial infections such as sexually transmitted diseases and respiratory infections. Doxycycline has a half-life of 20 hours. Digoxin is an antiarrhythmic used in the treatment of heart failure and dysrhythmias. It has a long half-life of 40 hours.

12. C: Formoterol (Foradil) is a bronchodilator used in the long-term treatment of asthma. Its mechanism of action is bronchodilation to allow relaxation and airflow through the respiratory passages. Formoterol is administered through a metered dose inhaler in order to reach the lungs. The first image is the oral route. Formoterol is not supplied as an oral liquid. The third image is a topical application. Formoterol works in the lungs and must be inhaled to produce its action. The last image is a syringe and needle used for intramuscular or subcutaneous administration. This is not the route used for formoterol administration.

13. 13 milliliters: The algebraic method is used to solve for compounded volumes. The following formula solves for the volume of the highest concentration of the stock dose: desired final volume × (smallest concentration available − final desired concentration) ÷ (smallest concentration available − highest concentration available). Using the information provided, the formula should be as follows: 40 mL × (2% − 3%) ÷ (2% − 3.5%). The answer to this equation is 26.6. This is the volume required of the 3.5% stock dose. To find the volume required of the 2% ointment, 26.6 needs to be subtracted from the desired volume of 40 milliliters:

$$40 \text{ mL} - 26.6 \text{ mL} = 13.4 \text{ mL}$$

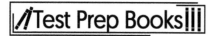

13.4 rounded to the nearest whole number is 13.

14. 0.2 milligrams: To find the total micrograms per dose, the patient's weight needs to be converted to kilograms. 1 kilogram = 2.2 pounds. The patient weighs 68.18 kg: $150 \div 2.2 = 68.18$. The patient's weight is multiplied by the ordered dose of 0.3 micrograms: $0.3 \times 68.18 = 20.45$. The patient will receive 20.45 micrograms per dose (minute). The order states the medication can be given for a maximum of 10 minutes. The amount per dose needs to be multiplied by 10 to find the maximum dose: $10 \times 20.45 = 204.5$. The maximum dose is 204.5 micrograms. The question asks for the dose in milligrams. 1 mg = 1,000 mcg. The maximum dose in milligrams is 0.20:

$$204.5 \div 1,000 = 0.20$$

0.20 milligrams rounded to the nearest tenth is 0.2 milligrams.

15. 9 milliliters: To find the total dose per day, the patient's weight is converted to kilograms. 1 kg = 2.2 lbs. The patient weighs 59.09 kilograms: $130 \div 2.2 = 59.09$. The weight is multiplied by 0.5 to find the total units per day: $0.5 \times 59.09 = 29.54$. The patient will receive 29.54 units per day. The question asks for a 30-day supply. The daily dose needs to be multiplied by 30 to find the total dose: $30 \times 29.54 = 886.2$. The patient will require 886.2 units over 30 days. The medication is supplied as 100 units/mL. To find the total volume needed, the total dose is divided by 100:

$$886.2 \div 100 = 8.86$$

The total volume required over 30 days is 8.86 milliliters. Rounded to the nearest whole number, 8.86 milliliters is 9 milliliters.

16. C: Ciprofloxacin is a first-generation fluoroquinolone used primarily in the treatment of urinary tract and intra-abdominal infections. It has a short half-life of 3–5 hours. Gemifloxacin is a second-generation fluroquinolone used in the treatment of chronic bronchitis and community acquired pneumonia. It is used as an alternative to more commonly used fluoroquinolones. Its half-life is 7 hours. Levofloxacin is a commonly used second-generation fluoroquinolone used in the treatment of various acute bacterial infections. It has a half-life of 8 hours. Moxifloxacin is a second-generation fluoroquinolone used in the treatment of skin, sinus, and respiratory bacterial infections. Its half-life is between 10–15 hours.

17. 4 tablets: The available formulation will provide 25 milligrams of medication for every milliliter of solution. To find the total milligrams in the supplied formulation, the dose/mL is multiplied by 40: $40 \times 25 = 1,000$. The suspension will include 1000 milligrams of medication. Each tablet has 250 milligrams of medication. To find the total number of tablets required for a 40 milliliter suspension, the total milligrams is divided by 250: $1,000 \div 250 = 4$. The pharmacist will require 4 tablets to create a 40 milliliter suspension. Rounded to the nearest whole number, 4 remains as 4 tablets. The patient's ordered dose is not relevant to the question in this scenario.

18. 10 milliliters: The available formulation will provide 20 milligrams of medication for every milliliter of solution. To find the total volume to be taken, the ordered dose is divided by 20:

$$200 \text{ mg} \div 20 \text{ mg} = 10 \text{ mL}$$

The patient will need to take 10 milliliters of the oral suspension with each dose. Rounded to the nearest whole number, 10 remains as 10 milliliters. Compounding the tablets into an oral suspension is irrelevant to the question being asked.

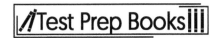

19. D: Nasoduodenal (ND) tubes are inserted through the nose and passed into the duodenum. The duodenum is the first part of the small intestine that is responsible for the absorption of fat-soluble vitamins, glucose, and minerals such as calcium and iron. Choice *A* is not correct. Nasogastric (NG) tubes are inserted through the nose and passed into the stomach. Absorption of nutrients takes place in the small intestine. The stomach secretes gastric acid that begins the digestive process. Choice *B* is not correct. A jejunostomy tube involves an invasive procedure that requires insertion of the feeding tube through the skin into the jejunum. The jejunum is the middle part of the small intestine and is responsible for absorbing proteins, amino acids, and fat. Choice *C* is incorrect. A percutaneous endoscopic gastrostomy (PEG) tube involves an invasive procedure that requires insertion of the feeding tube through the abdominal wall into the stomach. The stomach begins the digestive process. Nutrients are absorbed further down in the gastrointestinal tract.

20. B, C, D, & E: Sterile processes require maximum protection. Pharmacists should ensure that body surfaces are covered as much as possible and only sterile-gloved hands come in contact with the medication supplies. An autoclave is a container that is heated and works with very high temperatures to sterilize materials that can be reused. Hair covers are required when handling sterile products to ensure hair strands do not fall into the sterile field. Goggles are essential to ensure no eye tears come into contact with the sterile field. It also protects the pharmacist's eye membranes from noxious fumes. A face mask prevents saliva particles from falling into the sterile field and contaminating medication products. Choice *A* is incorrect. Gloves should be obtained from a sterile package. Boxed gloves are provided in bulk, remain open after initial use, and are not considered sterile.

21. 6 tablets: Every milliliter of solution will provide 30 milligrams of the medication. To find the total milligrams in the supplied formulation, the dose/mL is multiplied by 20: $20 \times 30 = 600$. The suspension will include 600 milligrams of medication. Each tablet has 100 milligrams of medication. To find the total number of tablets required for a 20 milliliter suspension, the total milligrams is divided by 100:

$$600 \div 100 = 6$$

The pharmacist will require 6 tablets to create a 20 milliliter suspension. Rounded to the nearest whole number, 6 remains as 6 tablets. The patient's medication order and the frequency are not relevant to the question.

22. A, C, E, & F: Ergotamine is an alpha-adrenergic blocker used in the treatment of vascular headaches. Ergotamine causes vasoconstriction of the dilated vessels in the area of tension. Ergotamine is 32% absorbed when administered intranasally. Intranasal administration requires a spray into the nasal cavity. Intravenous administration produces a rapid onset and lasts 8 hours in the bloodstream. The subcutaneous route has a rapid absorption and peaks within 15 minutes to 2 hours. Subcutaneous administration requires an injection into the third layer of the skin. Oral therapeutic effects can be enhanced with the concurrent administration of caffeine. The onset varies between 1–2 hours. Choices *B* and *D* are not routes of administration for ergotamine. The ophthalmic route requires drops administered into the eye. Intraosseous administration requires an injection into the bone.

23. 2 milliliters: The ordered dose is in micrograms. The supplied medication is in milligrams. The ordered dose needs to be converted to milligrams. 1 mg = 1000 mcg. The patient will need to receive 0.2 milligrams of medication:

$$200 \div 1,000 = 0.2$$

151

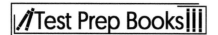

For every milliliter of medication, the supplied dose is 0.1 milligrams. The ordered dose is divided by the supplied dose to find the volume: $0.2 \div 0.1 = 2$. The patient will need to receive 2 milliliters of medication. Rounded to the nearest whole number, 2 remains as 2 milliliters.

24. 35 mL: The patient's weight (11 pounds) needs to be converted to kilograms; 2.2 kg = 1 lb (11 ÷ 2.2 = 5 kg). To determine how many milligrams the patient will require in 1 day, the weight in kilograms needs to be multiplied by 50 mg (5 kg × 50 mg = 250 mg a day). The patient requires the medication to be administered for 7 days. To determine the total number of milligrams required for the entire duration of treatment, the daily dose needs to be multiplied by 7 days (250 mg × 7 days = 1750 mg). The concentration of the medication is 50 mg/mL. To determine how many milliliters are needed, the total dose should be divided by 50:

$$1,750 \div 50 = 35 \text{ mL}$$

25. 1.2 mL: The patient will receive a total of 1.2 mL in 1 day. To find out how many milliliters the patient will receive in 1 day, the weight needs to be converted to kilograms; 2.2 kg = 1 lb. The patient weighs 12.2 kg (27 lb ÷ 2.2 kg = 12.2 kg). To find out how many total milligrams of medication the patient will receive, the weight needs to be multiplied by 5 (5 mg × 12.2 kg = 61 mg). The medication is available in 50-mg/mL vials. To find the total volume, the available dose needs to be divided into the ordered dose:

$$61 \text{ mg} \div 50 \text{ mg} = 1.22 \text{ mL}$$

The question asks to round to the nearest tenth (1.22 mL rounds down to 1.2 mL). The fact that the daily medication will be divided into 2 doses is not relevant to the question.

Developing or Managing Practice or Medication-Use Systems to Ensure Safety and Quality

1. A: Insulin lispro is a short-acting insulin that has an onset of 15 minutes and a peak of 30–90 minutes. Short-acting insulins require the patient to eat within 15 minutes of administering the medication to prevent hypoglycemic effects. Insulin administration without food can lead to diaphoresis, restlessness, and diabetic coma. Choice *B* is not correct. Short acting insulins are administered before meals to maintain adequate serum glucose levels. Long-acting insulins, such as insulin glargine, are administered at bedtime to maintain adequate glucose levels over a 24 hour period. Choice *C* is incorrect. Insulins are administered subcutaneously to enhance absorption. Choice *D* is incorrect. Insulins are administered subcutaneously at a 45–90 degree angle. A 15 degree angle is used for intradermal administration.

2. 2 tablespoons: The ordered dose is for 30 milliliters. The dose needs to be converted to a household measurement (1 tablespoon = 15 ml). The ordered dose needs to be divided by 15 to find the total number of tablespoons. The patient should be instructed to take 2 tablespoons of medication daily (30 ml/15 ml = 2).

3. B: According to the Centers for Disease Control and Prevention, the immunization schedule for childhood vaccinations recommends the first dose of the hepatitis B vaccine to be administered at birth. The administration of the first dose of the *Haemophilus influenzae* type B vaccine is recommended at 2 months of age. The influenza vaccine is recommended at 6 months of age and annually after the initial

152

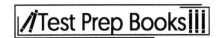

dose. The administration of the first dose of the measles-mumps-rubella (MMR) vaccine is recommended at 12 months of age.

4. C: Continuity of care is a longstanding process that involves an ongoing relationship between a patient and their providers, with shared goals to establish the most effective care. Continuity of care retains a focus on maintenance and wellbeing with cost-effective approaches in mind. The key to this relationship is longevity with health-maintenance engagements. Choice *A* signifies minimum standards, while Choice *B* and Choice *D* focus on reducing risks and improving care.

5. D: Electronic prescribing, or e-prescribing, allows physicians and other medical personnel to send prescriptions to a pharmacy electronically. This technology is quickly replacing other modes of prescription transmission such as written, faxed, or called-in prescriptions. E-prescribing has the advantage of providing the ability to transmit accurate, error free, and understandable prescriptions. As a result, it can decrease medication errors.

6. D: Using abbreviations increases the chance of errors due to misinterpretation. For example, some abbreviations are particularly risky like writing "u" for unit or adding a tailing "0" on the dosage (e.g. 1.0 mg).

7. C: Fragmentation of care occurs when the patient's case is shifted from one health care environment to another, in such a way that ambiguity over who is responsible for the patient's overall case results. This leads to errors and prolonged inaction as well as patient frustration. Continuity of care is the opposite of fragmentation of care and is the ideal. Continuity of care means the plan of care stays consistent across many different health care environments that the patient may find themselves in. Choices *B* and *D*, fluidity and division, are not terms used for these concepts.

8. A: Value-driven health care is now the operating framework for most major medical systems. The goal of a value-driven health care system is to increase positive outcomes for the patient by increasing the quality of services provided at a lower cost. Cost not only includes actual financial expenditure, but also the cost of medical errors, time spent, product waste, and so on. Ideally, quality should increase as overall cost over time decreases. Since the goal is not to have cost increase while quality decreases, Choice *B* can be eliminated. Although safety is related to quality, and revenue is related to cost, they are small parts of a bigger context when discussing value. Additionally, safety increasing is a positive outcome, but a consistent decrease in revenue could make it difficult for the medical facility to sustain itself. Therefore, Choice *C* can be eliminated. Increasing the number of providers offering services while decreasing reimbursement could also impact operations and is not widely recognized in value-driven health care. Therefore, Choice *D* can be eliminated.

9. D: The Pharmacy Quality Alliance is a national organization that has established quality standards for pharmacies and has partnered with the Centers for Medicare and Medicaid Services to increase value-driven pharmacy practices. Their standards are rigorous and focus on ensuring the continuous improvement of patient experience, safety, and outcomes. The Centers for Disease Control and Prevention focus on identifying and mitigating public health threats. They may work in partnership with pharmacies to initiate public health programs, but they do not establish pharmacy quality standards. Choice *A* can be eliminated. The Institute for Healthcare Improvement is a leading driver of continuous quality improvement in healthcare settings. They provide some recommendations for pharmacies but do not focus solely on pharmacy operations in the intensive manner performed by the Pharmacy Quality Alliance. Choice *B* can be eliminated. The federal Drug Enforcement Agency primarily specializes in criminal investigations and negligence relating to all drugs, including prescription drugs. They may audit

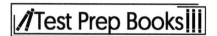

pharmacies for safety compliance and legal practices but are not a primary driver of quality standards. Choice *C* can be eliminated.

10. A, D, E: Continuity of care refers to a patient-centric approach where the patient's health care team works in collaboration to ensure that the patient receives the most comprehensive, accurate, and high-quality care. Benefits of this approach include improved health equity, meaning that socioeconomic factors do not place unfair barriers to health for some patients. Continuity of care has also been shown to decrease costs over time, as patients are less likely to relapse or experience secondary health conditions that are overlooked. Patients are also more likely to adhere to their prescribed medication regimen, which also improves patient outcomes. Therefore, Choices *A*, *D*, and *E* can be selected. However, since health data is stored electronically and shared across an interdisciplinary team, there is a higher risk of a breach of personal health information. Patients are also less likely to experience readmission into a clinical setting.

11. A, B, C: Pharmacists can play an important role in public health, a field which focuses on promoting health and preventing disease in a community of people. Immunizations, health education, and health coaching all promote health, reduce illness burden, and prevent additional disease in communities. Therefore, Choices *A*, *B*, and *C* can be selected. Selling over-the-counter medications and accepting certain tax-incentivized funds do not directly impact public or community health, so Choices *D* and *E* can be eliminated.

12. C: Pharmacy informatics is the field of reviewing various parts of patient and medication data. People in this role usually have a pharmacy background and often use data sets to track trends and examine gaps. Emmie's role uses data to examine how medication is being used within her pharmacy. Lois is primarily in a teaching role, so Choice *A* can be eliminated. Although Tai is publishing information, it is health promotion information and not related to data. Choice *B* can be eliminated. Isaac is in a purely administrative role, so Choice *D* can be eliminated.

13. B: A collaborative practice agreement is a legal agreement between a provider and pharmacist that outlines specific patient care that the pharmacist can deliver. These are usually specific tasks in specific settings, and these details are outlined in the agreement. A 1099 contract is a written agreement between an organization and a self-employed person, so Choice *A* can be eliminated. A memorandum of understanding is an agreement between two parties to carry out specific transactions; however, it usually applies to business interactions (rather than health care delivery) and is non-binding. Choice *C* can be eliminated. A non-compete agreement prevents employees or contractors from competing with an entity by which they are or were employed. This does not pertain to the type of agreement outlined between providers and pharmacies, so Choice *D* can be eliminated.

14. C: In pharmaceutical terms, stewardship focuses on efforts to effectively use antibiotics and minimize their misuse to decrease antibiotic resistance. Educating pharmacists and other pharmacy staff on antibiotic prescription, new therapeutics, optimizing use, and how to educate patients is an important component of stewardship. Value-based healthcare is a framework in which health care quality and outcomes drive cost and reimbursement. This does not pertain to the case presented, so Choice *A* can be eliminated. The pharmacy staff is not focused on purchasing or selling medicine during this training, so Choice *C* can be eliminated. Scope of practice refers to what is legal and ethical for a practitioner to perform. While training and continuing education could expand and guide a provider's scope of practice, the other details provided in the case align more closely with stewardship. Consequently, Choice *D* can be eliminated.

154

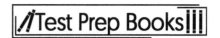

15. A: Compounding is a method in which medications are made in the pharmacy itself and are tailored for individual needs. A prescription is required; however, compounded medications can be particularly helpful for vulnerable populations, such as pediatric, elderly, injured, or immunocompromised patients. These patients are more likely to have allergies, difficulty swallowing, or other special needs that cannot necessarily be met by mass manufactured retail drugs. Compounded drugs can remove allergens, improve taste, combine multiple medications into a single dose, and customize active pharmaceutical ingredients in myriad ways that can help the patient with medication access and adherence. An ambulatory pharmacy provides medications to patients who are in transit (e.g., moving from hospital to hospice). They may or may not be part of a vulnerable population, and medication is usually not customized. Choice *B* can be eliminated. Retail pharmacy encompasses only mass manufactured pharmaceuticals, so Choice *C* can be eliminated. Pharmacology is a broad area of pharmacy that focuses on drug interactions and how a person may be affected. It does not necessarily focus on the actual manufacturing of a drug. Therefore, Choice *D* can be eliminated.

16. A: Screening initiatives are becoming more common in community pharmacies, as many pharmacists and pharmacy support staff are trained in primary care methods such as taking blood pressure, testing blood glucose levels, and collecting other metrics associated with chronic disease. Research indicates that screening initiatives in pharmacies can increase preventive screenings and support early disease detection. Screening initiatives tend to focus on chronic disease prevention, rather than acute illness. Although many pharmacies offer rapid infectious disease testing, Choice *B* can be eliminated. Since screening initiatives focus on community health, and not demographic information or patient satisfaction, Choices *C* and *D* can also be eliminated.

Practice Test #2

Obtaining, Interpreting, or Assessing Data, Medical, or Patient Information

1. How would you diagnose type 2 diabetes mellitus?
    a. One fasting blood glucose level of $\geq$ 126 mg/L
    b. An A1c value of > 7.5%
    c. Two random blood glucose levels $\geq$ 150 mg/L
    d. Two fasting blood glucose levels $\geq$ 126 mg/L

2. Which serologic test for infection detection involves coating the wells with the antigen and testing if the patient's blood contains the antibody?
    a. Enzyme immunoassay
    b. Immunofluorescent assay
    c. Complement fixation
    d. Dilution test

3. Which of the following statements is correct about troponin?
    a. Troponin is a compound injected into the patient to determine glomerular filtration rate.
    b. Troponin is a cardiac biomarker.
    c. Troponin is a diagnostic marker for acute heart failure.
    d. Troponin is a diagnostic marker for liver function.

4. A forty-year-old patient presents with behavior changes including lack of emotion, difficulty concentrating, memory lapses, and changes in mood. A PCR test and direct genetic test was conducted and tested positive for > 40 expanded CAG repeat nucleotides in the HTT gene. What disease state is most likely suspected?

5. What screening tool(s) can be used to assess cognitive function? (Select all that apply.)
    a. Montreal Cognitive Assessment (MoCA)
    b. Confusion Assessment Method (CAM)
    c. Mini-Mental State Examination (MMSE)
    d. Patient Health Questionnaire

6. A patient has been prescribed topical benzoyl peroxide for acne, but states that they have not been taking it as often as they should because the gel does not feel great on their hairy chest. Which of the following would you recommend to help with patient adherence?
    a. Tell the patient that the gel form is the best for them and recommend shaving the area.
    b. Tell the patient that benzoyl peroxide only comes in gel form, and they will need to deal with the uncomfortable feeling.
    c. Tell the patient that they can switch to a lotion form to help.
    d. Tell the patient to switch to a foam solution.

156

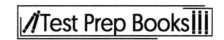

7. A patient presents to the ER; as the pharmacist, you collect their information when they arrive. They state that they are feeling like "their head is going to explode." You obtain more information regarding diet, medication history, and family history. In what section would you place diet information?
   a. Chief complaint
   b. Diet history
   c. Social history
   d. Socioeconomic background

8. While verifying a patient's new prescription for "Tramadol 120 mg: Take one tablet three times a day as needed for pain #90 tablets with zero refills," you notice they picked up the same prescription two weeks ago at another pharmacy. Both prescriptions are written from two different doctors, and both appear to be valid. What is your next action?
   a. Contact the prescriber and reverify that the prescription is valid.
   b. Nothing; both are valid prescriptions so the new one should be filled.
   c. Don't fill the prescription, but call the police.
   d. Contact the prescriber and relay the patient's medication history.

9. A patient, who appears to be homeless, has been diagnosed with uncomplicated urinary tract infection (cystitis). There are three guideline recommendations in the order of most preferred to least preferred:
       1. Bactrim: one tablet twice a day for three days
       2. Macrobid: one capsule twice a day for five days
       3. Fosfomycin: one tablet x one dose
Which of the following medications would be prescribed?
   a. Bactrim
   b. Macrobid
   c. Fosfomycin
   d. None of the above, as the patient is homeless and would not be able to afford the medication

10. You are working at a local retail pharmacy when a patient comes to pick up their medication. They state, "I really don't want to pick up this medication. It's really hard to remember taking all these pills and I already forget to take my current meds sometimes." What is your initial approach?
   a. Ask the patient why they have not been taking their medication.
   b. Demand the patient to take their medication as prescribed.
   c. Prescribe the patient a combination pill.
   d. Increase the dose to compensate for missed doses.

11. When collecting a patient's family history, what topic is most important to ask about?
   a. Past therapy regimens
   b. Medication allergies
   c. Past or current medical conditions
   d. Diet intake

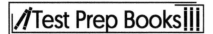

12. Isoniazid and rifapentine are commonly prescribed medications for patients with latent tuberculosis. The instructions are to take one tablet once a week for three weeks. Due to the inconsistency of a weekly medication regimen, what is the best method to ensure that your patient is adherent?
    a. Watch them take it every week.
    b. Tell them to set an alarm.
    c. Tell them to get a pill box.
    d. Tell them to keep it in their car so that they can see it every day.

13. Which of the following statements would be a chief complaint?
    a. "I'm allergic to penicillin and I get rashes and hives when I take it."
    b. "I smoke one pack a day, which may be contributing to my nauseousness."
    c. "My leg feels weird."
    d. "I am homeless."

14. A patient's family history would be important for which medication plan?
    a. Atorvastatin
    b. Warfarin
    c. Byetta
    d. Dapagliflozin

15. In a patient's medication history, what does PRN stand for?
    a. Per recommended need
    b. Postoperative nausea
    c. Pro re nata
    d. Prior refused narcotics

16. What does SOAP note stand for?

17. Which of the following lab parameters would indicate that a patient taking epoetin (Procrit) is achieving the goals of therapy? (Select all that apply.)
    a. Hematocrit, 34%
    b. Eosinophils, 3%
    c. Neutrophils, 61%
    d. Hemoglobin, 12 g/dL
    e. Red blood cells (RBCs), 5.1 million/mm^3

18. Which of the following signs correctly matches the disease state or cause?
    a. Weight loss—hyperthyroidism
    b. Increased heart rate—heart block
    c. Fatigue—amphetamine use
    d. Diarrhea—opioid abuse

19. Which of the following is a function of the liver? (Select all that apply.)
    a. Reabsorption of solutes
    b. Bile synthesis
    c. Drug metabolism
    d. Secretion of insulin

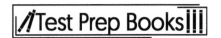

20. A patient presents with heartburn, dysphagia, and nausea. Which disease state would you most likely suspect?
    a. GERD
    b. Liver failure
    c. Heart failure
    d. Constipation

21. A family history of diabetes would have a strong correlation for developing which type of diabetes?
    a. Type 1
    b. Type 2
    c. Type 3
    d. Gestational

22. A "frequent, exaggerated TH2 response to harmless environmental allergens" describes which disease state?
    a. Chronic obstructive pulmonary disease (COPD)
    b. Allergic reaction
    c. Asthma
    d. Pulmonary embolism

23. What is the primary cause of type 1 diabetes?
    a. High blood glucose levels
    b. High sugar intake
    c. Decreased insulin production
    d. Insulin resistance

24. What is the underlying cause of rheumatoid arthritis?
    a. Genetic predisposition
    b. Wear and tear of joints
    c. Autoimmune response
    d. Infection with bacteria

25. The CHADSVASC score is used to determine the risk of what?

26. A patient presents to you with severe leg pain. Which of the following disease states would you be concerned about? (Select all that apply.)
    a. Hyperthyroidism
    b. Deep vein thrombosis
    c. Pulmonary embolism
    d. Acute kidney failure

27. Which of following statements is correct regarding the morphology of genital herpes?
    a. It is a double-stranded DNA virus.
    b. It is a gram-negative diplococcus.
    c. It is an obligate intracellular parasite.
    d. It is a single-stranded DNA virus.

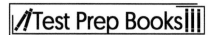

28. Which of the following signs/symptoms would you see in a patient with tuberculosis? (Select all that apply.)
    a. Night sweats
    b. Hemoptysis
    c. Weight gain
    d. Decreased WBC

29. Which of the following is NOT a risk factor for getting influenza?
    a. Pregnancy or postpartum
    b. BMI > 35
    c. Less than two years old or greater than sixty-five years old
    d. Chronic aspirin use in patients > nineteen years old

30. Which of the following is a major risk factor for aspergillosis?
    a. Travel to Africa, South Asia, or the Caribbean
    b. Unprotected intercourse
    c. Prolonged neutropenia
    d. Sarcoidosis

31. Which of the following is a risk factor for osteomyelitis? (Select all that apply.)
    a. Uncontrolled diabetes
    b. Orthopedic hardware
    c. Peripheral vascular disease
    d. Low albumin level

32. Which of the following is considered a structural risk factor for infective endocarditis?
    a. Injection drug use
    b. Healthcare exposure
    c. Poor dentition
    d. Pacemaker

33. Which catheter type has the highest risk of causing a catheter-related bloodstream infection (CRBSI)?
    a. Peripherally inserted central catheter
    b. Non-tunneled central vein catheter (CVC)
    c. Tunneled CVC
    d. Peripheral line

34. Cochlear implants, CSF shunts, community settings, and travel exposure are risk factors for which disease?
    a. Intra-abdominal infections
    b. Acute otitis media
    c. Meningitis
    d. Septic shock

35. Which of the following is a risk factor for urinary tract infections (UTI)? (Select all that apply.)
    a. Urethral catheter
    b. Menopause
    c. Diabetes mellitus
    d. Use of pilocarpine

36. Which of the following is a method of treating hypoactive sexual desire disorder (HSDD)?
    a. Oral combined hormonal contraceptives
    b. Clonidine
    c. Cognitive behavioral therapy
    d. Benzodiazepines

37. For a biologic to be classified as bioequivalent to another biologic, the 90 percent confidence interval must fall between what range?
    a. 85–130 percent
    b. 90–100 percent
    c. 80–125 percent
    d. 80–100 percent

38. Which of the following describes a Type II error?
    a. Accepting the null hypothesis and it is true
    b. Accepting the null hypothesis and it is false
    c. Rejecting the null hypothesis and it is true
    d. Rejecting the null hypothesis and it is false

39. Lexicomp is a common tool used for drug facts. It is considered to be which type of reference?
    a. Primary
    b. Secondary
    c. Tertiary
    d. Quaternary

40. A resource that is mainly in the form of searchable databases that allow for more efficient and expedient searching is which type of literature?
    a. Expert
    b. Primary
    c. Secondary
    D. Tertiary

41. Place the following types of resources in order of most reliable to least reliable: Primary, expert, secondary, tertiary.

Identifying Drug Characteristics

1. Which of the following over-the-counter heartburn relief medications is used for rapid relief of symptoms?
    a. Pepto-Bismol
    b. Famotidine
    c. Omeprazole
    d. Sodium bicarbonate

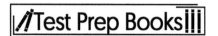

2. What class of medications is first line for constipation in most situations?

3. Which medication increases the "wetness" of the intestine and soften fecal mass?
    a. Colace
    b. PEG 3350
    c. Dulcolax
    d. Magnesium citrate

4. Which class of medications soften fecal contents by coating them, prevents absorption of water, and is not recommended for laxative use?

5. Which benign prostate hyperplasia (BPH) medication reduces prostate size?
    a. Tadalafil
    b. Finasteride
    c. Terazosin
    d. Tamsulosin

6. Which medication is first line for stress urinary incontinence?
    a. Oxybutynin
    b. Tamsulosin
    c. Dutasteride
    d. Duloxetine

7. What is the name of the calcineurin inhibitor used for renal transplants that has an adverse effect of nephrotoxicity, hyperglycemia, and alopecia?

8. What is the maximum number of doses of nitroglycerin 0.4 mg sublingual tablets that can be taken as needed for chest pain?
    a. One
    b. Two
    c. Three
    d. Four

9. What is the brand name for simethicone?
    a. Gas-X
    b. Beano
    c. Florastor
    d. Prevacid

10. Which of the following antiplatelet medications is for intravenous use only?
    a. Plavix
    b. Effient
    c. Brilinta
    d. Kengreal

11. What color can be observed when mixing dobutamine hydrochloride in 5 percent D5W?
    a. Light blue
    b. Pink
    c. Light orange
    d. Yellow

12. Which form of insulin below is supposed to be a cloudy solution?
    a. Lantus
    b. Humalog
    c. NPH
    d. Tresiba

13. Which of the following medications can NOT be placed in a polyvinylchloride (PVC) container? (Select all that apply.)
    a. Lorazepam
    b. Tacrolimus
    c. Vancomycin
    d. Nitroglycerin

14. What is the brand name of pyrimethamine?

15. Which of the following medications has a commercially available prescription and non-prescription strength option?
    a. Ibuprofen
    b. Naproxen
    c. Amlodipine
    d. Aspirin

16. Which Class III antiarrhythmic drug must be verified by the REMS program?
    a. Amiodarone
    b. Dofetilide
    c. Flecainide
    d. Propafenone

17. Which of the following is a black box warning for Depo-Provera?
    a. Causes sickle cell crisis
    b. Increases risks of seizures
    c. Can cause endometriosis
    d. Loss of bone mineral density

18. What is the maximum number of refills allowed for isotretinoin, an acne medication that requires verification through the REMS program?
    a. One
    b. Two
    c. Three
    d. None

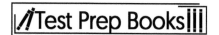

19. Which medication has a black box warning for being teratogenic and must be discontinued three years prior to trying for pregnancy?
    a. Tretinoin
    b. Tazarotene
    c. Adapalene
    d. Acitretin

20. Gray baby syndrome and a fatal blood dyscrasia black box warning are characteristics of which medication?

21. Which class of medications carry a black box warning for thyroid C-cell tumors?
    a. GLP-1 receptor agonists
    b. ACE-inhibitors
    c. Sulfonamides
    d. DPP-IV inhibitors

22. Why does Zyprexa Relprevv require a REMS program?
    a. It can induce medullary thyroid carcinoma.
    b. Is severely teratogenic.
    c. It can induce severe sedation, coma, or delirium.
    d. It can pass through milk during breastfeeding.

23. What is the first-line option for treatment of psychiatric disorders throughout pregnancy? (Select all that apply.)
    a. Paroxetine
    b. Benzodiazepine
    c. Selective serotonin reuptake inhibitors (SSRI)
    d. Tricyclic antidepressants (TCA)

24. Which anticonvulsant is NOT safe to use during breastfeeding and pregnancy?
    a. Keppra
    b. Topamax
    c. Phenytoin
    d. Depakote

25. Which cold/allergy medication CAN be used in pregnancy but CANNOT be used in breastfeeding?
    a. Loratadine
    b. Guaifenesin
    c. Pseudoephedrine
    d. Dextromethorphan

26. What is the generic name of the antidepressant used for postpartum depression that consists of a sixty-hour continuous infusion?

27. How do levothyroxine doses change in patients who become pregnant?
    a. Increase
    b. Decrease
    c. Remain the same
    d. Discontinued due to toxic effects.

28. Which medications should be avoided in pregnancy? (Select all that apply.)
    a. Warfarin
    b. Simvastatin
    c. Paroxetine
    d. Sulfasalazine

29. What is an infant at risk for developing if the mother was taking an oral corticosteroid in the first trimester?
    a. Termination
    b. Cleft lip
    c. Neural tube defects
    d. Floppy baby syndrome

30. You are working in the hospital pharmacy and receive a prescription for a Cervidil insert. Which of the following conditions is being treated?
    a. Preterm labor
    b. Cervical ripening
    c. Labor induction
    d. Group B streptococcus infection

31. What are the first line options for gestational hypertension? (Select all that apply.)
    a. Labetalol
    b. Nifedipine ER
    c. Nifedipine IR
    d. Hydrochlorothiazide

32. Which of the following antibiotics is the safest in all stages of breastfeeding?
    a. Minocycline
    b. Cephalexin
    c. Bactrim
    d. Nitrofurantoin

Developing or Managing Treatment Plans

1. JW, a fifty-year-old male, was recently admitted to the hospital for a myocardial infarction. He also has a past medical history (PMH) of type 2 diabetes mellitus (T2DM) with a hospital admission blood glucose of 340, no seasonal influenza vaccination, and uncontrolled asthma. Which of the following is the correct triage order (from first to last) that these medical conditions should be treated?
    a. Myocardial infarction, asthma, influenza vaccine, T2DM
    b. T2DM, myocardial infarction, asthma, influenza vaccine
    c. Myocardial infarction, T2DM, asthma, influenza vaccine
    d. Influenza vaccine, asthma, T2DM, myocardial infarction

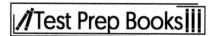

2. A patient walks into a community pharmacy and states that they have been constipated for the last twenty days, and they have not yet tried any over-the-counter (OTC) medication yet. What should the pharmacist do?
   a. Suggest polyethylene glycol 3350 to help relieve constipation.
   b. Ask the patient more questions about what led to their constipation.
   c. Suggest bisacodyl as a stool softener to help with constipation.
   d. Refer to another medical provider.

3. A patient walks into the pharmacy needing help with a cough that has not gone away after a month. He has no other symptoms, just "an annoying cough that won't go away." He has taken Sudafed for the last month. What should the pharmacist's recommendation be?
   a. Stop Sudafed and suggest dextromethorphan.
   b. Suggest Mucinex DM and to continue the Sudafed.
   c. Suggest Allegra along with the Sudafed.
   d. Refer to another medical provider.

4. A pharmacist is at an ambulatory clinic in a cardiology office. A new patient walks in with comorbid hypertension (HTN), hyperlipidemia (HLD), and nerve pain. Lab values are listed below:

Blood Pressure (BP)	160/100 mmHg
Total Cholesterol	240 mg/dL
LDL	160 mg/dL
HDL	80 mg/dL
Triglycerides	150 mg/dL

In order from first to last, which issues should they work on addressing?
   a. Hypertension, hyperlipidemia, nerve pain
   b. Hyperlipidemia, hypertension, nerve pain
   c. Nerve pain, hypertension, hyperlipidemia
   d. Whatever the patient would like to address first

5. A patient comes into the pharmacy asking for medicine to help with the pain of a two-day-old canker sore. What should be the first recommendation to help specifically with pain?
   a. Topical benzocaine 5%
   b. Ibuprofen capsules
   c. Carbamide peroxide wash
   d. Refer to another medical provider

6. Which patient should be referred to another medical provider?
   a. A sixteen-year-old patient who has impacted cerumen and signs of infection
   b. A three-year-old patient who needs treatment for ant bites
   c. A forty-five-year-old patient who has a wart, a six-month history of recurring warts, and has not tried any treatment yet
   d. A two-month-old infant who has refused to eat for the last twenty-four hours

7. What is the primary goal of a GLP-1 (glucagon-like peptide 1) agonist in T2DM?
   a. Decrease risk of heart attack
   b. Increase insulin secretion
   c. Decrease body weight
   d. Decrease pancreatitis risk

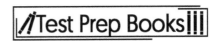

8. Which of the following is NOT a therapeutic goal for Hashimoto's disease?
   a. Restore a normal TSH between 0.4 to 4.0 µIU/mL.
   b. Provide symptomatic relief to the patient.
   c. Lower T4 levels.
   d. Avoid over-medication.

9. Which of the following that are clinical goals for a fourteen-year-old type 1 diabetes mellitus patient? (Select all that apply.)
   a. A1C under 7%
   b. A1C under 6%
   c. Pre-prandial blood glucose between 90–130 mmol/L
   d. Bedtime blood glucose between 90–150 mmol/L

10. Which of the following is a therapeutic goal outcome for community-acquired pneumonia (CAP)?
    a. Respiratory rate over 30 breaths/min
    b. WBC under 4,000 cells/µL
    c. Can breathe without mechanical ventilation
    d. Respiratory rate under 24 breaths/min

11. Which of the following is NOT a goal of therapy for osteoarthritis?
    a. Cure the patient of osteoarthritis.
    b. Maintain or improve joint mobility.
    c. Relieve pain and/or stiffness.
    d. Avoid side effects of therapy.

12. After a patient has received tPA for an ischemic stroke, which blood pressure goal should the patient be maintained at for the first twenty-four hours?
    a. Under 200/100 mmHg
    b. Under 250/105 mmHg
    c. Under 135/90 mmHg
    d. Under 180/105 mmHg

13. Which of the following is NOT a treatment goal for generalized anxiety disorder (GAD)?
    a. Improve patient's quality of life.
    b. Treat comorbid disorders.
    c. Cure the patient of generalized anxiety disorder.
    d. Reduce the symptoms of generalized anxiety disorder.

14. Which medication would be considered a duplication of therapy in a patient also taking budesonide?
    a. Fluticasone
    b. Salmeterol
    c. Umeclidinium
    d. Albuterol

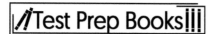

15. Which of the following medications would be considered a duplication of therapy if the patient is taking sertraline? (Select all that apply.)
   a. Buspirone
   b. Ibuprofen
   c. Citalopram
   d. Sildenafil

16. Which medication is used off-label to treat narcolepsy, or excessive daytime sleepiness (EDS)?
   a. Xywav
   b. Ritalin
   c. Provigil
   d. Strattera

17. Which patient has the most appropriate FDA approved use for semaglutide, specifically Ozempic?
   a. MJ, a sixty-year-old patient with a BMI of 35 kg/m2 who is looking for a weight loss option
   b. HF, a fifteen-year-old patient with a BMI of 40 kg/m2 who is looking to lose weight from hypothyroidism
   c. MC, a forty-five-year-old patient with a BMI of 30 kg/m2 and an average fasting blood glucose of 250 mg/dL
   d. KR, a fifty-five-year-old patient with a BMI of 20 kg/m2, a PMH of T2DM for the last 20 years, and an average fasting blood glucose of 150 mg/dL

18. Several different patients come up to the pharmacist to ask about medication interactions. Which patients would benefit most from a medication reconciliation? (Select all that apply.)
   a. A patient who takes a multivitamin daily and is now taking OTC medication for a cold
   b. A patient taking four prescription medications daily and is now picking up two more daily medications
   c. A caregiver picking up their eighty-five-year-old mom's monthly prescription medications, which include twelve different medications
   d. A nurse picking up her own medications for a new chronic condition

19. An intern is now ready to do their own medication reconciliations, and this is their first one to do solo. Before the intern gives their recommendations, the pharmacist is reviewing all the information that the intern collected from the patient.

   PQ, a sixty-five-year-old female, has a PMH of T2DM, hyperlipidemia, gout, and diabetic neuropathy. The patient currently takes atorvastatin 20 mg once daily, allopurinol 400 mg daily, gabapentin 300 mg three times daily, semaglutide injection 0.5 mg once weekly, ibuprofen 800 mg three times daily, and metformin 1 g twice daily. She reports that her nerve pain has not improved since starting the gabapentin. She also says her gout flare-ups have reduced to once a year. She has noticed a new loss of appetite and is concerned she has an infection. She has never smoked, drinks one glass of wine a week, and is up-to-date on all her current vaccines.
What other questions should the intern have asked? (Select all that apply.)
   a. How long have you had each condition?
   b. Do you take any OTC medications, vitamins, or supplements?
   c. How adherent are you to taking these medications?
   d. When did you start taking each medication?

168

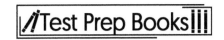

20. Which medications do NOT match their FDA-labeled indication? (Select all that apply.)
    a. Ciprofloxacin, COVID-19 infection
    b. Fluoxetine, generalized anxiety disorder
    c. Diclofenac sodium, hip strain
    d. Adapalene, acne vulgaris

21. Using the table below for vancomycin dosing with specific CrCl (creatinine clearance), what is the best loading dose for a fifty-nine-year-old male who has Stage 2 chronic kidney disease (CKD)?

CrCl (mL/minute)	Suggested loading dose	Suggested initial maintenance dose	Suggested dosing interval
Over 90	25 to 30 mg/kg	15 to 20 mg/kg	8 to 12 hours
50 to 90	20 to 25 mg/kg	15 to 20 mg/kg	12 hours
15 to 50	20 to 25 mg/kg	10 to 15 mg/kg	24 hours
Less than 15	20 to 25 mg/kg	10 to 15 mg/kg	48 to 72 hours

    a. 10 to 15 mg/kg
    b. 15 to 20 mg/kg
    c. 20 to 25 mg/kg
    d. 25 to 30 mg/kg

22. Which medication does NOT require dose adjustment for impaired renal function?
    a. Ciprofloxacin
    b. Gabapentin
    c. Acyclovir
    d. Guaifenesin

23. How long should an acute urinary tract infection be treated in a woman who is six months pregnant?
    a. Three days
    b. Five days
    c. Seven days
    d. Fourteen days

24. If a patient is on probenecid for gout prophylaxis, how long will the patient be on this medication?
    a. Two weeks after a gout attack
    b. Until serum urate level is under 6 mg/dL
    c. For two years after the last gout attack
    d. Indefinitely

25. Why do most renally excreted medications need adjustment?
    a. Accelerated renal function can cause quicker elimination of renally excreted drugs.
    b. Some medications rely on the kidneys to excrete them, and, with slower kidney function, drugs will accumulate, leading to toxicity.
    c. In patients with chronic kidney disease, protein binding increases, leading the patient to need an increase in doses of renally excreted drugs.
    d. The pH of the body decreases and breaks down the medications before they even reach the kidney.

169

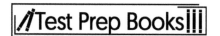

26. A patient has been recently diagnosed with HIV and has a CD4 count of 35. What is the medication and correct dose for prophylaxis for pneumocystis jirovecii pneumonia (PJP)? Select the only first-line treatment mentioned.
   a. One Bactrim double-strength tablet daily
   b. Dapsone 50 mg twice daily
   c. Augmentin 500 mg every 12 hours
   d. No prophylaxis needed

27. A type 1 diabetic patient weighs 40 kg and needs to start an insulin regimen. Which regimen would be appropriate?
   a. 5 units in the morning, 5 units at night, 1 unit before each meal
   b. 10 units in the morning, 10 units at night, 10 units before each meal
   c. 5 units in the morning, 5 units at night, 4 units before each meal
   d. 10 units in the morning, 10 units at night, 5 units before each meal

28. Which antidepressant is a nasal spray?
   a. Cymbalta
   b. Spravato
   c. Rexulti
   d. Prozac

29. An MMR vaccine needs to be administered. Which answer corresponds to where in the arm the vaccine should be administered?
   a. Epidermis
   b. Dermis
   c. Subcutaneous tissue
   d. Muscle

30. Which of these osteoporosis medications are injectable? (Select all that apply.)
   a. Ibandronate
   b. Denosumab
   c. Raloxifene
   d. Teriparatide

31. An eighty-year-old patient comes into an ambulatory clinic for joint pain management. Prior medical history includes hypertension, heart failure, and severe GERD. What would be the best option for them?
   a. Diclofenac sodium cream
   b. Ibuprofen capsules
   c. Liquid acetaminophen
   d. Fentanyl sublingual tablet

32. A mother comes in looking for an allergy medication for her son with autism. His symptoms include sensory processing issues with tastes and swallowing. What option should be recommended?
   a. Dissolvable cetirizine
   b. Liquid diphenhydramine
   c. Nasal spray oxymetazoline
   d. Liquid fexofenadine with grape flavoring added in

170

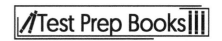

33. A newly diagnosed patient with Crohn's Disease has a past medical history of chronic constipation, glaucoma, and osteoporosis. Which of the following vitamin deficiencies is common in more than just Crohn's, and what route of administration should that supplement be taken?
    a. Vitamin B12, sublingual
    b. Vitamin C, topical
    c. Vitamin D, sublingual
    d. Vitamin K, topical

34. Which of these instructions are NOT correct for administering eye drops?
    a. Wash your hands before using eye drops.
    b. After putting the drops in, put pressure on the inside corner of your eye for one to two minutes.
    c. Tilt your head back to get the best angle for the drops to get into the eye.
    d. Make sure the tip of the container is touching the eye to ensure the drops get in the eye.

35. A patient comes in to fill a prescription from their cardiologist for nitroglycerin for angina. Which other disease state would warrant further questions to make sure the new prescription is not contraindicated in this patient?
    a. Pulmonary arterial hypertension
    b. Heart failure with preserved ejection fraction
    c. Asthma
    d. Generalized anxiety disorder

36. Which of the following antibiotics is a common allergen to patients?
    a. Gentamicin
    b. Metronidazole
    c. Clarithromycin
    d. Amoxicillin

37. Which of the following medications used to treat chronic migraines have a common adverse effect of dizziness? (Select all that apply.)
    a. Amitriptyline
    b. Ubrogepant
    c. Sumatriptan
    d. Butalbital

38. Hydroxyurea is a medication given to treat severe sickle cell disease in patients to decrease crises. What medication should NOT be given while a patient is on hydroxyurea?
    a. Varicella vaccine
    b. Pneumococcal vaccine
    c. Cardizem
    d. Wellbutrin

39. A forty-nine-year-old woman comes in experiencing severe hot flashes despite non-pharmacological therapy. She has a past medical history of a gravidity of 4 and a parity of 3, along with polycystic ovarian syndrome. Which medication would be her best option?
    a. Premarin
    b. Minivelle
    c. Estring
    d. Prefest

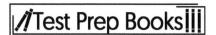

40. Which of the following can cause or worsen tachyarrhythmias? (Select all that apply.)
   a. Sotalol
   b. Ciprofloxacin
   c. Cocaine
   d. Fluconazole

41. A new medical assistant runs into the pharmacy, concerned that their patient "just turned as red as a tomato!" What is the most likely cause of this?
   a. A fever over 100 °F
   b. Vancomycin
   c. Norepinephrine
   d. Sulfamethoxazole/trimethoprim

42. A nineteen-year-old female comes into a community pharmacy and reports that she has had an increase in headaches. She is taking levocetirizine, a hormonal birth control pill (but does not remember which one), a fluticasone inhaler, and an albuterol rescue inhaler. Which medication is most likely causing the increase in headaches?
   a. Levocetirizine
   b. Hormonal birth control pill
   c. Fluticasone inhaler
   d. Albuterol inhaler

42. Which medicines have commercially available toxicology reversal medications? In other words, if someone overdoses on a medication or the effects need to be reversed, which medications can be reversed with an FDA approved medication? (Select all that apply.)
   a. Morphine
   b. Acetaminophen
   c. Apixaban
   d. Tobramycin

43. A thirty-five-year-old newly pregnant woman asks for help because she is not sure if she can stay on her current acid reflux medicine (omeprazole) now that she is pregnant. She states that she only takes it as needed, which is usually about once a month for "mild burning." Can she stay on omeprazole, and, if not, is there a better suggestion for what medication she should take?
   a. She can stay on omeprazole; it is safe in pregnancy.
   b. Recommend calcium carbonate or another antacid.
   c. Recommend bismuth subsalicylate.
   d. There is no medication that is safe for acid reflux in pregnancy; suggest non-pharmacological methods.

44. Which oncology medication does NOT match the correct adverse effect?
   a. Gemcitabine and pruritus with an allergic skin rash
   b. Paclitaxel and hypersensitivity
   c. Irinotecan and constipation
   d. Fluorouracil and cardiovascular issues

172

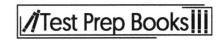

45. A patient arrives at the hospital with a rattlesnake bite. The patient's blood pressure is 80/40 mmHg, their heart rate is 180 bpm, and they are dyspneic. They have not yet received any treatment. What is the appropriate first step?
    a. Administer antivenom immediately.
    b. Discuss with the patient and the people with them the exact breed of snake to determine treatment.
    c. Treat only with fluids to treat the shock.
    d. Watch symptoms to see if antivenom and/or fluids are needed.

46. A thirty-six-year-old man is admitted unconscious to the ER. His vitals are 100/70 mmHg, 75 bpm, 96.5 °F, and 10 breaths/min. His ROS includes miotic pupils, decreased bowel sounds, and seizures. What is the most likely cause, and what should be the first step of treatment?
    a. Opioid overdose, naloxone
    b. Stroke, tPA
    c. Anxiety attack, midazolam
    d. Blood loss from a traumatic accident, blood transfusion

47. Which three drug classes are considered the renal "triple whammy"—three drugs that combined can cause worsening of renal diseases?
    a. Acetaminophen, ACE inhibitors, and calcium-channel blockers
    b. Corticosteroids, ARBs, and diuretics
    c. Non-steroidal anti-inflammatory drugs, ACE inhibitors, and diuretics
    d. Non-steroidal anti-inflammatory drugs, beta-blockers, and histamine antagonists

48. Which antiviral is a strong CYP3A4 inhibitor?
    a. Ritonavir
    b. Tenofovir
    c. Maraviroc
    d. Atazanavir

49. A pharmacist is precepting four new pharmacy students and has assigned them each to a different infectious disease case. Which student made the WORST recommendation?
    a. Student A recommended hydroxychloroquine for a malaria patient.
    b. Student B recommended oseltamivir for a mild influenza infection.
    c. Student C recommended echinocandin for a recurring candidemia infection.
    d. Student D recommended tenofovir for a hepatitis A infection.

50. A patient walks into an anticoagulant clinic and states that she heard her friend say she is taking Vitamin K with her warfarin, and she wants to know why she herself is not on Vitamin K with her warfarin. What could the pharmacist tell her?
    a. Vitamin K is given when warfarin is not doing as much as it needs to.
    b. Vitamin K is given when warfarin is working too well, and the effects need to be reversed.
    c. Vitamin K was given to her friend for something other than helping with the effect of warfarin.
    d. She was most likely taking Vitamin A instead with warfarin.

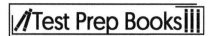

51. Which medication can interact with pseudoephedrine and worsen adverse effects?
   a. Adderall
   b. Mucinex DM
   c. Tylenol
   d. Benadryl

52. Below are common bipolar disorder medications and other medications for common comorbidities. Select all the medication pairs that are contraindicated.
   a. Lithium and lisinopril
   b. Divalproex and olopatadine
   c. Carbamazepine and ranolazine
   d. Lamotrigine and acetaminophen

53. A grandma and her five-year-old granddaughter walk into the pharmacy with a diagnosis of pediculosis and have no idea what that means nor what treatment to get. What should the recommendation be, and what disease is this?
   a. Athlete's foot, miconazole cream
   b. Lice, permethrin and a nit comb
   c. Allergic reaction rash, hydrocortisone cream 1%
   d. Dandruff, pyrithione zinc shampoo

54. A patient's labs come back unlabeled, and the pharmacist calls the lab for more information. The medical assistant, who is working her very first shift, answers and says, "I'm not sure which lab value is which, but I do know that the labs are within normal limits." Which of these lab values would fall in the normal range for carbon dioxide values?
   a. 140
   b. 87
   c. 24
   d. 0.9

55. Which is a correct SIRS criterion to determine if a patient is septic? Choose the answer with the most accurate description, even if it is technically correct.
   a. HR over 120 bpm
   b. RR under 20 breaths/min
   c. Temperature above 100.4 °F or below 96.8 °F
   d. Normal white blood cell count

56. Which test is most widely used for estimating the stage of chronic kidney disease with GFR?
   a. MDRD
   b. CKD-EPI
   c. Cockcroft-Gault
   d. Cystatin C

57. With which medications would a patient benefit from prior pharmacogenetic testing? (Select all that apply.)
   a. Antidepressants
   b. Anti-coagulants
   c. Proton pump inhibitors
   d. Statins

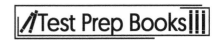

58. A patient is newly diagnosed with congenital heart disease and has an elevated troponin but no signs or symptoms of heart failure. What NYHA stage is the patient?
    a. Stage A
    b. Stage B
    c. Stage C
    d. Stage D

59. Which lab parameter is the major sign that a patient who recently underwent a renal transplant is rejecting the new kidney?
    a. Decreased BUN/SCr
    b. Increased BUN/SCr
    c. Leukopenia
    d. Thrombocytopenia

60. What does the half-life of a medication indicate?
    a. It indicates the time it takes to reach maximum plasma concentration.
    b. It indicates the time it takes for the drug to reach 50 percent of its original concentration.
    c. It indicates the time it takes the drug to reach 0 percent plasma concentration.
    d. It indicates the amount of the drug still in the plasma when it reaches its maximum plasma concentration.

61. A patient is on ibuprofen and fluoxetine, and they just recently added doxepin for insomnia. They come to the pharmacy three weeks later and state that it has not helped their insomnia at all. What is the most likely cause? (For more information, ibuprofen is not affected by or metabolized through CYP2D6, fluoxetine is a CYP2D6 inhibitor, and doxepin is metabolized by CYP2D6.)
    a. Doxepin does not treat insomnia.
    b. Ibuprofen is an inhibitor of the CYP450 enzyme that doxepin is metabolized through.
    c. Fluoxetine is an inhibitor of the CYP450 enzyme that doxepin is metabolized through.
    d. Fluoxetine is a strong inducer of CYP2D6, so the doxepin needs to be at a higher dose.

62. How long does it usually take for a schizophrenia patient to see decreased symptoms after they start taking haloperidol?
    a. Twenty-four hours
    b. Seventy-two hours
    c. One to two weeks
    d. One to two months

63. What is the duration of tadalafil in a patient with erectile dysfunction?
    a. One hour
    b. Three hours
    c. Twenty-four hours
    d. Thirty-six hours

64. Which epilepsy medications need to be closely monitored for pharmacokinetic and pharmacodynamic efficacy? (Select all that apply.)
    a. Phenytoin
    b. Primidone
    c. Carbamazepine
    d. Levetiracetam

175

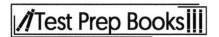

65. Below is a PK curve for Vyvanse and the metabolites lisdexamfetamine (LMX) and dexamphetamine (d-AMP). What is the best estimate for the time at which peak plasma concentration, C_{max}, is reached (which is t_{max} of d-AMP)?

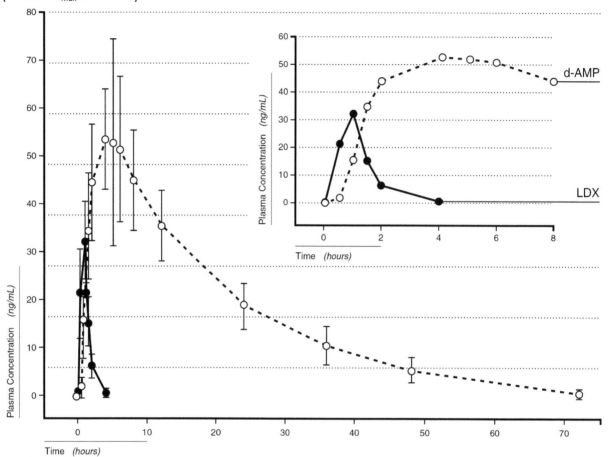

a. 2 hours
b. 5 hours
c. 11 hours
d. 72 hours

66. Below is a PK (pharmacokinetic) curve for different dosing of tamsulosin. What are these PK curves indicating? The right graph is a more zoomed-out picture of the left graph.

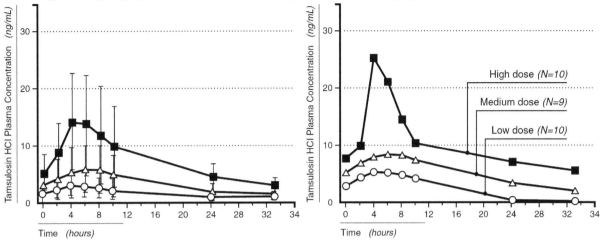

a. Each dose reached the same C_{max} in the trials.
b. The low dose most likely caused the most adverse anticholinergic effects.
c. The high dose most likely caused the most adverse anticholinergic effects.
d. The high dose most likely caused the most adverse antiemetic effects.

67. A female has a hemoglobin of 11 g/dL. According to the WHO guidelines, does this patient meet the criteria for anemia?
a. The patient does have anemia.
b. The patient is at risk for anemia.
c. The patient does not have anemia.
d. There is not enough information to know if she meets all the guidelines for anemia defined by the WHO.

68. According to the 2023 AHA Dyslipidemia guidelines, what is the HDL goal for a woman with type 2 diabetes mellitus?
a. Greater than 30 mg/dL
b. Greater than 40 mg/dL
c. Greater than 50 mg/dL
d. Greater than 60 mg/dL

69. What is the first-line treatment for pediatric patients who have cystic fibrosis for chronic Pseudomonas infections?
a. Azithromycin
b. Tetracycline
c. Gentamicin
d. Ampicillin

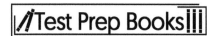

70. According to the National Comprehensive Cancer Network guidelines, with a Philadelphia chromosome-positive acute lymphoblastic leukemia in adolescents and young adults (AYA), what are the two first-line treatments?
    a. Multiagent chemotherapy and tyrosine kinase inhibitor
    b. Tyrosine kinase inhibitor and a corticosteroid
    c. Corticosteroid and multiagent chemotherapy
    d. No medication; only a stem cell transplant

71. According to the 2014 APA Guidelines, cholinesterase inhibitors are the mainstay of Alzheimer's treatment. Which of these medications is NOT a cholinesterase inhibitor?
    a. Exelon
    b. Razadyne
    c. Namenda
    d. Aricept

72. What is the first-line treatment for stable ischemic heart disease when the patient cannot take beta-blockers?
    a. Non-DHP calcium channel blockers
    b. DHP calcium channel blockers
    c. Nitrate
    d. Ranolazine

73. A seventy-two-year-old female says she has not had any vaccines since she was eighteen and would like to receive all the vaccines she is behind on. Which vaccines is she eligible for? (Select all that apply.)
    a. Gardasil
    b. Prevnar
    c. Boostrix
    d. Fluzone

74. Which of these eye drops are available OTC? (Select all that apply.)
    a. Olopatadine
    b. Cyclosporine
    c. Loteprednol
    d. Bromfenac

75. Which is a common supplement used to lower blood pressure?
    a. Cinnamon
    b. Turmeric
    c. Cranberry
    d. Garlic

76. Which OTC weight loss product is banned by the FDA?
    a. Orlistat
    b. Sibutramine
    c. Semaglutide
    d. Phentermine

77. Which patient would be a good candidate for nicotine replacement therapy such as nicotine gum?
    a. A fifty-year-old man with dentures
    b. A twenty-five-year-old lawyer
    c. A thirty-seven-year-old stay-at-home mom
    d. A sixty-five-year-old man who has TMJ

78. What is the first-line treatment for most patients with acute, mild allergic rhinitis?
    a. Diphenhydramine
    b. Ephedra
    c. Loratadine
    d. Promethazine

Performing Calculations

1. A fifty-year-old female patient who is 89 kg and 178 cm tall comes into a clinic with these lab values. What is her CrCl?

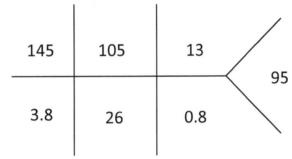

2. A patient with 2.4 mg/dL total bilirubin, 3.1 g/dL albumin, 1.4 INR, slight ascites, and Grade 3 encephalopathy needs to have his Child-Pugh score calculated for cirrhosis severity. What is his score and class?
    a. 6, Class A
    b. 8, Class B
    c. 10, Class C
    d. 12, Class C

3. A seventy-two-year-old male is admitted to the hospital for community-acquired pneumonia, and the team is wondering if he also needs to be monitored for stroke risk. He has a past medical history (PMH) of hypertension, T2DM, and peripheral artery disease. What is his CHA2DS2-VASC score?
    a. 2
    b. 4
    c. 6
    d. 8

4. A patient who just underwent ACL surgery on his knee needs an oxycodone prescription. What is the total daily dose that would need to be prescribed, in mg?

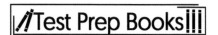

5. A patient with COPD is taking salmeterol (one inhalation twice daily) for a DPI (dry powder inhaler) with 50 mcg/actuation and needs a 90-day supply. There are 10,000 mcg of salmeterol in one canister. How many canisters will this patient need for 90 days?
    a. 1 canister
    b. 2 canisters
    c. 3 canisters
    d. 4 canisters

6. A patient has been admitted with an ischemic stroke that occurred not more than two hours ago. He is seventy-nine years old, weighs 210 lbs, and has a past medical history of T2DM and a current blood glucose of 150. He has Stage 1 hypertension with a current BP of 150/102 mmHg and hyperlipidemia. He is on atorvastatin, semaglutide, basal insulin, and lisinopril. Is he a candidate for tPA (IV alteplase), and what would be the dosage if so?
    a. Yes, 75 mg
    b. Yes, 86 mg
    c. Yes, 90 mg
    d. No

7. A patient with pulmonary arterial hypertension is on IV treprostinil. They weigh 62 kg, and the rate of administration is 40 ng/kg/min. What is the total dose they will receive over 24 hours of continuous infusion in mg?

8. Which of these rates of administration is the fastest?
    a. 0.1 mg/hr
    b. 58 mcg/hr
    c. 70 ng/min
    d. 100 ng/hr

9. A patient needs potassium chloride administered for hypokalemia. What would be an appropriate rate of administration?
    a. 5 mEq over 15 minutes via IV push
    b. 10 mEq over 1 hour via peripheral line
    c. 30 mEq over 1 hour via peripheral line
    d. 50 mEq over 1 hour via central line

10. A patient needs propofol at 15 mcg/kg/min, and they weigh 165 lbs. The stock bottle given is 1000 mg per 100 mL with a total volume of 100 mL. Calculate what the patient needs for 4 hours.
    a. 1.2 mL
    b. 2.6 mL
    c. 5.8 mL
    d. 6.7 mL

11. A five-year-old child is instructed to take EZPass for their constipation. The adult dose is 250 mg once daily. If the patient is 109 cm tall and weighs 19 kg, what is the dosing? Round to the nearest whole number.

12. A patient has to change medications from simvastatin to rosuvastatin due to insurance. If their previous simvastatin dose was 20 mg, what is their new rosuvastatin dose that would provide equal effects?

    a. 5 mg
    b. 20 mg
    c. 40 mg
    d. 50 mg

13. A 30 kg, nine-year-old patient needs to take Tylenol for their fever, but their father says they only have adult Tylenol available and do not know what dose to give their child. What would be the dose for the nine-year-old, and what is the dosing schedule?

14. A patient is admitted to the hospital for worsening acute heart failure and is taking furosemide 40 mg orally daily. What would be their bolus dose of IV bumetanide, and what would their new at-home dose be if switched to torsemide oral? For bumetanide bolus and torsemide oral, use 2 times the dose for the calculations.

    a. 1 mg bumetanide; 40 mg torsemide
    b. 2 mg bumetanide; 10 mg torsemide
    c. 2 mg bumetanide; 40 mg torsemide
    d. 1 mg bumetanide; 20 mg torsemide

15. What is the ratio strength of a medication with a 30% concentration? Round to the nearest hundredth.

16. What is the serum osmolality of a patient with 136 mmol/L sodium, 170 mg/dL blood glucose, and a BUN of 11 mg/dL?

    a. 100 mOsm/kg
    b. 165 mOsm/kg
    c. 202 mOsm/kg
    d. 285 mOsm/kg

17. What is the percent ionization of a drug with a pKa of 4.2 and a pH of 3.7? Round to the nearest whole number.

    a. 24%
    b. 32%
    c. 76%
    d. 100%

18. What is the milliosmolarity of a calcium chloride (molecular weight = 111 g) in 450 mL of a 20% calcium chloride solution? Round to the nearest whole number.

19. An order comes in for a 750 mL 25% solution of HappyRUs, but the solutions in stock are 15% and 40% concentrations. How much of the 15% stock solution is needed to make the 25%, 750 mL solution?

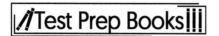

20. An eye drop for conjunctival edema due to allergies (olopatadine) has 0.1% of the active ingredient. What is the amount of the active ingredient in a preparation of 1 L in ounces (oz)?
    a. 0.0352 oz
    b. 1 oz
    c. 0.352 oz
    d. 0.1 oz

21. An order comes in for 200 mg of Vfend. The powder vial of 200 mg says to dilute with 19 mL of water to make a final concentration of 10 mg/mL. What is the powder volume of the Vfend?

22. A 40 mL preparation of 25% Rocephin needs to be made into 10% Rocephin. What is the amount of diluent added to the 25% Rocephin to achieve the desired concentration?
    a. 35 mL
    b. 45 mL
    c. 53 mL
    d. 60 mL

23. A TPN (total parenteral nutrition) order comes to the pharmacist to compound, and it needs 220 mL of 10% lipid emulsion formulation. How many grams of fat is this equal to?

24. A patient on TPN needs 25 g/day of protein. The stock solution provided is Amino Acids 15%. What is the amount in mLs of Amino Acids 15% that should be added to the patient's TPN bag?
    a. 58 mL
    b. 104 mL
    c. 167 mL
    d. 225 mL

25. A TPN order comes to the pharmacy with the following:
        350 mL dextrose 60%
        167 mL Amino Acids 15%
        220 mL lipid emulsion 10%
        80 mL 3% NS
        5 mL multivitamin
        789 mL sterile water
        x mL remaining electrolytes
        Total Volume: 1640 mL
What does x equal?
    a. 15 mL
    b. 29 mL
    c. 57 mL
    d. 80 mL

26. If the life expectancy of a colon cancer patient on a novel treatment extends their life by 5 years and has a quality of life score of 0.4, what is the quality-adjusted life year gained (QALY)?
    a. 1.5
    b. 2
    c. 3.5
    d. 5

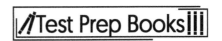

27. What is the percent risk of death in a population of 540 women in which 79 have a new strain of Covid-19? Round to the nearest whole percentage.
   a. 5%
   b. 15%
   c. 25%
   d. 45%

28. Which confidence interval (CI) is statistically relevant and supports the claim that a new treatment is superior to the placebo at preventing an adverse event?
   a. 1.92 (1.80–1.90)
   b. 1.04 (0.94–1.06)
   c. 0.45 (0.29–0.56)
   d. 1.34 (1.30–1.56)

29. If a medication's half-life is 3.5 hours and the dose was 20 mg/L, how long would it take to decrease to 5 mg/L in the patient? Assume first-order kinetics and round to the nearest hundredth.

30. What is the percent of steady state reached in a continuous infusion administered at 78 mg/h with an elimination rate constant of 0.453 h^{-1} and a time of 8.5 hours to reach steady state? Round to the nearest whole number.
   a. 3%
   b. 54%
   c. 98%
   d. 100%

31. What is the clearance of a medication in L/hr for oral administration with an AUC (area under curve) of 34 mg*h/L, F (oral bioavailability) of 0.93, and dose of 650 mg? Round to the nearest tenth.
   a. 17.8 mg/L
   b. 34.3 mg/L
   c. 52.0 mg/L
   d. 67.9 mg/L

32. What is the infusion rate needed to achieve a steady state concentration of 100 g/L in a medicine with a volume of distribution of 59 L and a half-life of 26.2 hours? Round to the nearest whole number.
   a. 74 g/hr
   b. 107 g/hr
   c. 153 g/hr
   d. 202 g/hr

Compounding, Dispensing, or Administering Drugs or Managing Delivery Systems

1. Which of the following is true when compounding a three-in-one total parenteral nutrition (TPN) solution?
   a. Always add the lipids first to prevent flocculation
   b. A 0.22-micron filter is required for administration
   c. Filters used for infusion should be changed every twelve hours
   d. Stabilizing a lipid emulsion requires a higher pH value

183

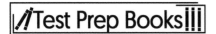

2. Patients who have the variant HLA-B*57:01 and take abacavir are at risk for what reaction?
   a. Hypersensitivity
   b. Stevens-Johnson syndrome
   c. Toxic epidermal necrolysis
   d. Malignant hyperthermia

3. Why do peptides NOT make good drug candidates? (Select all that apply.)
   a. Rapidly degraded in GIT
   b. Poor bioavailability
   c. Rapidly excreted
   d. Binds to a single receptor

4. Which of the following is FALSE regarding boronic acid bio-isosteres?
   a. They are bio-isosteres of carboxylic acids.
   b. They are toxic and not readily synthesized.
   c. They are proteasome inhibitors.
   d. Their target interaction involves hydrogen and covalent bonds leading to tighter binding and enhanced bioactivity.

5. Which of the following is true regarding prodrugs?
   a. They are active compounds that shield the active drug.
   b. They are used to provide solutions to membrane permeability.
   c. Carboxylic acids need ester groups to increase ionization.
   d. The more polar ester groups can cross the cell membrane.

6. What is the ISO Class requirement for primary engineering controls?
   a. Class 3
   b. Class 5
   c. Class 7
   d. Class 8

7. Which of the following pieces of equipment should NEVER be used for hazardous sterile compounding? (Select all that apply.)
   a. Laminar airflow workbench
   b. Horizontal laminar workbench
   c. Compounding aseptic containment isolator
   d. Biological safety cabinet

8. What is the minimum amount of air changes per hour (ACPH) required in a buffer room?
   a. Ten
   b. Twenty
   c. Thirty
   d. Fifty

9. Which of the following methods will help prevent precipitation between calcium and phosphorous?
   a. Add calcium first, then phosphate.
   b. Increase lipid concentration.
   c. Keep the preparation at a lower pH.
   d. Use calcium carbonate.

184

10. Which of the following excipients would you add to non-sterile dosage forms to protect them from microbial growth?
    a. Solubilizing agents
    b. Antioxidants
    c. Buffers
    d. Preservatives

11. Which of the following accurately describes a eutectic mixture?
    a. A mixture of compounds that has a lower melting point than the individual components
    b. A combination of powders that may react violently when mixed
    c. Dry aggregates of powder particles that are more stable physically and chemically
    d. A dry mixture that, when added to water, releases carbon dioxide and produces a fizzy effect

12. When compounding a sterile preparation, the rainbow method is used to prevent what?
    a. Accumulation of negative pressure
    b. Exposure to the compounder
    c. The blockage of airflow
    d. Accumulation of positive pressure

13. Which of the following is FALSE regarding gown use during hazardous compounding?
    a. Gowns should only close in the back.
    b. Isolation gowns are not acceptable for hazardous compounding.
    c. Gowns must be changed every four to five hours or immediately after a spill.
    d. Gowns must not be worn in other areas.

14. What is the name of the delivery system that provides pH-dependent delayed release for medications?

15. What is the name of the home infusion device that uses pressure to infuse medication at a consistent rate?
    a. Elastomeric infusion
    b. Ambulatory infusion
    c. Gravity-based infusion
    d. Enteral infusion

16. Elastomeric infusion devices commonly require the use of the specific technique prior to delivery to the patient. What is? Place the following steps in the proper order of operations: Attach pump, heparin flush, saline flush (1), saline flush (2).

17. Which of the following medications is NOT an intrauterine delivery system?
    a. Mirena
    b. Skyla
    c. Twirla
    d. Paragard

185

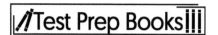

18. Which intrauterine contraceptive is non-hormonal?
    a. Paragard
    b. Liletta
    c. Skyla
    d. Mirena

19. How would you tell a patient to prepare a cocoa butter suppository to provide lubrication for insertion?
    a. Heat in microwave.
    b. Place in cold water for five to ten minutes before use.
    c. Rub suppository with the fingers.
    d. Cocoa butter suppositories are not used.

20. After the administration of a rectal suppository, how long should the patient withhold excessive movement and exercise?
    a. Fifteen minutes
    b. Thirty minutes
    c. One hour
    d. Two hours

21. Which of the following is NOT an instruction when using a spacer device?
    a. Shake the medicine.
    b. Insert mouthpiece of inhaler into the sealed end of the spacer.
    c. Spray medicine into the spacer and breath in fast and deep.
    d. Hold breath for five to ten seconds afterwards.

22. What is the most common type of container used for drugs that are sensitive to light?
    a. Amber glass
    b. Metal
    c. Clear glass
    d. Orange plastic

23. Which of the following is a disadvantage of using plastic packaging materials? (Select all that apply.)
    a. Permeation
    b. Leaching
    c. Sorption
    d. Flocculation

24. According to the revised USP <797>, what is the maximum beyond use date for Category 1 compounds at a controlled room temperature?
    a. Four hours
    b. Twelve hours
    c. Twenty-four hours
    d. Forty-eight hours

25. What is the name of the container where needles, broken glass, and open ampules should be discarded?

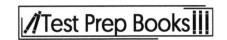

Developing or Managing Practice or Medication-Use Systems to Ensure Safety and Quality

1. A formal document that outlines patient care functions delegated to a pharmacist by a physician is known as what?
   a. Collaborative practice agreement (CPA)
   b.   Physician-pharmacist care release (PPCR)
   c. Clinical transfer agreement (CTA)
   d. Drug related problems agreement (DRPA)

2. Which of the following is FALSE regarding a collaborative practice agreement? (Select all that apply.)
   a. Specific drug names are required to be in the protocol.
   b. Specific training requirements for the pharmacist must be listed in the protocol.
   c. If the pharmacist is granted the ability to sign prescriptions, they must update their state board annually.
   d. The protocol will be posted on the board's website and will include license numbers of the pharmacists and physicians on the protocol.

3. Which of the following statements is correct regarding collaborative practice agreements?
   a. The protocols have no significant impact on patient care and outcomes. The existing roles and responsibilities of each professional are sufficient to provide optimal healthcare.
   b. Implementing these can lead to increased workload and administrative burden, resulting in decreased productivity and inefficient patient care.
   c. They are driven by profit-oriented motives and may compromise the quality of healthcare.
   d. They allow pharmacists and physicians to communicate their respective knowledge and skills during medication management decisions.

4. What is the name of the ASHP initiative that uses interprofessional efforts to standardize medications and decrease errors during transitions of care?

5. Which of the following methods is the most effective in promoting continuity of care for the patient in the outpatient, inpatient, and community settings?
   a. Medication action plan
   b. Letter to the patient
   c. Letter to the healthcare payer
   d. Telephone encounter

6. Which type of drug therapy focuses on disease prevention?
   a. Empiric
   b. Prophylactic
   c. Therapeutic
   d. Antimicrobial stewardship

7. The monofilament test screens for what condition?
   a. Peripheral edema
   b. Diabetic foot
   c. Neurological disorders
   d. Alzheimer's disease

187

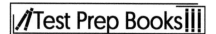
8. In addition to the Timed Up and Go (TUG) test, what is the name of the other test used to screen for risk of falls?

9. Which of the following pediatric screening programs assesses the first five years of life and analyzes five developmental areas including communication, gross motor and fine motor function, problem-solving, and personal-social skills?
   a. Ages and Stages Questionnaire (ASQ)
   b. Denver Developmental Screening Test (DDST)
   c. Early Screening Inventory (ESI)
   d. Bayley Infant Neurodevelopmental Screen (BINS)

10. Which steps during blood glucose testing are important to ensure quality and accuracy of the result? (Select all that apply.)
   a. Run a control test.
   b. Wipe the first drop of blood.
   c. Check only the expiration date.
   d. Place drop of blood on the test strip and then insert into the monitor.

11. Which of the following populations would NOT be eligible for the Vulnerable Population Assistance Program (VPAP)?
   a. Children
   b. Those who classify as homeless
   c. Veterans
   d. Those with limited English proficiency

12. The Americans with Disabilities Act of 1990 prohibited discrimination against qualified individuals with disabilities. Which of the following conditions is NOT considered a disability under this act?
   a. Deafness/blindness
   b. HIV
   c. Bipolar disorder
   d. Broken limbs

13. What is the acronym for the name of the department that provides recommendations for safety in the workplace?

14. Which of the following methods is used within pharmacy informatics? (Select all that apply.)
   a. CPOE
   b. BCMA
   c. Textbooks/ guidelines
   d. Clinical decision support

15. How does pharmacy informatics contribute to medication safety and quality assurance?
   a. By facilitating the detection and prevention of medication errors through automated systems
   b. By analyzing patient preferences to tailor medication formulations and flavors
   c. By designing aesthetically pleasing medication packaging for improved patient adherence
   d. By implementing virtual reality technology for patient education on medication usage

16. Fill in the blank: Pharmacy informatics is a subsection of _____ informatics.

188

Answer Explanations #2

Obtaining, Interpreting, or Assessing Data, Medical, or Patient Information

1. D: Type 2 diabetes mellitus (T2DM) is often diagnosed using a fasting plasma glucose test. The preferred method is to perform an overnight fast and measure the patient's glucose tolerance. The gold standard is to measure the blood on two separate occasions to prevent unnecessary diagnosis. If both fasting values are $\geq$ 126mg/L, this can indicate impaired glucose tolerance. Choice *A* is incorrect because it indicated only one test is sufficient for diagnosis. Choice *B* is incorrect because an A1c value of > 6.5 percent is the marker for T2DM. Choice *C* is incorrect because even though 150 mg/L is indicative of T2DM, the cutoff for diagnosis is 126 mg/L, not 150 mg/L.

2. B: An immunofluorescent assay is a technique used to detect if a patient's body made antibodies toward a specific antigen. The process involves coating the wells with the antigen and then placing the blood into the well. If binding occurs, the test result is positive. Choice *A* is incorrect because this describes the opposite. The antibody is coated on the well and the patient's blood is being tested for the antigen. Choice *C* is incorrect because complement fixation tests whether the complement system is activated and forms a complex. Choice *D* is incorrect because the dilution test is a method of determining an antibiotic's minimum inhibitory concentration.

3. B: Troponin is a regulator of skeletal muscle contraction. It is a biomarker for the heart to determine how much it is working. High levels of troponin indicate that the heart requires a lot of calcium-mediated actin and myosin contraction. Choices *A* and *D* are incorrect because troponin is not involved in kidney or liver function. Choice *C* is incorrect because although troponin is helpful in evaluating heart failure, it is not considered a diagnostic marker. High levels of troponin can be indicative of many issues.

4. Huntington's disease (HD): HD is an inheritable disease that causes the breakdown of nerve cells in the brain. The typical age of onset for HD is between thirty and fifty, and the first few signs seen include depression, difficulty concentrating, and memory lapses. The gold standard for diagnosis is a genetic test that analyzes CAG repeats. Any value $\geq$ 36 repeats is indicative of HD, whereas any values < 26 can rule it out.

5. A, C: MoCA and MMSE are used to assess cognitive impairment, such as issues with thinking or memory. Choice *D* is incorrect because the patient health questionnaire (PHQ) is a common diagnostic method for depression. Choice *B* is incorrect because the CAM is a screening tool to assess for delusion and delirium.

6. D: Benzoyl peroxide comes in many forms including lotion, cream, gel, pledget, and foam. Foams are the preferred method for patients with hairy areas, as this form can help with adherence and prevent patients from having to shave, which should be avoided if possible. Therefore, Choice *A* is incorrect. Choice *B* is incorrect because there are many forms of benzoyl peroxide. Choice *C* is incorrect because the lotion form would be preferred if the patient wanted a form that was more moisturizing.

7. C: Social history is part of the subjective information of a SOAP note and includes diet, smoking, alcohol, and occupational history. Choice *A* is incorrect because the chief complaint would contain the patient's feeling regarding their head. Choice *B* is incorrect because this there is not a formal section

189

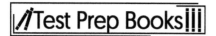
labeled "diet history." Choice *D* is incorrect because the socioeconomic background would be included in the demographic section.

8. D: Since the instructions were "take one tablet three times a day", a prescription with ninety tablets should last them thirty days. The prescriptions may be valid, but because they are from two different doctors, the patient's prescription history may not have been relayed to both prescribers. Choice *A* is incorrect because you not only need to verify that prescriptions are accurate, but also that there is no potential for abuse. Calling only to reverify but not to inform the prescribers would not be the best course of action. Choice *B* is incorrect because the patient should not have run out of medication two weeks early, and it is a pharmacist's duty to prevent abuse of drugs. Choice *C* is incorrect because calling the police would be an excessive next action, as the prescriptions appear to be valid and the patient is not confirmed to have broken any law.

9. C: Although the patient is homeless, health care should not be denied, and most hospitals have programs for patients who cannot afford services or prescriptions. Since Fosfomycin is a one-time dose, this would be the best option regarding treatment adherence. Choices *A* and *B* are incorrect because although they may be more preferred, these options would require the patient to take the medication multiple times a day for several days, which may be unlikely given their social background. Choice *D* is incorrect because, again, healthcare should not be denied due to lack of finances.

10. A: Before attempting to change the patient's medication regimen, try to understand why the patient is having difficulty with their current regimen. If the issue is too many bottles, a weekly pill planner may help. Choice *B* is incorrect because simply telling the patient to take their medication as prescribed does not address the underlying issue and could hurt the pharmacist-patient relationship. Choice *C* is incorrect because providing the patient with educational materials may be helpful, but it should be done after identifying and addressing their specific adherence barriers. Choice *D* should never be a solution to adherence issues.

11. C: Family members with medical conditions can alter the patient's medication plan. For example, a primary family member with a history of medullary thyroid carcinoma would prevent the patient from receiving a GLP-1 receptor agonist medication commonly used in type 2 diabetes mellitus. Choices *A*, *B*, and *D* are incorrect because these factors do not play a role in the patient's therapy regimen and are not important for documentation.

12. A: Direct observed therapy is a researched method of helping patients stay adherent to medications that are taken weekly, specifically with this regimen. Setting up a Zoom call once a week to watch them administer the medication has one of the highest success rates of therapy. Choice *B* is incorrect because patients can forget to set alarms or snooze them, and alarms doesn't assure the provider that the patient is adherent. Choice *C* is incorrect because a pill box may be too excessive for a once-a-week regimen, especially if the patient is not on other daily medications. Choice *D* is incorrect because medications should not be stored in the car due to overheating, and the patient may not own a vehicle. This method also does not assure the provider that the patient is adherent.

13. C: A chief complaint describes why the patient is in front of the provider. Choice *A* is incorrect because this information would be under the allergies section. Choice *B* is incorrect because this would be used under the social history section. Choice *D* is incorrect because this would be important socioeconomic information.

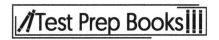

14. C: Byetta (exenatide) is a GLP-1 receptor antagonist used for type 2 diabetes. This class of medications has a black box warning for patients with a primary family history of medullary thyroid cancer. Choices *A*, *B*, and *D* are incorrect because all these medications have no family history component.

15. C: PRN stands for "pro re nata," which means "as needed." This term is used to indicate that a medication should be taken only when necessary, rather than on a fixed schedule. Often confused with "per recommended need," "postoperative nausea," and "prior refused narcotics."

16. Subjective, Objective, Assessment, Plan: The SOAP note format is a commonly used documentation method for healthcare providers. These notes can be comprehensive or targeted. Subjective information would consist of patient's home medication, signs/symptoms, and family history. Objective information would consist of vital signs taken and medication administered by a healthcare professional. The assessment section would include evaluation of a patient's current therapy for a specific disease state. The plan section would contain goals of therapy change, monitoring plans, and follow-up instructions.

17. A, D, and E: Epoetin (Procrit) is a hematopoietic agent used in the treatment of anemia. It stimulates the bone marrow to produce red blood cells (RBCs). The expected goal of therapy is to have an increase in RBC and its components. The normal RBC count is 4.2 to 6.2 million/mm^3. Hematocrit measures the volume of RBCs to the total circulating blood volume in the body. Patients taking epoetin will have their dose adjusted depending on the hematocrit percentage. The suggested value is between 30% and 36% to allow for maturation of RBCs. Hemoglobin is the concentration of oxygen saturation in RBCs. The normal value range is 12 to 18 g/dL. Choices *B* and *C* are components of white blood cells (WBCs) used in the immune response. Neutrophils are granulocytes that help resolve infections and repair damage to tissues by foreign bacteria. Eosinophils fight infection and play a part in the inflammatory process. Epoetin's main mechanism of action is stimulating the formation of RBCs.

18. A: Weight loss is a common symptom of hypothyroidism, which is caused by an overactive thyroid gland. Choice *B* is incorrect because heart block would cause bradycardia, or decreased heart rate. Choice *C* is incorrect because amphetamine use often has a side effect of being very alert. Choice *D* is incorrect because opioid use commonly causes constipation.

19. B, C: The liver is the main organ responsible for drug metabolism and plays a role in bile synthesis. Choice *A* is incorrect because the kidney is the organ responsible for reabsorption of solute. Choice *D* is incorrect because the secretion of insulin is primarily the responsibility of the pancreas, not the liver.

20. A: Heartburn is the most common symptom of GERD (gastroesophageal reflux disease), which occurs when stomach acid flows back up into the esophagus. Nausea and dysphagia (trouble swallowing) are also common signs. Choice *B* is incorrect because you would not experience heartburn or dysphagia with liver failure. Choice *C* is incorrect because heartburn might be relayed as chest pain, but more prominent effects of heart failure would also be present. Choice *D* is incorrect because constipation may cause nausea but would not affect a person's ability to swallow.

21. B: There are many risk factors for T2DM, including genetics, age, obesity, and lifestyle factors. However, a family history of diabetes is a strong correlation for a patient developing the disease, and genetic predisposition is more correlated than in Type 1 diabetes.

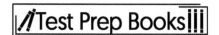

22. C: Asthma is a chronic respiratory disease characterized by airway inflammation and hyperresponsiveness that often presents as wheezing, coughing, and difficulty breathing. The fundamental abnormality in asthma is an exaggerated TH2 immune response to normal, environmental allergens. TH2 cells will activate, and B cells will produce eosinophils that then produce an allergic response. Choice *A* is incorrect because COPD occurs when there is a pathophysiological reason for obstruction in the airways. Choice *B* is incorrect because an allergic reaction occurs when the body responds to a particular substance that triggers the immune system. Choice *D* is incorrect because a pulmonary embolism describes a clot in the lung that is blocking blood flow.

23. C: Type 1 diabetes mellitus (T1DM) is an autoimmune disease that typically presents in childhood. With this disease, the body's immune system begins to attack the beta-1 cells of the pancreas, which are normally responsible for insulin production. Choice *A* and *B* are incorrect because these factors do not cause T1DM, but they can contribute to the worsening of the disease state. Choice *D* is incorrect because insulin resistance is a primary cause of type 2 diabetes mellitus.

24. C: Rheumatoid arthritis is a type IV autoimmune response in which the body's immune system attacks the synovial lining of the joints and eventually causes bone and cartilage destruction, as well as bone ankylosis. It presents as stiffness and swelling of the joint. Choices *A* and *B* are incorrect because while genetic factors and wear and tear of joints can contribute to the development of rheumatoid arthritis, autoimmune response is the primary driver of the disease. Choice *D* is incorrect because bacterial infections are not a cause of rheumatoid arthritis and cannot cause this autoimmune response.

25. Stroke: The CHADSVASC score considers a variety of factors like hypertension, age, diabetes, and gender to determine a patient's risk of stroke. The score consists of the following:

       C: Congestive heart failure = one point
       H: Hypertension or high blood pressure = one point
       A: Age greater than or equal to seventy-five years = two points
       D: Diabetes mellitus or type 2 diabetes = one point
       S: Prior stroke or TIA = two points
       V: Vascular disease = one point
       A: Age between sixty-five and seventy-four years = one point
       S: Female sex = one point

Scores ≥ 2 for females or ≥ 3 for males indicate the need for anticoagulation therapy.

26. B, C: Severe leg pain is often a symptom of severe deep vein thrombosis (DVT) and occurs when there is stagnant blood toward the bottom half of the body that causes that area to be more prone to clots. The clots can then embolize, move into the lung, and cause blockage—thus, a pulmonary embolism. Choice *A* and *D* are incorrect because these are not affected by blood flow, so a clot embolizing would not affect thyroid or renal function.

27. A: Genital herpes is a sexually transmitted infection that is lifelong and requires medications such as acyclovir and valacyclovir to treat its symptoms. Out of the most common sexually transmitted diseases, Choice *B* is incorrect because this describes gonorrhea and Choice *C* is incorrect because this describes chlamydia. Choice *D* is incorrect because it specifies single-stranded rather than double-stranded.

28. A, B: Night sweats, hemoptysis, productive cough, and fever are a few examples of symptoms a patient would experience with tuberculosis. Choice *C* is incorrect because patients would experience

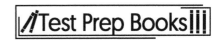

unintentional weight loss, rather than weight gain, and Choice *D* is incorrect because patients would experience elevated WBC with lymphocyte predominance.

29. B: Patients with BMI > 40 are considered at risk for the influenza virus. Choices *A*, *C*, and *D* are incorrect because these are risk factors for infection, in addition to having comorbidities and being in a nursing home.

30. C: Prolonged neutropenia, which means decreased neutrophils for > 7 days, is considered a major risk factor for this lung fungal infection. Choice *A* is incorrect because this would be considered a risk factor for malaria. Choice *B* is incorrect because this is a risk factor for various sexually transmitted infections. Choice *D* is incorrect because this is a risk factor for many disease states, including cryptococcus meningitis.

31. A, B, C: These are all risk factors for both hematogenous and contiguous osteomyelitis, which is a type of bone marrow infection. Choice *D* is incorrect because albumin levels do not affect risk of infection.

32. D: All the following are risk factors for infective endocarditis. However, there are two types, structural- vs bacteremia-based risk factors. Choice *D* is the only structural risk factor listed. Choices *A*, *B*, and *C* are bacteremia-based risk factors and are thus incorrect.

33. B: Catheter-related bloodstream infections are very serious. If not treated, they can lead to septic shock. Each catheter type has a risk of causing further issues; however, a non-tunneled CVC has the highest risk. The order of highest risk to lowest risk is as follows: Choice B > A > C > D.

34. C: All options listed are common risk factors of central nervous system infections. Community settings like schools and daycare, immunosuppression, and ages < two and > sixty-five are other risk factors. Choice *A* is incorrect because intra-abdominal infection risk factors would include low albumin and poor nutritional status. Choice *B* is incorrect because acute otitis media risk factors would be between six and twenty-four months old. Choice *D* is incorrect because septic shock risk factors include recent intravenous antibiotics and prolonged hospital stay.

35. A, B, C: Urinary tract infection (UTI) risk factors include increased entry of organisms, like through a catheter device, changes in the microbiota, like menopause, and an impaired immune function, like diabetes mellitus. Choice *D* is incorrect because another risk factor or UTI's would be the use of anticholinergic drugs that hinder the ability to urinate. Pilocarpine is a cholinergic drug that would produce the opposite effect.

36. C: Non-pharmacological methods are often a first-line therapy for various disorders, including hypoactive sexual desire disorder (HSDD). Cognitive behavioral therapy, sex/couples therapy, and pelvic floor training are all options. Choices *A*, *B*, and *D* are incorrect because these are medications that can cause HSDD and should be stopped if experiencing HSDD.

37. C: The FDA considers 90 percent of the reference value with a confidence interval of 80–125 percent to be bioequivalent. If the formulation falls outside of this range, it's considered non-therapeutically equivalent and will need to undergo revisions. The range of 80–125 percent is the FDA standard, so Choices *A*, *B*, and *D* are incorrect.

38. B: When you accept the null hypothesis as true, but it is false, that is considered a type II error and the researchers must reanalyze power. Choice *A* is incorrect because if you accept the null hypothesis

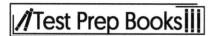
and it is true, this means there is no error. Choice *C* is incorrect because this would indicate a type I errors and the researchers need to reanalyze the alpha and p-value. Choice *D* is incorrect because this would indicate no error.

39. C: Databases like Lexicomp and Micromedex, as well as review articles and textbooks, are considered tertiary resources. They describe resources that are simple, understandable, and summarized by the author or editor. Therefore, Choices *A*, *B*, and *D* are incorrect.

40. C: Secondary literature is used to allow for more efficient searing and retrieval of primary resources. This can include EBSCOHost, Ovid MEDLINE, and PubMed.

41. Primary > Secondary > Tertiary > Expert: The description of each is as follows:

> Primary: Trial, studies, and most current information
> Secondary: Looks for potential sources of primary literature
> Tertiary: Basic background info and drug-disease state information
> Expert: Experts in the fields and guidelines

Identifying Drug Characteristics

1. D: Sodium bicarbonate is a commonly used antacid for the relief of heartburn and dyspepsia. It is short-acting, especially if taken on an empty stomach. Choice *A* is incorrect because Pepto-Bismol's mechanism for relieving heartburn has not been established. Choice *B* is incorrect because famotidine is a histamine 2 receptor antagonist that has a slower onset, but longer duration compared to antacids. Choice *C* is incorrect because omeprazole is a proton pump inhibitor that can take one to four days for complete relief.

2. Bulk laxatives: Bulk laxatives like psyllium and methylcellulose, or Metamucil, are often first-line treatments for constipation because they most closely approximate the physiologic mechanism in promoting evacuation.

3. A: Colace, also known as docusate sodium, is part of the emollient class of medications that is best used for patients who are proactively trying to avoid a painful defecation, such as in pre/post-surgery. They are commonly referred to as stool softeners and are typically taken one to three days prior to defecation complications. Choice *B* is incorrect because PEG 3350 is a hyperosmotic agent that causes an increased amount of water to be drawn into the rectum to allow for movement. Choice *C* is incorrect because Dulcolax (bisacodyl) is a stimulant laxative that irritate the intestinal mucosa to increase motility. Choice *D* is incorrect because magnesium citrate is a saline laxative that draws water into the rectum to increase movement.

4. Lubricants: Mineral oil is the only over-the-counter lubricant used to produce bowel movements; however, it should not be used because aspiration can lead to lipid pneumonia and can impair the absorptions of fat-soluble vitamins.

5. B: Finasteride is a 5-alpha reductase inhibitor that decreases intraprostatic and serum dihydrotestosterone levels. This medication is preferred in patients with signs of an enlarged prostate. Choice *A* is incorrect because tadalafil is a phosphodiesterase inhibitor that causes smooth muscle relaxation in the bladder and is not considered first line for this disease state. Choices *C* and *D* are

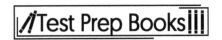

incorrect because both are first-line alpha-adrenergic antagonists; however, they do not reduce prostate size and only work by relaxing the intrinsic urethral sphincter.

6. D: Stress urinary incontinence is a result of the urethral sphincter insufficiently impeding urine flow. This condition is common in pregnancy, menopause, and in the elderly. The goal of pharmacological therapy is to target the adrenergic control of the internal sphincter, and duloxetine is considered first line. Choice *A* is incorrect because oxybutynin is typically used for urge urinary incontinence (UUI) to target muscarinic control. Choice *B* is incorrect because tamsulosin is an alpha-adrenergic antagonist commonly used for benign prostate hyperplasia. Choice *C* is incorrect because dutasteride is a 5-alpha reductase inhibitor used for enlarged prostates.

7. Tacrolimus: There are two calcineurin inhibitors used for renal transplants: tacrolimus and cyclosporine. While both medications cause nephrotoxicity, tacrolimus is the one that can also cause hyperglycemia and alopecia.

8. C: Nitroglycerin is a common medication given to patients with a history of acute coronary syndrome and is taken by the patient to relieve chest pain. The instructions state to take one sublingual tablet, wait five minutes, and if the chest pain has not subsided, take another tablet, and call 911. If the patient is still experiencing chest pain five minutes after the second dose, they may take a third tablet and then the medical team will assess for other treatment options.

9. A: Gas-X is a common over-the-counter treatment used for antiflatulence. Choice *B* is incorrect because Beano is also known as alpha-galactosidase. Choice *C* is incorrect because Florastor is a brand of probiotics that has many strands within it. Choice *D* is incorrect because Prevacid is also known as lansoprazole.

10. D: Kengreal (cangrelor) is a continuous infusion that is used if the team cannot reliably obtain an oral P2Y12 agent or if a coronary artery bypass graft (CABG) is expected soon. Choice *A, B,* and *C* are incorrect because these are all oral P2Y12 receptor antagonists.

11. B: The mixture of both medications causes a slight pink color due to minimal oxidation of dobutamine; however, this does not affect the potency or efficacy of the medication.

12. C: NPH is an intermediate-acting insulin that is an isophane mixture of the human-produced insulin. Most insulins are supposed to be clear; however, isophane insulins have a cloudy, white appearance that should be counseled to patients as normal. Choices *A, B,* and *C* are incorrect because each of these medications should be clear. If they are cloudy, they should be discarded.

13. A, B, D: The common acronym used to recall which medications should not be placed in a PVC container is LATIN—lorazepam, amiodarone, tacrolimus, insulin, and nitroglycerin. They can cause issues with sorption, or the drug leaking into the container, as well as leaching, or the container leaking into the drug. These medications can be placed in glass, polypropylene, or polyolefin containers. Choice *C* is incorrect because vancomycin has no incompatibility with PVC.

14. Daraprim: Commonly used for the treatment of toxoplasmosis infections.

15. A: Ibuprofen (Motrin, Advil) comes in 200 mg tablets over the counter and 400, 600, or 800 mg tablets as prescription-only strengths. Choices *B* and *D* are incorrect because these medications only have strengths that can be purchased without a prescription. Choice *C* is incorrect because amlodipine is a prescription-only medication.

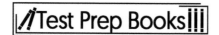

16. B: Dofetilide (Tikosyn) is a second-line option for conversion and maintenance of normal sinus rhythm, but it can cause prolonged QT segments (Torsades de pointes) which is a serious ventricular arrythmia. The REMS program ensures that the benefits outweigh the risks, and it is clearly documented and routinely followed up on. Choice A is incorrect because, although it is Class III, it does not have the adverse effect of QT prolongation. Choices C and D are incorrect because these are Class I medications and do not cause these adverse effects.

17. D: Depo-Provera is an injectable contraceptive administered every three months in a doctor's office. Its mechanism is intended to inhibit the production of estrogen, an important hormone in bone formation. Depo-Provera is preferred in patients who have sickle cell disease, endometriosis, a history of seizures, and who are obese; therefore, Choices A, B, and C are incorrect.

18. D: Isotretinoin is used for severe acne vulgaris but can cause significant teratogenic effects. Patients must undergo strict protocols to receive the medications, including the following:

1. A maximum thirty-day supply
2. No refills
3. A pregnancy test every month
4. iPledge REMS verification for each prescription
5. Must fill prescription within seven days of the office visit

19. D: Acitretin (Soriatane) is a second-generation retinoid used for severe, resistant acne vulgaris. It can metabolize into etretinate, which is highly teratogenic. It can linger for a long time, which is why it must be stopped three years prior to any attempts for conception. Choices A and B are incorrect because although they are teratogenic, they do not need to be stopped as far in advance. Choice C is incorrect because adapalene is not teratogenic and is considered the safer retinoid on the market, which is why it is available over the counter as Differin.

20. Chloramphenicol: This antibiotic medication is metabolized via glucuronic acid conjugation; however, babies lack this ability and will cause toxic metabolites to accumulate and cause a gray skin color. It can also cause fatal blood dyscrasias such as thrombocytopenia, granulocytopenia, and aplastic anemia.

21. A: GLP-1 receptor agonists, like Victoza and Ozempic, are used as non-insulin medications for the management of type 2 diabetes. Studies have linked this class of medications to an increased risk of dose- and duration-dependent thyroid C-cell tumors. Choices B, C, and D do not have this concern and therefore are incorrect.

22. C: Zyprexa Relprevv is a long-acting injection that is part of the antipsychotic drug class. It can cause excessive sedation, coma, or delirium within three hours after administration and requires a REMS program to ensure monitoring within three hours of every administration. Therefore, Choices A, B, and D are incorrect.

23. C, D: SSRIs and TCAs are commonly used to treat a variety of psychiatric disorders throughout pregnancy because they have been found to not cross the placenta and affect the fetus. Choice A is incorrect because it is recommended that paroxetine be avoided throughout pregnancy. Choice B is incorrect because benzodiazepines can cause floppy baby syndrome, which is when the baby becomes addicted to benzodiazepines in the womb and then shows withdrawal signs once delivery occurs and supply of the medication suddenly stops.

196

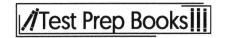

24. D: Depakote (Valproic acid) is considered an L4 category (Hale's lactation risk), which means it's possibly hazardous. If used, there is an increased risk for neural tube defects and neurodevelopmental pushbacks. Choices *A*, *B*, and *C* are incorrect because these medications are all considered to be in the L2 category, which states they are probably safe.

25. D: Dextromethorphan (Robitussin, Delsym) is a common cough medication that can be purchased over the counter. It does not cross the placental barrier and can be used during pregnancy; however, it can cross into the milk ducts in the breasts and be passed to the baby during breastfeeding. Choices *A* and *B* are incorrect because both medications can be used in pregnancy and breastfeeding, Choice *D* is incorrect because pseudoephedrine should be avoided in breastfeeding and before the first trimester of pregnancy.

26. Brexanolone: This medication is a second-line antidepressant for postpartum depression, after sertraline. Administration consists of the patient receiving a sixty-hour continuous infusion, a process described as taking a "very long nap." It can be very costly and thus is not used often.

27. A: Pregnant patients show increased clearance of levothyroxine and require higher doses than normal. It is common to increase the dose by up to 25 percent; thus, Choices *B*, *C*, and *D* are incorrect.

28. A, B, C: Warfarin is an anticoagulant that is recommended to be avoided and switched with enoxaparin; however, it can be used in patients with a mechanical heart valve. All statins and paroxetine are contraindicated in pregnant patients. Choice *D* is incorrect because sulfasalazine is considered the safe option for patients with rheumatoid arthritis instead of methotrexate.

29. B: There is an increased risk for developing cleft lip or cleft palate. The risk is higher during the first trimester, and administration should be limited to the control of severe symptoms of asthma. Choice *A* is incorrect because oral corticosteroids are not considered teratogenic. Choice *C* is incorrect because neural tube defects are a common issue with the use of valproic acid. Choice *D* is incorrect because floppy baby syndrome occurs if the mother was taking benzodiazepines.

30. B: Prostaglandin E2 analogs like Cervidil or Prepidil are used to induce cervical ripening. Choice *A* is incorrect because preterm labor induction would use agents such as terbutaline or nifedipine to prolong labor. Choice *C* is incorrect because labor induction typically requires used of oxytocin. Choice *D* is incorrect because Group B strep infections are treated with penicillin G IV every four hours.

31. A, B: Gestational hypertension is defined as elevated blood pressure without proteinuria around twenty weeks of pregnancy. Labetalol and nifedine ER are the most-used, first-line options to manage this disease state. Choice *C* is incorrect because intermediate release (IR) formulations are not recommended in pregnancy. Choice *D* is incorrect because thiazides, like hydrochlorothiazide, are considered second-line options.

32. B: Cephalosporins and penicillin are the safest antibiotics that can be administered during breastfeeding and can be used for various infections like mastitis and group B streptococcus. Choice *A* is incorrect because tetracyclines are strongly recommended to be avoided. Choice *C* is incorrect because Bactrim is only safe after the infant is ≥ 2 months old, otherwise there is risk for hyperbilirubinemia. Choice *D* is incorrect because nitrofurantoin is only safe in infants ≥ 1 month old, otherwise there is risk for hemolytic anemia.

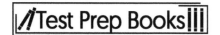

Developing or Managing Treatment Plans

1. C: Choice *C* is correct because the most critical disease states must be addressed first. The myocardial infarction is the most critical, and it is also probably causing the elevated blood glucose. Next, the T2DM should be addressed to control the glucose. His daily management of diabetes should also be checked to see if this increased his risk of myocardial infarction. The uncontrolled asthma would be next. Although getting his asthma under control is important, it is not critical to the current situation. It would, however, improve the patient's overall quality of life. After all of these are addressed, then recommending the influenza vaccine would be a good course of action.

2. D: Choice *D* is correct because the patient has had symptoms for over fourteen days, which excludes them from self-care. They need to be referred to a practitioner to have a full evaluation.

3. D: Choice *D* is correct because the cough has not improved and lasted longer than two to three weeks. Even though it may just be a lingering cough from a prior cold, it is better to be cautious and have a practitioner do a full workup.

4. A: Their BP is considered Stage 2 HTN, defined as a systolic BP over 140 mmHg and/or a diastolic BP over 90 mmHg. It is not yet a hypertensive crisis, which is a systolic BP over 180 mmHg and/or a diastolic BP over 120 mmHg. This is the most crucial disease state to treat because it can quickly lead to a hypertensive crisis, stroke, or heart attack if not addressed. Next, the hyperlipidemia should be addressed. Their LDL is high (over 100 mg/dL), and their total cholesterol is high (over 200 mg/dL). Their triglycerides are right on the border of high (over 150 mg/dL), and their HDL is optimal at 80 mg/dL (normal is 40 mg/dL and greater). These values are not terribly high, so they are important to treat for the prevention of heart diseases; however, they are not as crucial as the hypertension. The nerve pain, although distressing, is not life-threatening and should be addressed last. Choice *D* is incorrect; although the pharmacist should listen to which order the patient will actually want to follow, they need to stress to them the importance of treating in this triage order.

5. A: Choice *A* is correct because topical benzocaine is a local anesthetic often used for canker sore pain. Ibuprofen would help if the pain increased, and the carbamide peroxide wash would help with wound debridement and healing. There is no known indication to refer them to another medical provider.

6. A: At the first signs of infection (fever, chills, malaise), a patient needs further medical evaluation. Choice *B* is incorrect because self-care for ant bites can be done for three-year-olds and up. Choice *C* is incorrect because they have not yet tried any treatments, so it cannot be determined if it is treatment-resistant. Choice *D* is incorrect because referral to a practitioner would be after seventy-two hours of the infant refusing to eat.

7. B: GLP-1 agonists work by promoting insulin release from the pancreatic beta cells by stimulating cAMP release. Choices *A* and *C* are the results of the mechanism of action (MOA), not the primary goals of a GLP-1 agonist. The medicine was made to increase insulin in T2DM patients. Choice *D* is wrong because this medicine increases the risk of pancreatitis in patients, not decreases the risk.

8. C: The goal in Hashimoto's disease, or hypothyroidism, is to raise T4 because hypothyroidism leads to low T4. However, TSH is the main target for regulation and is what lab monitoring is based on. The other three answers are clinical goals for Hashimoto's.

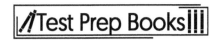
9. A, C, D: All ages for both T1DM and T2DM have an A1C goal of below 7%, and the blood glucose measurements vary for each age group. Choice *C* and Choice *D* are correct because these are the ADA recommendations for this patient population.

10. D: The respiratory rate should be under 24 breaths/min because a person's respiratory rate increases in pneumonia. Choices *A* and *B* are indicative of CAP, and Choice *C* does not mean that the CAP has completely healed. Not all CAP patients require mechanical ventilation, either.

11. A: Choice *A* is correct because there is no cure for osteoarthritis. Treatment is focused on providing symptomatic relief.

12. D: A patient needs to maintain a BP under 180/105 mmHg to ensure treatment efficacy and success. Choice *C* is incorrect. While 135/90 mmHg is lower, it is difficult to achieve with a patient who just had a stroke and is too strict of a goal. Choices *A* and *B* are too high of a blood pressure to even receive tPA (must be under 185/110 mmHg), and other treatment should be administered.

13. C: Choice *C* is correct because there is no cure for GAD. Treatment focuses on symptom relief and treating comorbidities.

14. A: Choice *A* is correct because budesonide is an inhaled corticosteroid (ICS), and fluticasone is also an ICS. If the patient took both, this would be considered a duplication of therapy because they are taking two medicines that have the same mechanism of action and act on the same disease and symptoms. Choice *B* is a long-acting beta agonist (LABA), Choice *C* is a long-acting muscarinic agonist, and Choice *D* is a short-acting beta agonist.

15. A, C: Choices *A* and *C* would be considered a duplication of therapy. Sertraline is an SSRI, and citalopram is also an SSRI. Buspirone is an anti-anxiety medication. Although sertraline is a different drug class than buspirone, the FDA indications are still to treat the same disease states (anxiety, depression, and other mood disorders).

16. D: Strattera (atomoxetine) does not have an FDA indication for treating narcolepsy or EDS, but all stimulants can be used by providers to treat these conditions. Xywav (sodium oxybate), Ritalin (methylphenidate), and Provigil (modafinil) all have FDA indications for treating narcolepsy and EDS.

17. C: Choice *C* is correct because semaglutide (Ozempic) does not yet have an FDA indication for just weight loss, which makes Choice *A* incorrect. Ozempic also does not have any pediatric FDA indications, so Choice *B* is incorrect. Choice *D* is incorrect because KR's BMI is under 27 kg/m2, which, along with more than one comorbid condition that is affected by weight, is the FDA indication for Ozempic for T2DM patients (even though her blood glucose is still elevated above goal). Choice *C* is the only patient that fits the high blood glucose and BMI criteria for Ozempic.

18. B, C, D: Choices *B*, *C*, and *D* would all benefit from a medication reconciliation. Medication reconciliation is when a provider reviews a patient's medication regimen in all aspects (adverse effects, interactions, effectiveness, adherence, disease states, effective use, patient's personal situations, patient's social situations, patient's work situations, and any other pertinent questions specific to a patient) to optimize a patient's medication regimen and health. Although every patient taking even just one supplement and/or medication would benefit from a medication reconciliation, patients on multiple medications, especially when picking up new prescriptions, largely benefit. Choice *A* is incorrect because the patient is only on a multivitamin, and OTC cold medications are not known to interact with any multivitamins. This patient should be able to manage this medication regimen on their own. Choice *B*

199

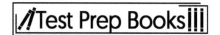

would benefit because they are already on medications and now have six total prescriptions. The patient should be checked for side effects, informed of the optimal timing of taking medications, questioned about therapeutic effectiveness, and asked if they are on any supplements. Choice *C* would benefit from the same questions because overmedicating is common in the geriatric population. In addition, the patient may not even need some of those medications or they may be causing more harm than good. Choice *D* would benefit; even though she is in the medical field, that does not mean she knows what side effects, drug interactions, or benefits this new medication has.

19. A, B, C, D: The intern covered patient demographics, past medical history, medications, some of the routes of administration, recent adverse reactions, medication effectiveness, and the patient's social and vaccine history. Being as in-depth as possible is crucial in medication reconciliations to understand how best to optimize the patient's health. All the answer choices would be helpful questions to understand the whole picture.

20. A, B, C: Ciprofloxacin does not have an FDA indication to treat COVID-19 infections. Fluoxetine, although commonly used for GAD, does not have a true FDA indication for GAD. Diclofenac sodium is a topical NSAID, and the hip is too deep into the body for a topical skin medication to absorb into the hip muscles. Choice *D* is accurate because adapalene, or Differin, is FDA approved to treat acne vulgaris.

21. C: The answer is 20 to 25 mg/kg because Stage 2 CKD can have an eGFR of 60–89 mL/min. That would fall into the 50 to 90 mL/minute category for this dosing chart, so 20 to 25 mg/kg would be correct.

22. D: Ciprofloxacin, gabapentin, and acyclovir all require dose adjustments for specific CrCl. Guaifenesin (Mucinex) does not have any renal adjustment guidelines.

23. C: No matter the medication, all pregnant women are treated for a urinary tract infection for seven days.

24. D: There is no set stop date or clinical measure to stop gout prophylaxis. Once someone is on gout prophylaxis, indicating they had more than one gout attack within a year, they should stay on medication indefinitely to prevent future attacks.

25. B: Choice *A* can be correct, but this does not usually cause as much concern because the drug is not having an effect (not accumulating and causing toxicity). Most of the well-known renally adjusted medications are adjusted because of accumulation. Choice *C* is incorrect because chronic kidney disease leads to reduced protein binding, which causes the drug to not bind to proteins properly. This does lead to an increase in dose usually, but because the protein binding is decreased. Choice *D* is incorrect. Although the pH will change in a patient with altered renal function, this is not the direct cause of needing to dose adjust medications.

26. A: The indication for treating prophylactically for PJP is a CD4 less than 200 or 14%, so Choice *D* is incorrect. The first-line treatment is Bactrim, one double-strength or one single-strength tablet daily. Choice *B* is a second-line treatment with incorrect dosing—it should be 50 mg daily. Choice *C* is incorrect because Augmentin is not used for PJP prophylaxis.

27. C: First, calculate the total daily dose, which is typically:

$$0.5 \text{ units/kg} - 40/0.5 = 20 \text{ units daily dose}$$

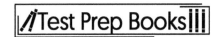

For type 1 diabetes, the starting insulin regimen is typically split into half in the morning and night, and the other half spread out preprandial (before meals). Half of 20 units is 10 units, and half of that is 5 units, so the patient needs 5 units in the morning and 5 units at bedtime. The remaining 10 units are divided equally by 3. Since that equals 3.33 units in this case (and that is not a typical dose), always round up to ensure they have enough insulin. This comes out to 4 units given preprandial.

28. B: Spravato (esketamine) is delivered intranasally and given in instructional settings. Cymbalta (duloxetine), Rexulti (brexpiprazole), and Prozac (fluoxetine) are not available as nasal sprays.

29. C: The MMR (measles, mumps, and rubella) vaccine is administered subcutaneously, which makes Choice *C* is the correct answer.

30. B, D: Ibandronate and raloxifene are given orally, and both denosumab and teriparatide are subcutaneous injections.

31. A: Due to the severe GERD (gastrointestinal reflux disease), taking anything other than an oral route would be preferred. Choices *B, C,* and *D* are all taken orally. Even though sublingual is not considered an oral route, it is still taken by putting it into the mouth, which could cause acid irritation. Choice *B* is also incorrect because patients with hypertension should not take NSAIDs (such as ibuprofen) because they could worsen the hypertension.

32. C: This is based solely on patient preference. If a patient (especially a pediatric patient) does not prefer a medicine, they will not be adherent. Oxymetazoline is an effective allergy medication that has the least taste and will not be orally delivered. Choices *A* and *B* would be incorrect because the son has sensory issues with taste and swallowing, so avoiding any oral or sublingual medications would be ideal. Choice *D* is incorrect because the mom did not state he liked flavorings more; some children will actually dislike the flavoring more than the unflavored.

33. C: Both Crohn's Disease and osteoporosis can lead to vitamin D deficiencies. Because Crohn's affects intestinal absorption, it is given sublingually to avoid the first-pass metabolism through the intestines.

34. D: All the other answer choices are good counseling points for eye drops, but the tip of the eye dropper should NOT touch the eye. It can cause scratches and further irritation.

35. A: Common pulmonary arterial hypertension treatments include PDE-5 inhibitors (such as tadalafil) which are agents contraindicated with nitrates such as nitroglycerin. These can cause a severe hypotension episode.

36. D: Amoxicillin is a penicillin medication, and penicillin allergies are common. A true penicillin allergy can affect all classes of penicillins, so non-penicillin agents should always be chosen over the other options in these patients.

37. A, C, D: Choices *A, C,* and *D* are all known for causing dizziness. Choice *B*, ubrogepant (Ubrelvy), does not have dizziness as a common side effect. It can happen, but not as often as with the other three medications.

38. A: The Varicella vaccine is a live vaccine, and hydroxyurea is an immunosuppressant. These two should not be given together. Choice *B*, pneumococcal vaccines, are not recommended. The hydroxyurea can diminish the effects of the vaccine, but it is not completely contraindicated. Choices *C* and *D* have no known interactions with hydroxyurea.

201

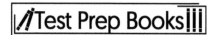

39. D. Prefest is estradiol and norgestimate together. Premarin, Minivelle, and Estring are all estrogen-only formulations, and since it is not listed that the woman has had a hysterectomy, she cannot take estrogen on its own.

40. B, C, D: Choices *B*, *C*, and *D* all can cause or worsen tachyarrhythmias (fast, irregular heart rates). Choice *A*, sotalol, is a beta-blocker. It can cause arrhythmias, but it is much more likely to cause bradycardia instead.

41. B: Vancomycin can cause extreme flushing, which is colloquially known as "red man syndrome." If someone turns uncharacteristically red while on vancomycin, it is most likely just a benign adverse event from the vancomycin.

42. B: While almost all medications have listed adverse effects as headaches, the estrogen in hormonal birth control is infamous for causing headaches. Lowering the estrogen dosing in her birth control should help decrease headache pain and frequency.

42. A, B, C: Choices *A*, *B*, and *C* all have readily available reversal agents in case of overdose. Morphine's overdose agent is naloxone, acetaminophen's reversal agent is N-acetylcysteine, and apixaban's reversal agent is andexanet alfa, or Andexxa. Tobramycin is an antibiotic that does not have a reversal agent.

43. B: First-line treatment is non-pharmacological therapy, such as sitting up for thirty minutes after eating and avoiding spicy foods. The first-line pharmacological therapy for acid reflux in pregnant women is calcium carbonate or other antacids. Choice *A* is incorrect because, although it is true, giving proton pump inhibitors like omeprazole is reserved for patients who cannot tolerate other agents approved in GERD for pregnancy. Choice *C* is wrong because bismuth salicylate, or Pepto-Bismol, is contraindicated in pregnancy. Choice *D* is incorrect because there are safe medications for GERD in pregnancy.

44. C: Irinotecan is well-known for causing diarrhea, not constipation.

45. A: In a snake bite situation where the patient is in critical condition and the type of snake is known or relatively certain, administering the appropriate antivenom for the snake breed is crucial. All the other answers imply a delay in treatment and, therefore, are incorrect.

46. A: The most important signs of overdose in this patient are lowered temperature, lowered respiratory rate, miotic pupils, decreased bowel sounds, and seizures. Another key piece of information is that the heart rate and blood pressure are lower but still considered normal—this is common with opioid overdoses. Administering naloxone promptly is crucial to this patient's treatment.

47. C: These three drugs together are considered the renal "triple whammy" and can worsen already present kidney diseases.

48. A: Ritonavir is a strong CYP3A4 inhibitor. Tenofovir, Choice *B*, has a weak association with CYP3A4. Maraviroc, Choice *C*, is a substrate of CYP3A4. Atazanavir, Choice *D*, is a CYP3A4 substrate but is a major inhibitor of UGT1A1.

49. D: With the given information, Choices *A*, *B*, and *C* are all correct treatments. Choice *D* is wrong because hepatitis A does not have any therapies; tenofovir is a treatment for chronic hepatitis *B* infection.

50. B: Vitamin K aids with blood clotting, and warfarin is an anticoagulant. When the warfarin dose is too high and causes abnormal amounts of blood thinning, Vitamin K is given to patients to return their blood to normal clotting. Choice *A* is wrong because the opposite is true. Choice *C* is incorrect because Vitamin K is only clinically given generally for blood clotting purposes. Choice *D* is incorrect because only Vitamin K is given for blood clotting, no other vitamin.

51. A: Adderall is a stimulant that can worsen the stimulant effects of pseudoephedrine and cause tachycardia, tachypnea, and increased anxiety and agitation. The other answer choices are given commonly with pseudoephedrine. Different disease states may cause interactions with Choices *B*, *C*, and *D*, but not for the general population.

52. C: Carbamazepine is a strong CYP3A4 inducer, which would decrease the serum concentration of ranolazine (which is metabolized by CYP3A4). This is the only contraindicated pair. For Choice *A*, ACE inhibitors like lisinopril can raise the serum concentration of lithium; it is advised to consider a therapy modification, but it is not contraindicated. For Choice *D*, acetaminophen may decrease the serum concentration of lamotrigine, but it is only advised to monitor therapy and not contraindicated. Choice *B* does not have any known interactions. They are safe to take together.

53. B: Pediculosis means lice of any kind, and the first-line treatment is permethrin and a nit comb to remove the lice and larvae.

54. C: Choice *C*, 24, falls in the normal carbon dioxide range of 22–26 mmol/L, 140 falls in the normal sodium range of 135–145 mEq/L, 87 falls in the normal blood glucose range of 60–120 mg/dL, and 0.9 falls in the normal range for creatinine of 0.7–1.3 mg/dL.

55. C: Choice *A* is wrong because the heart rate only has to be over 90 bpm to be considered septic. Choice *B* is incorrect because someone with sepsis will have a respiratory rate of over 20 breaths/min. Choice *D* is wrong because patients are septic due to an infection, and infections cause high or low white blood cell counts. Choice *C* is a correct SIRS criterion.

56. C: Although all are formulas for estimating creatinine clearance, only the Cockcroft-Gault formula is used globally to estimate GFR.

57. A, B, C, D: Choices *A*, *B*, *C*, and *D* would all benefit from pharmacogenomic testing. For Choice *A*, SSRIs interact with CYP2D6, CYP2C19, CYP2B6, SLC6A4, and HTR2A; tricyclic antidepressants interact with CYP2D6 and CYP2C19. For Choice *B*, clopidogrel interacts with CYP2C19. For Choice *C*, proton pump inhibitors also interact with CYP2C19. For Choice *D*, statins interact with SLCO1B1, ABCG2, and CYP2C9. All these medications would benefit from prior pharmacogenetics testing to avoid treatment failure or jumping between treatments to see what will work for each patient.

58. B: Stage A is everyone who does not have heart failure (no signs or symptoms). Stage B has no signs or symptoms but has structural heart disease, elevated cardiac troponin, and/or elevated BNP. Stage C is symptomatic heart failure for patients with current or previous signs and /or symptoms of heart failure. Stage D is advanced heart failure, where the heart failure interferes with daily life and causes recurrent hospitalizations.

59. B: Like other renal diseases, when the kidney stops functioning and filtering properly, the serum creatinine (SCr) and blood urea nitrogen (BUN) do not filter out and the levels are raised in the blood. This would be a sign that the transplanted kidney is not functioning properly nor adjusting to the new host.

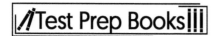

60. B: The half-life of a medication (or any substance) is the time it takes for the medication to reach 50 percent of its original concentration. Choice *A* is t_{max}, Choice *C* is not a known marker, and Choice *D* is C_{max}.

61. C: Because fluoxetine inhibits CYP2D6, the enzyme doxepin is metabolized by, concomitant use will keep doxepin from being able to properly function. It will just be excreted with no effect.

62. C: It normally takes one to two weeks to see clinically significant improvement in schizophrenia patients.

63. D: Tadalafil, or Cialis, is known as the "weekend pill" because, if stimulated, it can help men achieve an erection in a thirty-six-hour window after taking the medication.

64. A, C: Therapeutic drug monitoring needs to be done on phenytoin and levetiracetam due to their more unpredictable pharmacokinetic (PK) states. Choices *B* and *D* have more predictable and less fluctuating PK effects in a patient and do not need more consistent monitoring.

65. B: The C_{max} will be when the concentration of the medication is at its highest amount. That is at five hours, or where the peak of the curve is.

66. C: The highest concentration, or C_{max}, reached was with the high dose tamsulosin. A higher dose of an anticholinergic medication (such as tamsulosin) will cause more adverse effects related to the cholinergic pathways because it is being inhibited.

67. A: The WHO defines a hemoglobin level for a female under 12 g/dL (and a male under 13 g/dL) as anemia.

68. C: The new 2023 AHA Dyslipidemia guidelines state that the HDL target for women with concomitant T2DM is greater than 50 mg/dL, while the target for men is greater than 40 mg/dL.

69. A: Azithromycin is the recommended agent from the Cystic Fibrosis Foundation to treat Pseudomonas aeruginosa colonization in pediatric patients older than five years.

70. A: For this specific patient population, multiagent chemotherapy and a tyrosine kinase inhibitor are the first-line treatments. Choice *D* is incorrect. Although it is advised for this patient population to have a stem cell transplant if possible, they should also be on the two medicinal agents. Choices *B* and *C* are not first-line treatments for this patient population. A corticosteroid is not included.

71. C: Namenda is memantine, which is an NMDA receptor antagonist. It is often used in Alzheimer's patients but is not in the same class as the other three medications listed here. Exelon is rivastigmine, Razadyne is galantamine, and Aricept is donepezil. These are all cholinesterase inhibitors.

72. A: Non-DHP (dihydropyridine) calcium channel blockers (diltiazem and verapamil) are the next-line therapy if a patient cannot take beta-blockers. If the heart rate is under 60 bpm with either a beta-blocker or a non-DHP calcium channel blocker, then Choice *B* is added (a DHP calcium channel blocker). If the patient's blood pressure is under 130/80 mmHg, and they are still having symptoms and/or pain, adding a long-acting nitrate, Choice *C*, or ranolazine, Choice *D*, would be the last step.

73. B, C, D: Gardasil is only recommended for all patients under the age of twenty-five and conditionally recommended for those under forty-five; it is not recommended for individuals over the age of forty-five. Prevnar (pneumonia), Boostrix (Tdap), and Fluzone (influenza) would all be recommended.

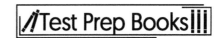
74. A: Cyclosporine (Restasis) for dry eyes, loteprednol (Lotemax) as a steroid, and bromfenac (BromSite) as a topical NSAID eye drop are all prescription only.

75. D: Garlic can also be used to improve hyperlipidemia and immune function. Cinnamon is used for lowering blood glucose, turmeric is used for arthritis, and cranberry is used for urinary tract health.

76. B: Sibutramine was banned by the FDA in 2010 for increased cardiovascular events. Orlistat, Alli, is still available OTC. Choices *C* and *D* are only available through prescription.

77. C: Choice *A* would likely benefit more from lozenges or patches so they do not have to chew constantly. Choice *B* would not be a good candidate because of their job. If they are constantly in front of others, chewing gum often may be seen as rude. They would benefit more from patch therapy. Choice *D* is incorrect because the patient has jaw pain, and they would not be adherent to chewing gum because it would increase pain. They would benefit from lozenges or patches instead.

78. C: Choice *A* is an effective antihistamine, but it can have other adverse effects such as somnolence and dizziness. Choice *B* was banned by the FDA for an increased risk of stroke. Choice *D* also has common side effects of sedation and dizziness. Choice *C*, loratadine, is a second-generation antihistamine, meaning it does not cause sedation as frequently and works just as effectively as first-generation antihistamines (such as diphenhydramine).

Performing Calculations

1. 102 mL/min: The formula for CrCl is:

$$CrCl\left(\frac{mL}{min}\right) = \frac{(140 - age) \times IBW\ (or\ AdjBW\ if\ IBW > 120\%\ of\ ABW)}{72 \times SCr} \times (0.85\ if\ female)$$

IBW stands for ideal body weight, and SCr stands for serum creatinine. First, calculate what the ideal body weight is. The formula for that is:

$$IBW\ (kg) = 45.5\ (50\ if\ male) + (2.3 \times inches\ over\ 5\ feet)$$

For this patient, she is female, so use 45.5. Convert centimeters to inches:

$$\frac{178\ cm}{2.54\ cm\ (2.54\ cm\ equals\ 1\ inch)} = 70.1\ inches$$

Taking the 70.1 inches and knowing that there are 12 inches in one foot, use multiples of 12:

$$12 \times 5 = 60\ inches$$

From this:

$$70.1\ inches - 60\ inches = 9.9\ inches, round\ to\ 10\ inches$$

This patient is 5'10", so this would be her IBW equation:

$$45.5 + (2.3 \times 10) = 68.5\ kg$$

If her ABW (actual body weight) is greater than 120% of her IBW, the AdjBW (adjusted body weight) formula should be used to calculate CrCl.

205

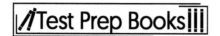

$$\frac{89}{68.5} \times 100\% = 130\%$$

Her ABW is 130% of her IBW, so the AdjBW formula must be used:

$$AdjBW\ (kg) = IBW\ (kg) + 0.4[ABW(kg) - IBW(kg)]$$

$$68.5\ kg + 0.4[\ 89\ kg - 68.5\ kg] = 76.7\ kg$$

For finding SCr, use the fishbone diagram. The fishbone diagram does not use labels or units, but this is how it would be filled in if it did:

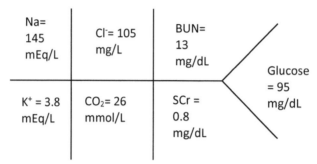

Na is sodium, K^+ is potassium, Cl^- is chloride, CO_2 is carbon dioxide, and BUN is blood urea nitrogen. The only value needed from this to calculate CrCl is the SCr.

Filling in the formula:

$$\frac{(140 - 50) \times 76.7\ kg}{72 \times 0.8\ mg/dL} \times (0.85) = 102\ mL/min$$

Therefore, the patient's CrCl is 102 mL/min.

2. C: Child-Pugh scores are calculated according to the table below:

Measurement	Total Bilirubin	Albumin	INR	Ascites	Encephalopathy
1 point	< 2 mg/dL	> 3.5 g/dL	< 1.7	Absent	None
2 points	2–3 mg/dL	2.8–3.5 g/dL	1.7–2.3	Slight	Grade 1–2 (minimal)
3 points	> 3 mg/dL	< 2.8 g/dL	> 2.3	Moderate	Grade 3–4 (advanced)

Class	Total Points
Class A	5–6 points
Class B	7–9 points
Class C	10–15 points

Add up his scores: 2 points for total bilirubin, 2 for albumin, 1 for INR, 2 for slight ascites, and 3 for Grade 3 encephalopathy. This equals 10 points and Class C Child-Pugh.

3. B: His age, which is between sixty-five and seventy-four, is one point. Hypertension is one point, T2DM is one point, and a vascular disease (peripheral artery disease) is another point. This equals four

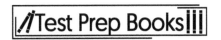

points total and a 4.0 percent stroke risk. The other points that can be earned for the CHA2DS2-VASC score are one point for congestive heart failure, two points for being seventy-five years old and over, two points for prior stroke/transient ischemic attack/thromboembolism, and one point for females. The maximum score a person could receive is nine.

4. 60 mg: The recommended dosing schedule for acute pain postoperatively is 5–10 mg every 4–6 hours as needed, and the prescription needs to be written for the maximum daily dose.

$$10 \ mg \ \times 6 \ times \ daily \ (every \ 4 \ hours) = 60 \ mg$$

It is not specified here, but if a patient is opioid-naïve, starting with the lower end of 5 mg would be more beneficial to reduce opioid dependence later on.

5. A: To calculate the number of canisters needed, first calculate the number of inhalations in one canister:

$$10,000 \ mcg \ per \ canister \div 50 \ mcg \ per \ inhalation = 200 \ inhalations \ per \ canister$$

Now, calculate how many inhalations this patient will need for 90 days:

$$1 \ inhalation \ \times 2 \ times \ daily \ \times 90 \ days = 180 \ inhalations$$

Since there are 200 inhalations in a canister, the patient will only need one canister for 90 days.

6. B: The patient does qualify. The stroke could not have occurred more than 4.5 hours prior to this moment of tPA administration, and none of his comorbidities are contraindicated with tPA. Uncontrolled hypertension would be contraindicated, but his chronic hypertension is only Stage 1 (which is 130–139 mmHg systolic BP or 80–89 mmHg diastolic) and his current BP is under 185/110 mmHg (which is the cutoff for the current blood pressure reading). His blood glucose is over 50 mg/dL, which is the cutoff for current blood glucose reading. This eliminates Choice *D*. IV alteplase (tPA) is dosed at 0.9 mg/kg, with a max of 90 mg. First, his weight must be converted to kilograms:

$$210 \ lbs \ \div 2.2 = 95.5 \ kg$$

Then, multiply by 0.9 to find the dosing:

$$\frac{0.9 \ mg}{kg} \times 95.5 \ kg = 85.9 \ mg, round \ up \ to \ 86 \ mg$$

In some cases, hospitals may round up to 90 mg because it is the simpler dose and not notably different; however, the exact dose would be 86 mg.

7. 35.7 mg: First, calculate the amount needed per minute for this patient:

$$40 \ ng * \frac{kg}{min} \times 62 \ kg = 2480 \ ng/min$$

Then, multiply this times the number of minutes in 24 hours:

$$\frac{2480 \ ng}{min} \times \frac{60 \ min}{1 \ hour} \times 24 \ hours = 3,571,200 \ ng \ per \ 24 \ hours$$

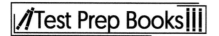

Converting this to mg:

$$3{,}571{,}200 \; ng \; \times \; \frac{1 \; mg}{100{,}000 \; ng} = 35.7 \; mg$$

Therefore, the patient will need 35.7 mg of treprostinil every 24 hours.

8. A: There are many different routes to take, but the simplest way to answer the question is to make all of the answers have common units. For this problem, the least amount of math would be converting each choice to ng/hr since those are the two most common units presented. For Choice A, the mg needs to be converted to ng:

$$\frac{0.1 \; mg}{hr} \times \frac{1000000 \; ng}{1 \; mg} = \frac{100{,}000 \; ng}{hr}$$

For Choice B, the mcg needs to be converted to ng:

$$\frac{58 \; mcg}{hr} \times \frac{1000 \; ng}{1 \; mcg} = \frac{58{,}000 \; ng}{hr}$$

For Choice C, the minutes need to be converted to hours:

$$\frac{70 \; ng}{min} \times \frac{60 \; min}{1 \; hr} = \frac{4{,}200 \; ng}{hr}$$

For Choice D, nothing needs to be changed to make them similar units.

Ranking these in order of smallest to largest: Choice D, Choice C, Choice B, then Choice A. Choice A is the fastest rate of administration because it delivers the most medication the quickest.

9. B: Choice B is the only correct option. Potassium chloride should NEVER be administered via IV push because it can cause fatal cardiac arrest, so Choice A is incorrect. Choice C is incorrect because the safest maximum peripheral rate is 10 mEq/hour. Choice D is incorrect because the maximum rate for a central line is 40 mEq/hour. Therefore, Choice B is the only appropriate answer.

10. D: First, find the dose needed for this patient based on their weight:

$$165 \; lbs \; \div 2.2 = 75 \; kg$$

$$\frac{15 \; mcg}{kg} \times 75 \; kg = 1125 \; mcg \; per \; min$$

Then, take this number and convert it to mg (like the stock bottle is in):

$$\frac{1124 \; mcg}{min} \times \frac{1 \; mg}{1000 \; mcg} = \frac{1.124 \; mg}{min}$$

With the 1.124 mg/min, find how much is needed for 4 hours:

$$\frac{1.124 \; mg}{min} \times \frac{60 \; min}{1 \; hr} \times 4 \; hours = 269.76 \; mg \; per \; 4 \; hours$$

Now, calculate how many mL of the propofol stock solution is needed:

$$\frac{269.76 \, mg}{4 \, hours} \times \frac{100 \, mL}{1000 \, mg} = 6.744 \, mL \, for \, 4 \, hours, round \, to \, 6.7 \, mL$$

Therefore, Choice *D* is correct.

11. 110 mg: To calculate for an unknown drug for a pediatric dosage, use the BSA Pediatric Dosing/Nomogram method. First, calculate the BSA of the patient with this formula:

$$BSA \, (m^2) = \sqrt{\frac{[height \, (cm) \times weight \, (kg)]}{3600}}$$

Substitute the values in:

$$0.76 \, m^2 = \sqrt{\frac{[109 \, cm \times 19 \, kg]}{3600}}$$

Knowing that the BSA is 0.76 m², insert that into the Nomogram formula:

$$pediatric \, dose \, (mg) = \frac{patient's \, BSA \, (m^2)}{1.73 \, m^2} \times adult \, dose \, (mg)$$

$$109.6 \, mg = \frac{0.76 \, m^2}{1.73 \, m^2} \times 250 \, mg$$

Rounding this answer to the nearest whole number, the answer is 110 mg.

12. A: Simvastatin 20 mg is considered a moderate-intensity statin, and a dose of rosuvastatin from 5 to 10 mg is also considered a moderate-intensity statin. Therefore, Choice *A* is the only correct option.

13. 300 mg to 450 mg every 4 to 6 hours: Acetaminophen is a weight-based dosing for pediatrics, and it is 10 to 15 mg/kg every 4 to 6 hours, with nothing exceeding 5 doses in 24 hours, 75 mg/kg, or 4,000 mg/day. For this patient:

$$30 \, kg \times 10 \, mg = 300 \, mg$$

$$30 \, kg \times 15 \, mg = 450 \, mg$$

The answer should be anything between 300 mg to 450 mg every 4 to 6 hours.

14. C: The conversion between each drug is as follows:

$$1 \, mg \, bumetanide = 20 \, mg \, torsemide = 40 \, mg \, furosemide$$

So, if they are on 40 mg furosemide orally at home, this would mean they take the equivalent of 1 mg bumetanide orally. From there, convert that to the IV dose, which is 2 times the normal at-home daily dose:

$$1 \, mg \times 2 = 2 \, mg \, bumetanide$$

209

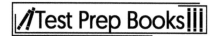

For the purposes of this problem, 2 times was used, so it would be 2 mg daily of bumetanide for the bolus dose in the hospital. For the transition to at-home dosing of torsemide, convert the previous furosemide at-home dose to torsemide:

$$40 \ mg \ furosemide = 20 \ mg \ torsemide$$

The total daily dose is 1 to 2.5 times the previous total daily dose:

$$20 \ mg \ torsemide \times 2 = 40 \ mg \ torsemide$$

Therefore, they should take 40 mg torsemide when they are discharged for their new at-home dose. Choice C is correct.

15. 1:3.33: Set up this problem as a ratio of the percent equal to 1/x parts, which is the number being asked for:

$$\frac{30\%}{100\%} = \frac{1}{x \ parts}$$

$$x \ parts = 3.33$$

Then, to make it a ratio, put the numerator before the colon and the dominator after the colon: 1:3.33.

16. D: Osmolality is the milliosmoles of solute per kg of solvent. For serum osmolality, a specific formula is used:

$$serum \ osmolality = \left[Na^+(\frac{mmol}{L}) \times 2\right] + \left[\frac{BUN \ (\frac{mg}{dL})}{2.8}\right] + \left[\frac{glucose \ (\frac{mg}{dL})}{18}\right]$$

Filling in the numbers given:

$$\left[136 \ \frac{mmol}{L} \times 2\right] + \left[\frac{11 \ \frac{mg}{dL}}{2.8}\right] + \left[\frac{170 \ \frac{mg}{dL}}{18}\right] = 285 \ mOsm/kg$$

17. A: Choice A is correct. Use the Henderson-Hasselbach equation for percent ionization of an acid:

$$pH = pKa + log \frac{salt \ or \ ionized}{acid \ or \ un - ionized}$$

(If this was for a base, the numerator and denominator would be flipped.)

Add in what is given:

$$3.7 = 4.2 + log \frac{salt \ or \ ionized}{acid \ or \ un - ionized}$$

$$0.316 = \frac{salt \ or \ ionized}{acid \ or \ un - ionized}$$

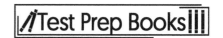

This number is then converted to a ratio:

$$\frac{0.316}{1 + 0.316} = \frac{ionized}{un - ionized}$$

The denominator is 1 + 0.316 because it is the percent ionized plus the percent un-ionized to get a correct ratio. The denominator for a ratio needs to have the total, not just the remaining part. That equals 0.24, and that has to be multiplied by 100 to get a percentage:

$$0.24 \times 100 = 24\%$$

The drug is 24 percent ionized, Choice *A*. Choice *B* is if 0.316 was not added to the denominator when making it a ratio. Choice *C* is if the pKa and pH were flipped. Choice *D* would mean the pKa and the pH equal each other.

18. 2432 mOsmol: Osmolarity is the milliosmoles of solute per L of solvent. To set up the formula:

$$\frac{mOsmol}{L} = \frac{concentration\ of\ the\ substance\ (\frac{mg}{L})}{molecular\ weight\ (mg)} \times number\ of\ species\ \times 1000$$

The 20% calcium solution equals 20 g per 100 mL, so convert that to g/L:

$$\frac{20\ g}{100\ mL} \times \frac{1000\ mL}{1\ L} = 200\ g/L$$

The only number not expressly given in the problem is the number of species. To find the number of species, count the number of particles (or species) that the compound will dissociate into. For $CaCl_2$:

$$1\ Ca^{2+} + 2\ Cl^- = 3\ species$$

(For non-electrolytes, the species would equal 1 because they do not dissociate in solution.)

Enter the numbers in the osmolarity equation:

$$\frac{mOsmol}{0.45\ L} = \frac{200\ \frac{g}{L}}{111\ g} \times 3\ \times 1000$$

The osmolarity of this 450 ml 20% calcium chloride solution is 2432 mOsmol.

19. 450 mL: This is an alligation question, where there are two concentrations and the desired concentration is in the middle. First, start by filling out a table with what is known:

Higher strength: 40%		Parts of higher:
	Desired strength: 25%	
Lower strength: 15%		Parts of lower:

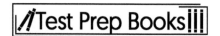

Subtract across the diagonals:

Higher strength: 40%		Parts of higher: 10 p
	Desired strength: 25%	
Lower strength: 15%		Parts of lower: 15 p

Then, the parts represent the strengths they are horizontally across from. This means that 10 parts of 40% HappyRUs and 15 parts of 15% HappyRUs make the 25% HappyRUs solution. To solve for the separate amounts, add the total number of parts:

$$10\,p + 15\,p = 25\,p\ total$$

Use this to set up a proportion:

$$\frac{750\ mL\ total}{25\ p\ total} = \frac{x\ mL\ 15\%}{15\ p\ 15\%}$$

X equals 450 mL, which means that in order to make this solution with these two solutions, 450 mL of the 15% HappyRUs stock solution is needed.

20. C: Using the %w/v proportion, set the proportion up to find the grams of olopatadine in the solution:

$$0.1\%\frac{w}{v} = \frac{x\ g\ olopatadine}{100\ mL\ solution}$$

Solving for x, there is 1 gram olopatadine for every 100 mL of solution. The last step is converting this to ounces as the question asked:

$$\frac{1\ g}{1} \times \frac{1\ kg}{1000\ g} \times \frac{2.2\ lb}{1\ kg} \times \frac{16\ oz}{1\ lb} = 0.0352\ oz$$

Set up a new proportion to figure out the %w/v in 1 L of olopatadine solution, knowing that 1 L equals 1000 mL:

$$\frac{0.0352\ oz}{100\ mL\ solution} = \frac{x\ oz}{1000\ mL\ solution}$$

X would equal 0.352 oz, so 0.352 oz per 1000 mL would be the correct answer.

21. 1 mL: Set this up first as a proportion with the final concentration needed and the concentration per the amount in the vial, 200 mg:

$$\frac{200\ mg}{x\ mL} = \frac{10\ mg}{1\ mL}$$

X then equals 20 mL, which equals the total volume of the Vfend solution. To find the powder volume, subtract the amount of diluent (water) added:

$$20\ mL - 19\ mL = 1\ mL$$

The powder volume of the Vfend is 1 mL.

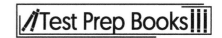

22. D: This is a dilution question, so $C_1V_1=C_2V_2$ should be used to find the answer.

$$25\% \times 40\ mL = 10\% \times V2$$

V_2 equals 100 mL, which is the FINAL volume needed of the 10% Rocephin. To get the diluent added to make the solution:

$$100\ mL - 40\ mL = 60\ mL\ diluent$$

60 mL diluent added to 40 mL of 25% Rocephin makes 100 mL of the concentration of 10% Rocephin.

23. 22 g: Set this up as a proportion, with the concentration in g/mL on one side and the amount of fat (what is being solving for) over the mL ordered:

$$\frac{10\ g}{100\ mL} = \frac{x\ g\ fat}{220\ mL}$$

Solving this, x equals 22 grams of fat.

24. C: Set this up as a proportion. Put the amount needed daily in grams over what that would be equal to in mL (x, the missing number) and make this equal to the concentration of the stock solution, 15 percent. This translates to 15 grams over 100 mL:

$$\frac{25\ g}{x\ mL} = \frac{15\ g}{100\ mL}$$

X = 166.67 mL, or, rounded, 167 mL needed per day.

25. B: Choice *B* is correct. The total volume is given, as well as all of the other values. Take the total and subtract all the other known mL from 1640 mL:

$$1640\ mL - 350\ mL - 167\ mL - 220\ mL - 80\ mL - 5\ mL - 789\ mL = 29\ mL$$

There are 29 mL of remaining electrolytes that are in this TPN solution.

26. B: This is the formula used to calculate QALY:

$$quantity\ of\ life\ extended\ (years) \times quality\ of\ life = QALY$$

The quality of life score is calculated in many different ways and by different measures (such as patient scores, costs, burden, etc.) depending on the treatment and disease. This is the formula for this specific patient:

$$5\ years \times 0.4 = 2.0\ QALYs$$

This score helps look at the value of providing treatment for a patient and understanding if the cost is worth the utility of the treatment.

27. B: To calculate this, use a ratio:

$$\frac{79\ with\ disease}{540\ total\ women} \times 100\% = 14.6\%\ risk$$

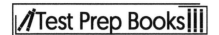
28. C: First, eliminate which CI would not be relevant without even looking at the data. Choice *B* is not relevant because the interval crosses 1, which indicates that there is no statistically significant difference between the treatment and the placebo. This does not give us any helpful data. Choice *A* is ruled out because the hazard ratio, the first number not in parenthesis, is not between the predicted 95% CI. Choice *D* is incorrect. Although the hazard ratio falls into the CI, a number greater than 1 suggests that the treatment caused more adverse effects than the placebo caused adverse effects. This leaves Choice *C*, which does not cross 1 and also favors the treatment over the placebo. If the question had asked if the treatment was superior to the placebo in lowering blood glucose levels to below 100 mg/dL, Choice *D* would be the correct answer. In that scenario, a number greater than 1 would be favored. Always pay attention to exactly what the question is asking for in statistics.

29. 4.63 hours: Assuming first-order kinetics, the equation needed is:

$$C = C_0 \times e^{-kt}$$

C equals the desired concentration, C_0 equals the initial concentration, k equals the rate, and t is the time it takes. To find k:

$$t_{1/2} = 0.693/k$$

$$3.5 \ hours = 0.693/k$$

K equals 0.198 hours^{-1}. Using this:

$$5 \ mg/L = 20 \ mg/L \times e^{-0.198t}$$

$$\ln \ln \left(0.4 \frac{mg}{L} \right) = \ln \ln \left(e^{-0.198t} \right)$$

$$-0.916 = -0.198t$$

T equals *4.63 hours.*

30. C: The equation for finding steady state in a continuous infusion is:

$$F_{ss} = 1 - e^{-kt}$$

F_{ss} equals the steady state, and k is the elimination rate constant in this equation. Fill it in with all the known variables. (The h^{-1} and the h for the elimination rate constant and time to steady state, respectively, cancel each other out.)

$$F_{ss} = 1 - e^{-0.453 \times 8.5}$$

F_{ss} is equal to 0.9788, and, to find the percentage, multiply by 100:

$$0.9788 \times 100 = 97.88\%$$

97.88% steady state is reached at 8.5 hours with this drug. Rounded to the nearest whole number, it is 98%, so Choice *C* is correct.

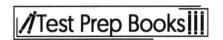

31. A: The formula for clearance of an oral administered drug is:

$$Cl\left(\frac{mL}{h}\right) = \frac{F \times dose\ (mg)}{AUC\ (mg \times \frac{h}{L})}$$

Fill in the formula:

$$\frac{0.93 \times 650\ mg}{34\ mg \times \frac{h}{L}} = 17.8\frac{mg}{L}$$

32. C: The equation to calculate steady state concentration is:

$$C_{SS}\left(\frac{g}{L}\right) = \frac{R\left(\frac{g}{hr}\right)}{k\ (h^{-1}) \times V_d\ (L)}$$

C_{ss} is steady state concentration, R equals infusion rate, k is the elimination rate constant, and V_d is the volume of distribution. Since k is not given in the problem, use the half-life to calculate k:

$$t_{1/2} = 0.693/k$$

$$26.2\ h = 0.693/k$$

The variable k equals 0.026 h^{-1}. Put this into the equation:

$$100\frac{g}{L} = \frac{R\left(\frac{g}{hr}\right)}{0.026\ h^{-1} \times 59\ L}$$

R equals 153.4 g/hr, which is the infusion rate needed to achieve a steady state concentration of 100 g/L. Choice *C* is correct if rounded to the nearest whole number.

Compounding, Dispensing, or Administering Drugs or Managing Delivery Systems

1. D: Lipid emulsions are more stable when they are at a higher pH, have a low dextrose and protein concentration, and have low amounts of divalent cations. Choice *A* is incorrect because lipids must be added last to prevent flocculation, creaming, coalescence, and so on. Choice *B* is incorrect because a three-in-one emulsion should be a minimum of 1.2-micron filter, whereas a two-in-one solution requires a 0.22-micron filter. Choice *C* is incorrect because the CDC recommends changing of the filters every twenty-four hours.

2. A: Abacavir is a nucleoside RT inhibitor commonly used in HIV therapy. HLA-B is present on the surface of almost all cells and is involved in recognizing self vs non-self-molecules to produce an immune response accordingly. The variant HLA-B*57:01 can increase hypersensitivity reactions towards abacavir and is recommended to be avoided. Choices *B* and *C* are incorrect because the conditions can be caused when combining HLA-B*15:02 and carbamazepine. Choice *D* is incorrect because this is a common adverse effect in patients with RYR1 variants who use volatile anesthetics like halothane.

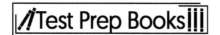

3. A, B, C: Peptides are important endogenous molecules used in various pathways such as those of neurotransmitters, hormones, and neuromodulators. Peptidomimetics is the process of making a compound that mimics peptides' effects. Since peptides are bad drug candidates due their poor bioavailability, rapidly excretion, and short half-life, the new compound must adjust the structure to remove those effects. Choice *D* is incorrect because peptides bind multiple receptors, which is undesirable when the goal is to produce a specific response.

4. B: Boronic acid bio-isosteres are non-toxic and readily synthesized; the first FDA-approved compound is Bortezomib. Choice *A* is incorrect because they do mimic carboxylic acids. Choice *C* is incorrect because they do act as proteasome inhibitors through hydrogen and covalent bonds between boron and the active site of an amino acid, which means Choice *D* is also incorrect.

5. B: Prodrugs are functional groups that shield the active drug because the active compound would be too toxic if released directly. Prodrugs are used for a variety of reasons, including to increase acid sensitivity and membrane permeability, decrease drug toxicity, and increase duration of action. Choice *A* is incorrect because prodrugs are inactive and non-toxic. Choice *C* is incorrect because the issue with carboxylic acid is that it can ionize and prevent crossing into the membrane, so ester groups act to prevent that. Choice *D* is incorrect because the less polar groups are going to cross the membranes.

6. B: The primary engineering control is the main area for sterile compounding products. It can include biological safety cabinets or compounding aseptic containment isolators. There are a set of acceptable cleanliness standards that each compounding facility must abide by, measured through air quality. Choice *A* is incorrect because ISO Class 3 is the highest level of cleanliness that exists, but it is not considered the minimum. Choice *C* is incorrect because ISO Class 7 is the minimum standard for secondary engineering controls. Choice *D* is incorrect because Class 8 is the minimum standard for anterooms.

7. B, C: Horizontal airflow workbenches have air that flows in the direction toward the compounder, which is not the preferred direction, especially when handling hazardous compounds. Compounding aseptic containment isolators are also known as glove boxes and are used for low risk compounding only. Choices *A* and *D* are incorrect; these are the safest and most preferred pieces for hazardous compounding because they decrease the risk of exposure to the compounder.

8. C: ACPH are set by the ISO and each compounding area has its own requirements. The buffer room is a secondary engineering control with a minimum standard of ISO Class 7 and requires thirty ACPH. ISO Class 5 requires fifteen ACPH. Therefore, Choices *A*, *B*, and *D* are incorrect.

9. C: Calcium and phosphorous are often mixed in total parenteral nutrition (TPN) bags. Various steps ensure prevention of precipitation. Acidic conditions can increase the absorption of phosphorous, which decreases the chance of interaction with calcium. Choice *A* is incorrect because phosphate should be added first. Choice *B* is incorrect because lipids can increase pH, which is not preferred, so decreasing the total lipid concentration is recommended. Choice *D* is incorrect because calcium gluconate is the preferred form and will have less precipitation than calcium carbonate.

10. D: Excipients are any substance other than the active drug or prodrug that is included into a product during the manufacturing process. Each excipient serves a purpose; preservatives are used to prevent microbial growth in a formulation that is often used in oral preparations, multidose ophthalmias, and most products that are not used immediately. Choice *A* is incorrect because solubilizing agents help increase bioavailability. Choice *B* is incorrect because antioxidants help prevent chemical degradation.

216

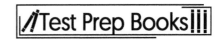

Choice *C* is incorrect because buffers are used to change the pH to help increase availability, prevent toxicity, and so on.

11. A: A eutectic mixture consists of two or more powder substances together that liquefy when combined and have a lower melting point than that of the individual substances. It's advised that the components be dispensed as separate sets of powders to avoid forming a eutectic mixture. Choice *B* is incorrect because this describes an explosive mixture and occurs when mixing an oxidizing and reducing agent together. Choice *C* is incorrect because dry aggregates describe granules. Choice *D* is incorrect because this describes effervescent granules.

12. C: The rainbow method is used when flipping the vial upside down to prevent blockage of airflow. The needle shaft and top of the vial are examples of critical sites that should constantly receive HEPA-filtered airflow. Blocking the airflow can result in contamination within the preparation. Choices *A* and *D* are incorrect because pressure within the vial depends on the amount of air pushed into the vial in comparison to the amount of fluid coming out. Choice *B* is incorrect because the rainbow method is not involved in the level of exposure on the compounder.

13. C: Gowns must be changed every two to three hours throughout the hazardous preparation process or immediately after a spill or splash. Choices *A*, *B*, and *D* are incorrect because these are all processes that must be incorporated.

14. Enteric coating: Enteric coating is used to make sure the drug dissolves in a basic environment and not an acidic one, like the stomach. An enteric coating implies extended release or delayed release of medications.

15. A: Elastomeric infusion devices look like an inflatable ball and come in different sizes depending on the fluid volume. They can be useful because they are simple, portable, and have no cords or batteries; however, they can't be used for large volumes or for delivery of pain medications. Choice *B* is incorrect because these are battery-powered devices that can be used to deliver a drug at a set rate. Choice *C* is incorrect because these systems must be held above the infusion site and use tubes of various sizes to deliver the drug. Choice *D* is incorrect because enteral infusion is only to deliver nutrients into the gastrointestinal tract.

16. Saline flush (1) > Attach pump > Saline flush (2) > Heparin flush: The SASH system involves flushing the IV line/lumen with saline before and after prevents mixture of antibiotics in the line and ensure full delivery of all medication. Heparin flushes prevent the formation of blood clots within the line.

17. C: Twirla is a transdermal combined hormonal contraceptive. Choices *A*, *B*, and *D* are all intrauterine options and thus are incorrect.

18. A: ParaGard is a copper formulation device that is non-hormonal and thus does not contain progestin and estrogen. Copper works by interfering with sperm transportation and implantation. Choices *A*, *B*, and *D* are all hormonal options and thus are incorrect.

19. C: Cocoa butter suppositories are a fatty and ideal base because they melt just below the body temperature and can keep solidity at a normal room temperature. Cocoa butter exists in several polymorphic forms that can differ depending on the temperature. The preferred heating temperature is between 35 and 37 °C. That means it should not be microwaved or kept in cold temperatures, so Choices *A* and *B* are incorrect. Choice *D* is incorrect because cocoa butter suppositories are the preferred base and are commonly used.

217

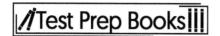

20. C: Rectal suppositories should be inserted, and the buttocks should be held together until the feeling to expel has passed. Afterward, excessive movement should be avoided for one hour, and emptying the bowels should be avoided for one hour as well. Thus, Choices *A*, *B*, and *C* are incorrect.

21. C: The purpose of spacer devices is to allow easier inhalation of the medication, reduce oropharyngeal deposition, and increase the distance between the mouth and aerosol generation. It also helps prevent fast moving particles from hitting the mouth, which is why the instructions are to breath in slowly and deeply, typically over 3-5 seconds. Choices *A*, *B*, and *D* are incorrect because these are all the correct steps to take when utilizing a spacer.

22. A: Some medications, like nitroglycerin tablets, are sensitive to photolysis, or the degradation of drug in normal sunlight or room light. Amber glass protects against the ultraviolet rays; however, the iron oxide within the amber glass may react with drug products, so make sure not to use any iron-reactive compounds.

23. A, B, C: Permeation is the transmission of gases through packaging materials. Leaching is the migration of package components into the drug. Sorption is when the drug migrates into the container, which can result in a loss of drug. Choice *D* is incorrect because flocculation is the formation of light and fluffy conglomerates that are thermodynamically unstable. This occurs during the mixing process, rather than resulting from the use of plastic packaging.

24. B: The revised USP <797> chapter split the compounds into Category 1, 2, or 3, whereas prior compounds were split into low-, medium-, and high-risk. At controlled room temperature, Category 1 medications should have a maximum of twelve hours beyond use date (BUD); anything past that date should be discarded. Therefore, Choices *A*, *C*, and *D* are incorrect.

25. Sharps: The sharps container is a red puncture-proof container that provides a safe destination for used needles, opened ampules, and broken glass. This helps prevent accidental needlesticks, cuts, and transmission of various diseases.

Developing or Managing Practice or Medication-Use Systems to Ensure Safety and Quality

1. A: CPAs are protocols written by the pharmacist and collaborating physician to delegate specific responsibilities to the pharmacist that extends their scope of practice. These protocols will have specific statements regarding which disease states, drugs, therapy management steps, and documenting procedures that the pharmacist will have.

2. A, B: Specific drug names are not required to be in the protocol; the pharmacist can recommend any drug indicated for the disease states listed in the protocol. Although training requirements are not required to be listed in the protocol, it is highly recommended that they are included. Choices *C* and *D* are a required component and are therefore incorrect.

3. D: Collaborative practice agreements are a great method of expanding pharmacist roles and responsibilities to enhance clinical decisions for the patient. Choice *A* is incorrect because these protocols are found to be incredibly helpful with patient care outcomes, especially regarding communication between healthcare providers. Choice *B* is incorrect because although the workload may be increased, the patient outcomes are not decreased. Choice *C* is incorrect because the protocols are patient-driven to improve outcomes, rather than finance-driven.

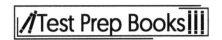

4: Standardize 4 safety (S4S): The S4S initiative is the first interprofessional resource that helps in all areas of care transitioning, including standardizing adult & pediatric continuous infusions, orally compounded liquids, and epidurals.

5. D: Telephone encounters are a great method of communication between healthcare providers regarding the encounters held between patient and pharmacist to ensure continuity of care. Choices *A* and *B* are incorrect because these are primarily used in the community setting to provide actions and reminders for the patient, but they may not be the most effective system. Choice *C* is incorrect because this is a method for reimbursement or medication approval.

6. B: Prophylactic therapy is used for patients who are at high risk for developing a specific disease state, so they are prescribed medications to help prevent the progression. Choice *A* is incorrect because empiric therapy is utilized for patients who have an infection, but the pathogen is unknown. Empiric therapy is also known as disease-based therapy. Choice *C* is incorrect because therapeutic, or definitive, therapy describes treatment based on a known pathogen. Choice *D* is incorrect because antimicrobial stewardship focuses on using the narrowest spectrum medication for the pathogens indicated.

7. B: The monofilament test consists of applying a thin, plastic stick on the patient's foot in various locations to assess the ability to sense touch. If the patient cannot feel the stick, this can indicate diabetic foot or another type of peripheral vascular disease. Choice *A* is incorrect because peripheral edema is often tested using the pitting technique. Choices *C* and *D* are incorrect because the monofilament test would not be an indicator for any neurological disorder, including Alzheimer's.

8. Romberg: The Romberg test consists of instructing the patient to stand up with their feet together, place their arms at their sides, and close their eyes for thirty to sixty seconds. If the patient has significant swaying, that is considered a positive result for the Romberg test and shows increased risk of falling.

9. A: The ASQ is a thirty-item questionnaire completed by the parent based on observations and includes questions such as "Does your child name at least three items from a common category?" Choice *B* is incorrect because the DDST screens children between one month to six years and measures four different areas of functioning. Choice *C* is incorrect because the ESI is designed to identify any special education considerations. Choice *D* is incorrect because the BINS tests children between three and twenty-four months to assess for neurodevelopmental skills.

10. A, B: Control tests are important to perform when there is a new vial of test strip, if the meter is suspected to be damaged, or if the vial was exposed to extreme temperatures. This ensures the accuracy of both the strips and the meter. Wiping the first drop of blood is recommended to reduce any discrepancies from the contaminants on the surface of the skin. Choice *C* is incorrect because you should check both the expiration date on the test strip vial and the date first opened, since air exposure may alter the quality. Choice *D* is incorrect because the correct steps would be to insert the strip into the meter and then touch the end of the strip to the blood.

11. A: Children do not qualify for the program unless they are children with disabilities. Other populations that would qualify are anyone less than sixty-five years old, those with mental illness, and those recently released from incarceration. The program is dedicated to hiring specific vulnerable population liaisons that can provide quality and compassionate care to these individuals. Choices *B*, *C*, and *D* are incorrect because all of these are considered a vulnerable population and would qualify.

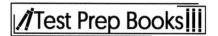

12. D: Under the American Disabilities Act (ADA), broken limbs, concussions, appendicitis, and common colds are not considered a disability and would not qualify for any workplace accommodations. Choices A, B, and C are incorrect because these are all considered disabilities, as well as autism, cancer, diabetes, and post-traumatic stress disorder.

13. OSHA: OSHA (Occupational Safety and Health Administration) provides recommendations and regulations regarding workplace safety to protect employees from hazardous situations.

14. A, B, D: A key role of a pharmacist informatic includes information management, which requires the pharmacist's medication knowledge to set up a barcode medication administration system (BCMA) or a computerized provider order entry system. In addition, another role includes knowledge delivery, which is important during the clinical decision support method. This method provides physicians, pharmacists, staff, and patients with information and patient-specific knowledge to enhance the health experience. Choice C is incorrect because pharmacy informatics specializes in the integration of technology and clinical knowledge rather than writing textbooks and guidelines.

15. A: Pharmacy informatics focuses on technological advances in the healthcare system to improve medication management, administration, and quality. Automated systems such as electronic health record (EHR) systems, barcode medication administration (BCMA) systems, and computer provide order entry (CPOE) all increase health outcomes and patient care. Choices B and C are incorrect because they don't focus on medication related data analysis through technology. Choice D is incorrect because virtual reality has not currently been proven to increase medication adherence.

16. Health: Health informatics is a broad specialty that focuses on various inputs of data that can be analyzed to develop technological programs to increase patient care and understand trends, as well as used for financial purposes. It's a multidisciplinary specialty that makes use of pharmacy, nursing, and public health fields for information, but is not limited to those fields. End

Index

Dear NAPLEX Test Taker,

We would like to start by thanking you for purchasing this study guide for your NAPLEX exam. We hope that we exceeded your expectations.

Our goal in creating this study guide was to cover all of the topics that you will see on the test. We also strove to make our practice questions as similar as possible to what you will encounter on test day. With that being said, if you found something that you feel was not up to your standards, please send us an email and let us know.

We have study guides in a wide variety of fields. If you're interested in one, try searching for it on Amazon or send us an email.

Thanks Again and Happy Testing!
Product Development Team
info@studyguideteam.com

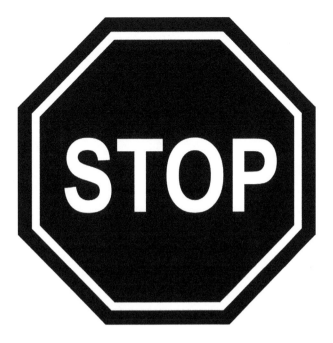

FREE Test Taking Tips Video/DVD Offer

To better serve you, we created videos covering test taking tips that we want to give you for FREE. **These videos cover world-class tips that will help you succeed on your test.**

We just ask that you send us feedback about this product. Please let us know what you thought about it—whether good, bad, or indifferent.

To get your **FREE videos**, you can use the QR code below or email freevideos@studyguideteam.com with "Free Videos" in the subject line and the following information in the body of the email:

    a. The title of your product

    b. Your product rating on a scale of 1-5, with 5 being the highest

    c. Your feedback about the product

If you have any questions or concerns, please don't hesitate to contact us at info@studyguideteam.com.

Thank you!